Antidepressant Therapy

at the Dawn of the Third Millennium

This publication was prepared with the aid of an unrestricted educational grant from Pierre Fabre Médicament

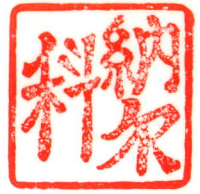

Antidepressant Therapy

at the Dawn of the Third Millennium

Mike Briley
Parc Industriel de la Chartreuse
Castres, France

Stuart A Montgomery
Imperial College of Medicine at
St Mary's Hospital
London, UK

Martin Dunitz

© Martin Dunitz Ltd 1998

First published in the United Kingdom in 1998 by
Martin Dunitz Ltd
The Livery House
7-9 Pratt Street
London NW1 0AE

A CIP catalogue record for this book is available from the British Library.

ISBN 1-85317-517-X

Composition by Wearset, Boldon, Tyne and Wear
Printed and bound in Great Britain by
Biddles Ltd, Guildford and King's Lynn

Contents

Contributors

Jules Angst
Zurich University Psychiatric Hospital, Lenggstrasse 31, PO Box 68, CH-8029 Zurich, Switzerland

Lotta Arborelius
Department of Physiology and Pharmacology, Division of Pharmacology, Karolinska Institutet, S-171 77 Stockholm, Sweden

David S Baldwin
Senior Lecturer, University Department of Psychiatry, Royal South Hants Hospital, Graham Road, Southampton, Hants SO14 0YG, UK

Otto Benkert
Department of Psychiatry, University Hospital of Mainz, Untere Zahlbacher Strasse 8, D-55101 Mainz, Germany

Richard Bergeron
Neurobiological Psychiatry Unit, McGill University, 1033 Pine Avenue West, Montreal, Quebec H3A 1A1, Canada

Kerstin Bingefors
Department of Psychiatry, University Hospital, Uppsala University, S-751 85 Uppsala, Sweden

Jon Birtwistle
Research Nurse, Mental Health Group, Faculty of Medicine, Health and Biological Sciences, University of Southampton, Graham Road, Southampton, Hants SO14 0YG, UK

Gérard Blanc
INSERM U.114, College de France, 11 Place Marcelin Berthelot, 75005 Paris, France

Pierre Blier
Neurobiological Psychiatry Unit, McGill University, 1033 Pine Avenue West, Montreal, Quebec H3A 1A1, Canada

Alexandre Bonnin
Unite de Pharmacologie Neuro-Immuno-Endocrinienne, Institut Pasteur, 75724 Paris, France

Mike Briley
Project Evaluation Manager, Institut de Recherche Pierre Fabre, Parc Industriel de la Chartreuse, 81100 Castres, France

Martin Burkart
Department of Psychiatry, University Hospital of Mainz, Untere Zahlbacher Strasse 8, D-55101 Mainz, Germany

Isabelle Cloëz-Tayarani
Unite de Pharmacologie Neuro-Immuno-Endocrinienne, Institut Pasteur, 75724 Paris, France

J Craig Nelson
Professor of Psychiatry, Yale University School of Medicine, USA

Philip J Cowen
University Department of Psychiatry, Littlemore Hospital, Oxford OX4 4XN, UK

Laurent Darracq
INSERM U.114, College de France, 11
Place Marcelin Berthelot, 75005 Paris,
France

J Dee Higley
Laboratory of Clinical Studies,
National Institute on Alcohol Abuse
and Alcoholism, Room 3C-103,
Building 10, Bethesda, MD 20892-
1256, USA

Pedro L Delgado
Department of Psychiatry, College of
Medicine, The University of Arizona
Health Sciences Center, 1501 N
Campbell Avenue, Tuscon, AZ 85724,
USA

Gilles Fillion
Unite de Pharmacologie Neuro-
Immuno-Endocrinienne, Institut
Pasteur, 75724 Paris, France

Marie-Paule Fillion
Unite de Pharmacologie Neuro-
Immuno-Endocrinienne, Institut
Pasteur, 75724 Paris, France

Alan J Gelenberg
Department of Psychiatry, College of
Medicine, The University of Arizona
Health Sciences Center, 1501 N
Campbell Avenue, Tuscon, AZ 85724,
USA

David G Grahame-Smith
Rhodes Professor of Clinical
Pharmacology, Department of Clinical
Pharmacology, University of Oxford
and the Oxford University SmithKline
Beecham Centre of Applied
Neuropsychobiology, Radcliffe
Infirmary, Woodstock Road, Oxford
OX2 6HE, UK

Brigitte Grimaldi
Unite de Pharmacologie Neuro-
Immuno-Endocrinienne, Institut
Pasteur, 75724 Paris, France

Martine Jasson
Department of Pharmacology, Groupe
Hospitalier Pitie-Salpetriere, 47-83
Boulevard de l'Hopital, 75013 Paris,
France

Siegfried Kasper
Professor and Chairman, Department
of General Psychiatry, University of
Vienna, Wahringer Gurtel 18-20,
A-1090 Vienna, Austria

Lars von Knorring
Professor and Head, Department of
Psychiatry, University Hospital,
Uppsala University, S-751 85
Uppsala, Sweden

Brian E Leonard
Pharmacology Department, University
College, Galway, Ireland

Love Linnér
Department of Physiology and
Pharmacology, Division of
Pharmacology, Karolinska Institutet,
S-171 77 Stockholm, Sweden

Markku Linnoila
Laboratory of Clinical Studies,
National Institute on Alcohol Abuse
and Alcoholism, Room 3C-103,
Building 10, Bethesda,
MD 20892-1256, USA

Olivier Massot
Unite de Pharmacologie Neuro-
Immuno-Endocrinienne, Institut
Pasteur, 75724 Paris, France

Luc Mequies
Department of Pharmacology, Groupe Hospitalier Pitie-Salpetriere, 47-83 Boulevard de l'Hopital, 75013 Paris, France

Stuart A Montgomery
Imperial College of Medicine at St Mary's Hospital, Praed Street, London W2, UK

Claude de Montigny
Neurobiological Psychiatry Unit, McGill University, 1033 Pine Avenue West, Montreal, Quebec H3A 1A1, Canada

Francisco A Moreno
Department of Psychiatry, College of Medicine, The University of Arizona Health Sciences Center, 1501 N Campbell Avenue, Tuscon, AZ 85724, USA

Chantal Moret
Centre de Recherche Pierre Fabre, 17 Avenue Jean Moulin, 81100 Castres, France

Alexander Neumeister
National Institute of Mental Health, Clinical Psychobiology Branch, Bethesda MD, USA

Rebecca Potter
Department of Psychiatry, College of Medicine, The University of Arizona Health Sciences Center, 1501 N Campbell Avenue, Tuscon, AZ 85724, USA

Alain J Puech
Department of Pharmacology, Groupe Hospitalier Pitie-Salpetriere, 47-83 Boulevard de l'Hopital, 75013 Paris, France

Jean-Claude Rousselle
Unite de Pharmacologie Neuro-Immuno-Endocrinienne, Institut Pasteur, 75724 Paris, France

S Paul Rossby
Department of Psychiatry and Pharmacology, Vanderbilt University School of Medicine, Nashville, TN 37232, USA

Laure Seguin
Unite de Pharmacologie Neuro-Immuno-Endocrinienne, Institut Pasteur, 75724 Paris, France

Jean-Christophe Seznec
Unite de Pharmacologie Neuro-Immuno-Endocrinienne, Institut Pasteur, 75724 Paris, France

Claudine Soubrie
Department of Pharmacology, Groupe Hospitalier Pitie-Salpetriere, 47-83 Boulevard de l'Hopital, 75013 Paris, France

Fridolin Sulser
Department of Psychiatry and Pharmacology, Vanderbilt University School of Medicine, Nashville, TN 37232, USA

Torgny H Svensson
Professor, Department of Physiology and Pharmacology, Division of Pharmacology, Karolinska Institutet, S-171 77 Stockholm, Sweden

Jean-Pol Tassin
Chaire de Neuropharmacologie, INSERM U.114, College de France, 11 Place Marcelin Berthelot, 75005 Paris, France

Fabrice Trovero
Psypharm, BP 5, 53410 La Brulatte, France

Matti Virkkunen
Department of Psychiatry, University
of Helsinki, POB 33, 00014 Helsinki,
Finland

Hermann Wetzel
Department of Psychiatry, University
Hospital of Mainz, Untere Zahlbacher
Strasse 8, D-55101 Mainz, Germany

Preface

The discovery of tricyclic antidepressants and monoamine oxidase inhibitors in the 1950s led, on the one hand, to the widespread pharmacotherapy of depression that we know today and, on the other hand, to the monoamine hypothesis of their mechanism of action and by extrapolation a possible biological basis for depression. Although the development of more selective and better tolerated drugs such as the selective serotonin reuptake inhibitors has not led to superior therapeutic efficacy, it has enabled millions to benefit from efficacious antidepressant therapy without uncomfortable, distressing and often dangerous adverse effects. This evolution from the 'dirty' tricyclic drugs to the highly (possibly overly) selective serotonin reuptake inhibitors (SSRI) has taught us a lot about the neurochemical substrate of depression. This understanding is now being put into practical terms with the availability of new classes of compounds such as the selective serotonin and noradrenaline reuptake inhibitors (SNRI), the reversible inhibitors of monoamine oxidase A (RIMA) and others. Conceptually based but non-pharmacological therapeutic approaches, such as light therapy and sleep deprivation are now being seriously exploited. 'Intelligent' drug combinations are being increasingly used to improve speed of onset and the extent of therapeutic efficacy.

This book sets out to present an overview of the current and near future advances in antidepressant therapy. Important new concepts of how the monoamine systems are regulated are being developed through in vitro and animal research. Experimental clinical pharmacology is making major fundamental advances using the only real model for depression – the depressed patient. Sophisticated drug trials are determining with ever greater precision the qualitative and quantitative differences between therapeutic approaches. Finally community-based and epidemological studies are highlighting areas where current therapies are still inadequate and where new conceptual approaches, social as well as pharmacological, will be required.

Antidepressant therapy is becoming increasingly multidisciplinary. The contributors of this book have thus been chosen not only for their active engagement at the cutting edge of research in antidepressant therapy but also for their ability to express their ideas and enthusiasm in a way that they can be understood by those outside of their specific field.

Mike Briley
Stuart Montgomery

1
Integrating the monoamine systems

Jean-Pol Tassin, Laurent Darracq, Gérard Blanc and
Fabrice Trovero

The concept that specific neurons modulate information processing rather than convey sensory or motor signals seems generally accepted. In any representation of the primary pathways responsible for the processing of sensory stimuli or motor outputs, it is notable that these pathways include neurons releasing GABA and excitatory amino acids, and possibly acetylcholine or neuropeptides, whereas noradrenergic (NA), dopaminergic (DA) or serotonergic (5-HT) neurons do not appear to be involved.

Since the demonstration by Vetulani and Sulser (1975) that most antidepressants decrease β_1-adrenergic receptor transduction in the cerebral cortex, this parameter has generally been considered as a good biochemical correlate of a therapeutic activity. This observation is noteworthy not only because it seems to be a common consequence of chronic treatments with most antidepressants whatever their mechanism, but also because its development parallels clinical improvements. Indeed, in animal studies, downregulation of β_1-adrenergic receptors only appears following 10–20 days of chronic treatment.

Not all antidepressants, however, induce desensitization of β-adrenergic receptors. A reactivation of 5-HT transmission, which can be obtained by some antidepressants, can hamper the development of β-adrenergic receptor desensitization even when NA transmission is also reactivated. This lack of response of β-adrenergic receptors is proposed to be due to past receptor events at the level of phosphorylations mediated by phosphokinases A and C (Chapter 5).

β_1-Adrenergic receptors are not the only receptors desensitized by antidepressants. A 5-HT receptor subtype, 5-HT_2, is also frequently affected (Peroutka and Snyder, 1980). This should not imply, however, that an upregulation of β_1-adrenergic or 5-HT_2 receptors is responsible for the disease and that, consequently, downregulation of these receptors is the goal to achieve. These observations rather suggest that both types of receptors, β_1-adrenergic and 5-HT_2, are very sensitive to any modification of their respective neurotransmissions and that an activation of these occurs following chronic treatment with antidepressants. According to that view, a deactivation of 5-HT and/or NA neurons is probably the main biochemical characteristic of depression.

The role of DA neurons in depression should not, however, be overlooked. Subcortical DA systems are known to play a crucial role in the processing of reward-related information and in the selection and elaboration of motivated behaviour. More precisely, the inability to experience pleasure (anhedonia) as well as emotional blunting are two symptoms which are frequently associated with depression and are very sensitive to DA agonists (Lisoprawski and Jouvent, 1989). Moreover, the co-occurrence of depression and Parkinson's disease seems well established (review: Randrup et al, 1975) and antidepressants have also been shown to modify different behavioural and biochemical parameters of the DA transmission (review: Willner, 1983). For example, repeated treatment with antidepressants increases the behavioural response to small doses of apomorphine (Maj et al, 1984) and decreases the number of D_1 binding sides in the rat striatum and limbic system (Klimek and Nielsen, 1987), thus indicating a rise in DA transmission. However, with the exception of the fact that some antidepressants block DA reuptake activity with good affinities (Randrup and Braestrup, 1977; Bolden-Watson and Richelson, 1993), most of the evidence implicating DA in depression is indirect. It is therefore possible that the effects of antidepressants on DA parameters are the consequence of modifications of NA and/or 5-HT transmission.

We have previously proposed that antidepressants could aim to re-establish a sufficient DA transmission in limbic structures, whatever their biochemical mode of action and specificity (Tassin, 1994, 1995). This hypothesis originates from different observations concerning the interactions between the three monoamine systems and will be tentatively reviewed in this chapter.

Interactions between 5-HT and DA neurons

Dopaminergic cells of the ventral tegmental area (VTA) project to limbic structures such as the nucleus accumbens, amygdala and lateral septum and receive convergent afferents from several parts of the brain, including the mesencephalic dorsal raphe nucleus (Phillipson, 1979; Steinbusch, 1981). Endogenous 5-HT, as well as synapses immunoreactive for 5-HT, can be found in the VTA (Saavedra, 1977; Hervé et al, 1987). These 5-HT fibres contact dendrites of cells which may or may not contain tyrosine hydroxylase, the DA synthetic enzyme (Hervé et al, 1987). In vitro electrophysiological studies indicate that 5-HT, via the stimulation of 5-HT$_2$ receptors, increases the firing of a large proportion of DA cells located in the VTA (Pessia et al, 1994). However, the overall effects may be more complex, since indirect changes in DA cell-firing can result from 5-HT exciting or inhibiting local GABA-containing interneurons (Pessia et al, 1994). Others have found that the systemic (IV) administration of ritanserine, a 5-HT$_2$ antagonist, increases the firing rate of DA neurons (Ugedo et al, 1989). This discrepancy between the effects of 5-HT$_2$ agonists and antagonists, which both increase DA cell-firing, is interesting, since it emphasizes that complex neuronal loops interfere when compounds are injected systematically.

An illustration of such a complexity has been obtained in experiments showing that, in mice, the amphetamine-induced locomotor hyperactivity can be blocked by systemic administration (IP) of specific and selective 5-HT$_2$ antagonists, MDL 100,907 and amperozide, respectively (Sorensen et al, 1993). MDL 100,907 is an extremely potent antagonist of 5-HT$_{2A}$ receptors ($K_i = 0.36$ nM) and amperozide exhibits the greatest affinity for 5-HT$_{2A}$ receptors ($K_i = 26$ nM) when compared to other monoaminergic receptors, including other 5-HT receptor subtypes (Haskins et al, 1987). If, as generally accepted, amphetamine-induced locomotor hyperactivity is due to an increased release of DA in the nucleus accumbens, the blockade of 5-HT$_2$ receptors may hamper this increased DA release. This possibility was confirmed by Ichikawa and Meltzer (1992), who showed that systemic injection of amperozide inhibits the ability of D-amphetamine to increase DA extracellular levels in the nucleus accumbens. However, these authors also found that amperozide injected alone could increase DA basal extracellular levels in the nucleus accumbens. This effect of amperozide on DA release seems even higher in the prefrontal cortex than in the nucleus accumbens (Pehek et al, 1993; Nomikos et al, 1994). Moreover, MDL 100,907, a 5-HT$_2$ antagonist, also increases DA release in the prefrontal cortex (Schmidt and Fadayel, 1995). In summary, 5-HT$_2$ antagonists decrease the reactivity of DA neurons to pharmacological stimulation but increase their basal activity.

Finally, although D-amphetamine increases DA release in the nucleus accumbens, it is well known that it also reduces DA cell-firing in the VTA (Wang, 1981). However, different 5-HT$_2$ antagonists, including MDL 100,907 (Sorensen et al, 1993), can block this slowing effect of amphetamine on DA cells. If we assume that 5-HT$_2$ antagonists do not act directly on DA presynaptic terminals, which is very likely, we have to consider that an increased neuronal activity can be associated with a decreased release of the corresponding neurotransmitter.

Altogether, these findings suggest that 5-HT neurons exert both direct and indirect, excitatory and inhibitory, controls on DA neurons. It is possible that 5-HT$_2$ receptors regulate, through indirect neuronal loops, the activity of DA cells with respect to the level of DA release. In other words, the stimulation of brain 5-HT$_2$ receptors may contribute to the 'efficacy' of DA release in subcortical structures such as the nucleus accumbens.

There is some indication that NA neurons may contribute to the link between these 5-HT and DA cells.

Interactions between 5-HT and NA neurons

General considerations

Most of the studies concerning interactions between 5-HT and NA neurons have initially been performed by Aghajanian and his colleagues. Two main findings can be emphasized. First, NA neurons exert, through the stimulation of α_1-adrenergic receptors located in the dorsal raphe nucleus, a tonic excitatory action on 5-HT neurons (Aghajanian, 1985). Second, 5-HT agonists, such as mescaline or LSD, decrease cell-firing of locus coeruleus NA neurons and facilitate the activation of these neurons by peripheral stimuli (Aghajanian, 1980). More recently, Chiang and Aston-Jones (1993) have further confirmed and refined these latter findings. A systemic injection of DOI, a 5-HT_2 agonist, increases the responses of NA neurons to peripheral sensory stimuli and decreases the basal activity of NA neurons. Both phenomena are blocked by ketanserin, a 5-HT_2 antagonist. Moreover, these effects are not due to a direct action on NA neurons, since they are no longer observed when DOI is injected locally in the locus coeruleus (Chiang and Aston-Jones, 1993).

It has been proposed that the regulation of basal activity of locus coeruleus NA neurons by 5-HT_2 receptors involves the prepositus hypoglossal nucleus and not the prefrontal cortex, a structure which nevertheless presents a high density of 5-HT_2 receptors (Gorea et al, 1991). However, since DOI exhibits a potent inhibitory activity on prefrontocortical cells (Ashby et al, 1990), the possibility cannot be excluded that the 5-HT_2 receptors of the prefrontal cortex, which do not seem to be implicated in the regulation of basal activity of NA neurons, intervene in the increased reactivity of NA neurons to peripheral stimuli.

Finally, it is interesting to note that amperozide, a 5-HT_2 antagonist, increases the basal firing rate of locus coeruleus NA neurons (Haskins et al, 1987). This effect may be associated with the activity of DA cells obtained with amperozide (Grenhoff et al, 1990) and with the selective increased release of DA in the prefrontal cortex induced by 5-HT_2 antagonists (Nomikos et al, 1994; Schmidt and Fadayel, 1995).

As well as in the case of 5-HT–DA interactions, 5-HT_2 receptors obviously play a major role in the regulation of the activity and the reactivity of locus coeruleus NA neurons. Although the precise site(s) of these interactions remain unknown, the prefrontal cortex seems to be among the good candidates, at least with regard to the reactivity of NA neurons. In any case, the blockade of 5-HT_2 receptors induces, for NA as well as for

DA neurons, an increased activity and a decreased reactivity, thus suggesting a common regulation of catecholaminergic neurons.

Therapeutic efficacy of SSRIs

Serotonergic transmission is generally considered as being the main target of antidepressants. This is due to the recent development of specific serotonin reuptake inhibitors (SSRIs) which have been shown to possess clear therapeutic efficacy. Affinity constants (K_is) for the blockade of the 5-HT reuptake system of the different compounds of this class vary from 0.4 nM to 40 nM, which corresponds to a 100-fold factor (Figure 1.1). However, SSRI clinical doses recommended by drug companies range from 20 to 75 or 100 mg per day. Moreover, a drug such as fluoxetine, which has a modest affinity for the 5-HT reuptake system, exhibits a clinical therapeutic efficacy as low as 20 mg/day, a dose which is not different from that of paroxetine, which presents, however, an affinity for the 5-HT reuptake system 25-fold higher than that of fluoxetine (Figure 1.1). Even if one considers the possible variations in bioavailability, these observations suggest that the modification of the 5-HT transmission is not the sole factor which can explain SSRIs' therapeutic efficacy.

Among the different possibilities, the affinities for the NA reuptake system appear very similar from one SSRI to the other (from 25 nM to 200 nM), with the exception of citalopram, which is the only SSRI with a K_i higher than 200 nM for the NA reuptake system (Figure 1.1). There is, however, some indication in the literature that citalopram could interfere with catecholaminergic transmission through other, still unknown, mechanisms (De Deurwaerdere et al, 1995). Altogether, these observations suggest that, in addition to their effect on 5-HT neurons, a modification of NA transmission might also be an important factor in the therapeutic efficacy of SSRIs. To test this hypothesis we have perfused various concentrations of fluoxetine through a microdialysis probe located in the rat prefrontal cortex and analysed extracellular variations of the three monoamines (5-HT, NA and DA) with an HPLC column coupled to an electrochemical (Coulochem II) detector.

Fluoxetine was perfused through the microdialysis probe to avoid any interference with the stimulation of 5-HT$_{1A}$ somatodendritic receptors (Artigas et al, 1996). Concentrations of fluoxetine ranged in the probe from 1 to 50 μM, thus corresponding to a range of 0.1–5 μM in the extracellular environment, assuming a 10% gradient through the membrane. Perfusions of fluoxetine quickly increased 5-HT extracellular levels to a plateau at 320% of the control values for concentrations ranging from 5 to 50 μM fluoxetine in the probe (Figures 1.2 and 1.3). Simultaneously, NA extracellular levels increased regularly, from above 500% of the control values at 5 μM of fluoxetine, to reach 1800% at 50 μM of fluoxetine in the probe (Figures 1.2 and 1.3). DA extracellular levels were not affected

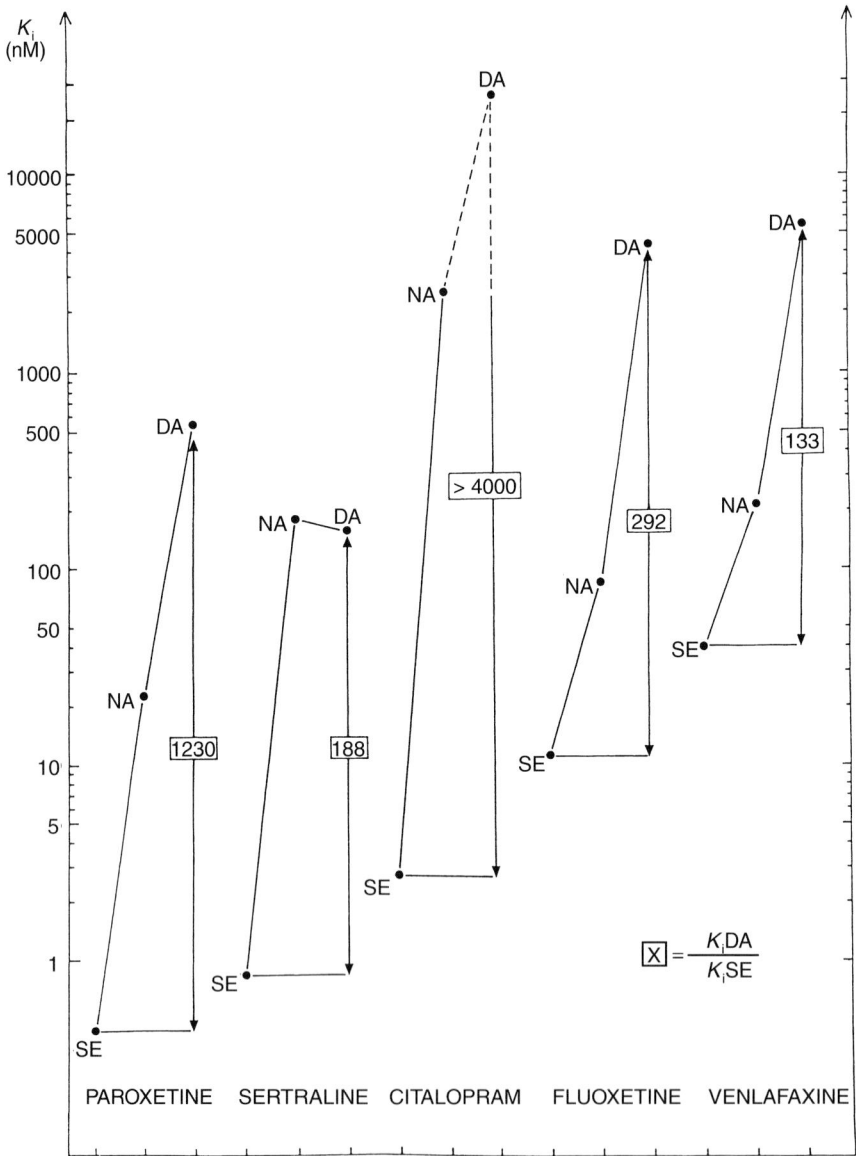

Figure 1.1

Representation of inhibition constants (K_i) of antidepressants selective for the blockade of the 5-HT reuptake in the three monoamine reuptake systems. K_i values are taken from Bolden-Watson and Richelson (1993) and from indications given by the drug companies. Slight variations from other published data may occur. They are due to differences in methodologies and to the nature of the cerebral tissues chosen for K_i determination. Note that the scale for the ordinates is logarithmic. SE, serotonin.

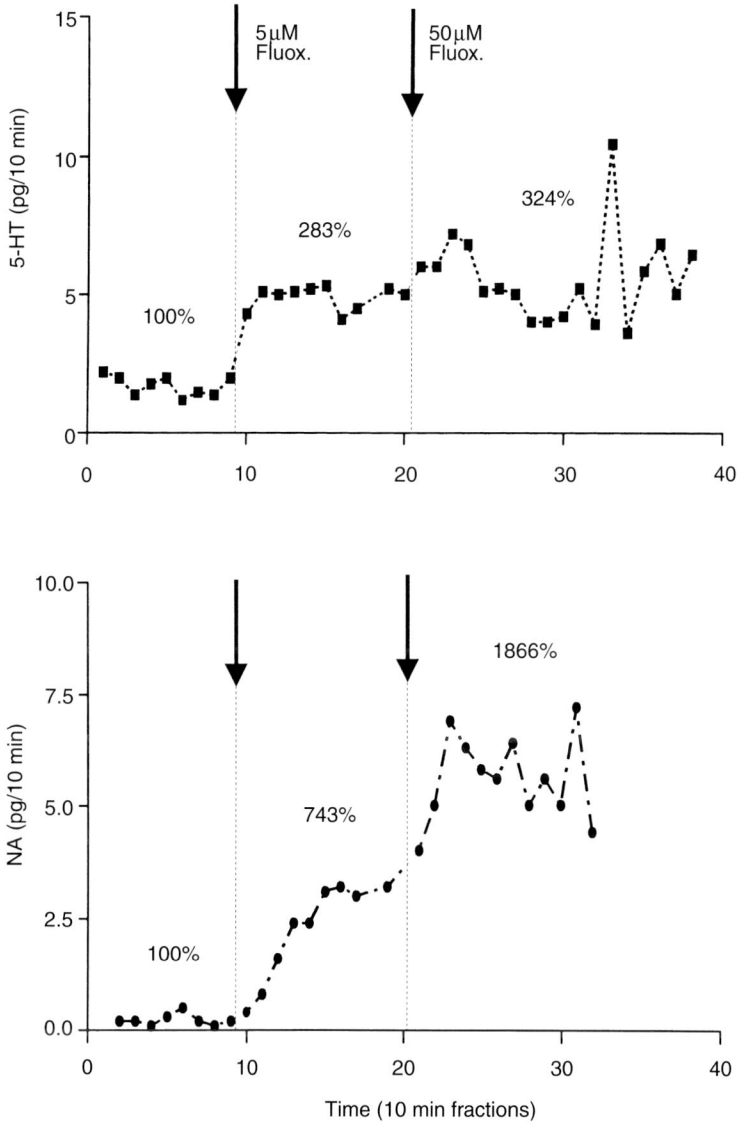

Figure 1.2

Example of effects of two doses of fluoxetine on the extracellular levels of 5-HT and NA in the prefrontal cortex of freely moving rats. Animals are perfused in the prefrontal cortex with artificial cerebrospinal fluid (2 μl/min) 2 h before the sampling of the first microdialysis fraction. Fractions are then collected every 10 min, and 5 or 50 μM fluoxetine are added in the perfusate in order to obtain corresponding fractions where indicated by arrows. When two doses of fluoxetine are given in the same experiment, they always differ by at least a 10-fold factor, the lower concentration being perfused first. Each sample (20 μl) is injected randomly in the HPLC column and monoamine levels are quantified with a Coulochem II detector (Eurosep, France) allowing a 0.2 pg sensitivity for each monoamine. Upper diagram: 5-HT levels. Lower diagram: NA levels.

until a concentration of 50 µM fluoxetine was obtained in the probe.

These data indicate that, for almost all the concentrations tested, fluoxetine affects the NA relatively more than the 5-HT transmission in the prefrontal cortex (Figure 1.3). This is probably due to the extreme sensitivity of NA neurons to external stimuli (Aston-Jones and Bloom, 1981), a slight effect on the NA reuptake system inducing important modifications of NA extracellular levels. Although it is difficult to determine precisely the concentration of fluoxetine attained in the clinical context, data based on fluoxetine and norfluoxetine concentrations in plasma of chronically treated patients indicate that these would correspond to brain levels obtained with concentrations ranging from 2 to 4 µM fluoxetine in the probe (Dailey et al, 1992).

This effect of fluoxetine on NA transmission has already been described (Jordan et al, 1994; Hughes and Stanford, 1996). However, these latter authors obtained only an 80% increase of NA extracellular levels in the prefrontal cortex following a 5 µM perfusion of fluoxetine in the probe. This relatively small effect may be due to the sensitivity of NA neurons to anaesthesia. Hughes and Stanford (1996) have indeed performed their microdialysis experiments the day following the anaesthesia necessary for the probe implantation, whereas, in our experiments, animals

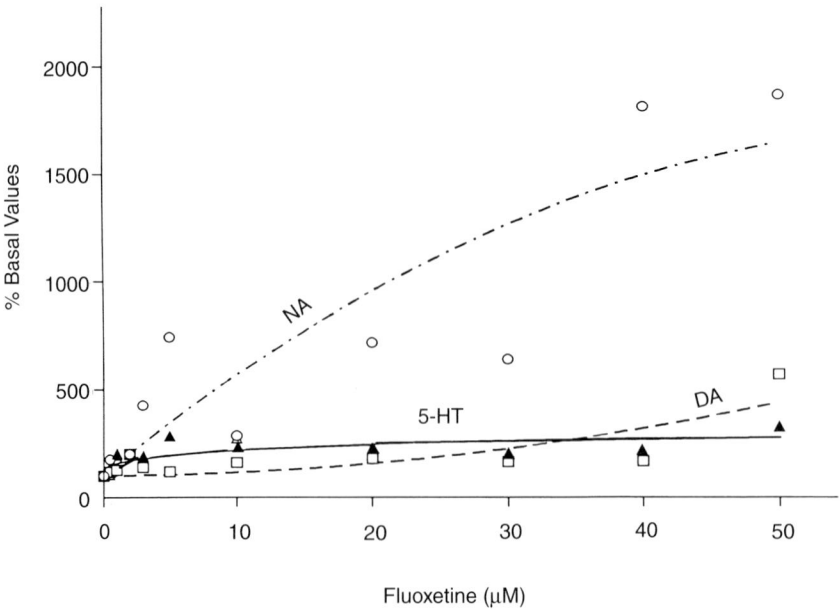

Figure 1.3

Effects of increasing doses of fluoxetine on the extracellular levels of the three monoamines in the prefrontal cortex of freely moving rats. Methods are described in the legend of Figure 1.2. 5-HT (▲), NA (○) and DA (□) levels are expressed as percentages of basal values.

were allowed to recover for at least 7 days and up to 3 weeks after the fixation of the guide.

There is, however, no clear evidence that the effect of fluoxetine on NA transmission is only due to the blockade of the reuptake system. Fluoxetine may directly block some receptors such as the central nicotinic (Garcia-Colunga et al, 1997) or the 5-HT$_{2C}$ (Ni and Miledi, 1997) receptors, or, alternatively but not exclusively, it may be the increased extracellular 5-HT which affects NA release, either locally (Blandina et al, 1991) or indirectly by increasing the reactivity of locus coeruleus NA neurons via the stimulation of 5-HT$_2$ receptors (Chiang and Aston-Jones, 1993). In any case, this example of fluoxetine shows that the concept that the clinical efficacy of an antidepressant is solely related to its effect on 5-HT transmission should be revisited. Perfusion of other SSRIs, in microdialysis experiments performed on freely moving animals having completely recovered from anaesthesia, may provide new and interesting data. In addition, besides their possible effects on cortical NA release, the possibility cannot be excluded that SSRIs modify DA subcortical transmission.

Interactions between NA and DA neurons

Assuming that a topographical proximity between NA and DA cell bodies and axons is necessary for direct interactions to occur, it is interesting to note that, although NA neurons located in the locus coeruleus innervate most of the structures of the forebrain, the DA nigrostriatal pathway seems to escape direct NA control. Indeed, the ventral part of the substantia nigra compacta lacks NA fibres (Swanson and Hartman, 1975; Gaspar et al, 1992) and the striatum is devoid of locus coeruleus axons (Room et al, 1981) or of NA terminals in both rats (Swanson and Hartman, 1975) and primates (Gaspar et al, 1985). In contrast, the VTA receives a significant NA innervation, although no ultrastructural study has been done to authentify direct connections (Swanson and Hartman, 1975; Simon et al, 1979; Gaspar et al, 1992). At the level of the DA target structures, which include the nucleus accumbens, septal nuclei, amygdala and cerebral cortex, there is also a significant NA terminal network but there is no complete overlap between NA and DA systems. DA and NA networks appear to innervate different subnuclei or territories within the amygdala (Sadikot and Parent, 1990) and the septum or the bed nucleus of the stria terminalis (Lindvall and Stenevi, 1978; Gaspar et al, 1985). Up to now, we have focused our attention on the VTA and the prefrontal cortex as putative sites of interactions between NA and DA neurons. In addition to the existence of NA–DA interactions in the VTA, we have obtained some indications that catecholaminergic interactions occurring in the prefrontal cortex may have some consequences on the DA subcortical transmission.

NA–DA interactions in the VTA

Initially, a specific destruction of the ascending NA neurons innervating the VTA was performed by injection of 6-OHDA in the vicinity of the NA pathway connecting the locus coeruleus to the VTA (Hervé et al, 1982). These lesions did not affect NA cortical innervation. Seven days later, a significant 38% decrease of the dihydroxyphelylacetic acid (DOPAC)/DA ratio was observed in the prefrontal cortex and no change in the nucleus accumbens. These data suggested that NA neurons exert a specific tonic excitatory control on mesocortical DA neurons. This was further confirmed in microdialysis experiments, performed on awake freely moving animals, where short-lasting abrupt physiological increases of NA extracellular levels in the prefrontal cortex were correlated with those of cortical DA extracellular levels ($N = 21$, $r = 0.91$; $p < 0.001$) (Gillibert, 1994).

Electrophysiological studies have indicated that prazosin, an α_1-adrenergic antagonist, dose-dependently decreases burst firing of VTA DA neurons (Grenhoff and Svensson, 1993). However, since prazosin was injected systemically, α_1-adrenergic receptors responsible for the modification of DA neuron activities may be located in other site(s) than the VTA. Recently, Pan et al (1996) have shown that the perfusion, through a microdialysis probe, of amphetamine in the VTA of anaesthetized animals increases DA release in the nucleus accumbens and the prefrontal cortex. These authors have also found that the perfusion, through the probe, of 0.1 µM phentolamine, an α_1-adrenergic antagonist, could block the VTA amphetamine-induced increased DA release in the prefrontal cortex but not in the nucleus accumbens. These data have therefore confirmed the presence of a specific tonic excitatory α_1-adrenergic input on DA mesocortical neurons.

NA–DA interactions in the prefrontal cortex

The first indication of the presence of interactions between NA and DA neurons in the prefrontal cortex was obtained when it was found that the 6-hydroxydopamine (6-OHDA) destruction of ascending NA neurons induces a collateral sprouting of mesocortical DA neurons (Tassin et al, 1979). Later on, it was shown that the denervation supersensitivity of cortical postsynaptic D_1 receptors only occurs if NA fibres are preserved by the lesion of mesocortical DA neurons. This permissive role of ascending NA fibres in the appearance of denervation supersensitivity of cortical D_1 receptors was finally demonstrated by showing that rats with an electrolytic lesion of the VTA exhibit increases in cortical DA-sensitive adenylyl cyclase activity, whereas rats with both electrolytic VTA lesions of DA neurons and 6-OHDA lesions of ascending NA neurons do not (Tassin et al, 1982, 1986).

Two groups of experiments were then performed to investigate what type of adrenergic receptor was responsible for the heteroregulation of cortical D_1 receptors by NA.

First, EEDQ, an irreversible antagonist of monoaminergic receptors, was injected into rats at a dose which induced a three-fold higher mean decrease of cortical α_1-adrenergic receptors than of cortical D_1 receptors. Four hours after EEDQ injection, we observed a significant increase (25%) of DA-sensitive adenylyl cyclase activity in the prefrontal cortex. This increase in cortical DA-sensitive adenylyl cyclase activity was abolished when rats were pre-injected with prazosin, an α_1-adrenergic antagonist (Trovero et al, 1992).

Second, the rate of resensitization of D_1 receptors in embryonic cortical cell cultures previously incubated with 50 µM DA was analysed. We found that the rate of resensitization of the DA-sensitive adenylyl cyclase activity was almost doubled when cultured cells were incubated in the presence of methoxamine, an α_1-adrenergic agonist. This effect was abolished in the presence of 1 µM prazosin (Trovero et al, 1994).

Both types of experiment indicate that the stimulation of cortical α_1-adrenergic receptors inhibits the cortical DA transmission mediated by D_1 receptors. Moreover, embryonic cell culture experiments suggest that α_1-adrenergic and D_1 receptors are, at least partly, located on the same neurons in the rat cerebral cortex.

Behavioural consequences of NA–DA interactions in the prefrontal cortex

Bilateral electrolytic lesions of the rat VTA induce deficits such as locomotor hyperactivity and disappearance of spontaneous alternation (Le Moal et al, 1977). Correlation studies have indicated that the amplitude of locomotor hyperactivity is proportional to the extent of destruction of the DA fibres innervating the prefrontal cortex and to the development of a D_1 receptor supersensitivity in this area (Tassin et al, 1978, 1982, 1995; Ashby and Tassin, 1995).

Since destruction of ascending NA pathways downregulates cortical D_1 receptor denervation supersensitivity induced by electrolytic lesion of the VTA, we have investigated whether the locomotor hyperactivity induced by this electrolytic lesion could be affected by chemical (6-OHDA) lesions of the NA innervation. Indeed, both deficits induced by the electrolytic lesion of the VTA, locomotor hyperactivity and disappearance of spontaneous alternation were abolished by a superimposed 6-OHDA lesion of ascending NA neurons (Taghzouti et al, 1988). This functional recovery provided new insights into the antagonistic properties of NA and DA neurons. A functional hierarchy may exist between these systems, since no significant modification of the locomotor activity or spontaneous alternation was observed in rats with NA lesions alone.

To confirm the hypothesis that the prefrontal cortex could be an important site of interaction between NA fibres and the target cells of the mesocortical DA neurons, two groups of experiments were performed with rats implanted with chronic bilateral cannulae in both the prefrontal cortex and the nucleus accumbens.

We first found that the locomotor hyperactivity induced by the infusion of amphetamine into the nucleus accumbens was inhibited when amphetamine was simultaneously injected into the prefrontal cortex. Complementary experiments have indicated that this cortical effect is mediated via D_1 receptors, since the injection of SCH 23390, a D_1 antagonist, into the prefrontal cortex, doubled the locomotor hyperactivity induced by the infusion of amphetamine into the nucleus accumbens. The injection of sulpiride, a D_2 antagonist, was without effect (Vezina et al, 1991). These results suggest that the inhibitory role of prefrontocortical DA innervation on locomotor behaviour is mediated by D_1 receptors when the DA transmission in the nucleus accumbens is activated. We then showed that the injection of prazosin or WB 4101, two α_1-adrenergic antagonists, into the prefrontal cortex completely reversed the locomotor hyperactivity induced by the injection of amphetamine into the nucleus accumbens. Neither antagonist had an effect on locomotor activity when injected alone (Blanc et al, 1994).

Altogether, these results not only confirm that NA and DA neurons exert opposite functional roles in the prefrontal cortex, but also demonstrate that the stimulation by NA of cortical α_1-adrenergic receptors is necessary for a functional subcortical DA transmission.

In recent experiments, performed with minute-by-minute sampling microdialysis, we have tried to study the influence of cortical α_1-adrenergic receptor stimulation on the DA release in the nucleus accumbens. It was found that the level of extracellular DA needed in nuclei accumbens to elicit a significant locomotor hyperactivity was about 10-fold higher when D-amphetamine (1 mM) was perfused locally in both nuclei accumbens than when it was injected systemically (0.5 mg/kg IP). Moreover, systemic prazosin (0.5 mg/kg IP) did not modify the increase of extracellular DA levels in the nucleus accumbens induced by the perfusion of a subthreshold concentration (3 µM) of D-amphetamine, a dose which increases by fivefold DA extracellular levels but which is not sufficient to elicit locomotor hyperactivity. However, when D-amphetamine was injected systemically (0.5 mg/kg IP) in animals previously perfused with 3 µM D-amphetamine in the nucleus accumbens, prazosin was able to block both the increased release of DA in the nucleus accumbens and the locomotor hyperactivity induced by the systemically injected amphetamine. The same blockade of DA release in the nucleus accumbens induced by systemic amphetamine was obtained when prazosin was injected locally into the prefrontal cortex (Darracq et al, 1997). These data indicate that, although amphetamine can release DA by a local action, it is the effect of amphetamine distal from the nucleus accumbens which is mainly responsible for the development of locomotor hyperactivity, i.e. the functional role of DA in the nucleus accumbens. Since the amphetamine-induced locomotor hyperactivity is more dependent on the route (systemic or local) chosen to inject amphetamine than to the amount of DA released in the nucleus accumbens, we propose that systemic D-amphetamine injections induce a synchronization of DA neurons via the stimulation of cortical α_1-adrenergic receptors.

Stimulation of cortical α_1-adrenergic receptors by NA would initiate, through an inhibition of cortical D_1 transmission, the phasic and synchronized release of DA in subcortical structures, thus inducing a functional subcortical DA transmission.

Conclusion

The aim of this chapter was to try to delineate some of the interactions between the three monoamine systems which could be relevant to the action of antidepressants. From a general point of view, it seems necessary to differentiate between modifications of neuronal activity and reactivity induced by pharmacological manipulations. More precisely, the stimulation of $5-HT_2$ receptors appears to decrease the basal activity and increase the reactivity to environmental stimuli of both NA and DA neurons. In so far as depression can be due to a decreased reactivity of catecholaminergic neurons, a reactivation of 5-HT cells by antidepressants may be the first step to achieve in order to obtain relief of depression. The links between $5-HT_2$ receptors and NA neurons as well as between α_1-adrenergic receptors and DA neurons seem well established, whereas those between $5-HT_2$ receptors and DA neurons appear more complex. We propose that NA neurons play the role of 'go-between' to couple 5-HT and DA cells (Figure 1.4).

It is clear that other interactions do occur, such as the NA tonic excitatory input to the 5-HT cells in the dorsal raphe nucleus. However, clinical data argue against the importance of such an interaction, a specific blocker of the NA reuptake system, desipramine, exhibiting a narrower antidepressive efficacy than other antidepressants which associate or are specific for the blockade of the 5-HT reuptake system.

Our hypothesis would therefore be that depression corresponds, depending on the patients, to an effect on one or more of the three neuromodulatory systems. Antidepressants would re-establish interactions between them in accordance with a physiological sequence: following the reactivation of 5-HT neurons, antidepressants would, through NA cells, reinstate functional subcortical DA transmission. The therapeutic delay usually observed in the pharmacological treatments of depression is probably due not only to the generally described desensitization of autoreceptors, but also to the time necessary to obtain this readjustment. Final relief would occur only following recoupling of monoaminergic neurons to neuronal networks responsible for sensory stimuli processing.

Cerebral Cortex

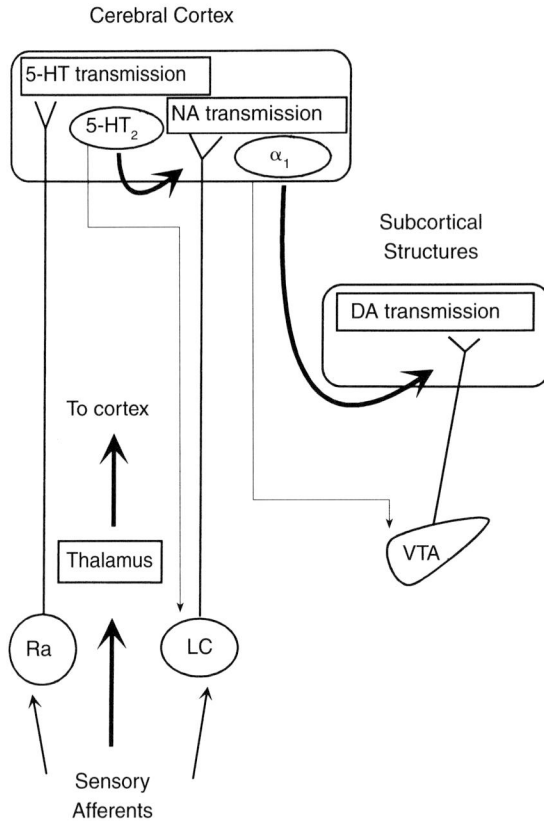

Figure 1.4

Schematic diagram of the putative monoaminergic cascade induced by antidepressants. The reactivation of the 5-HT transmission by antidepressants facilitates the stimulation of 5-HT$_2$ receptors and restores the sensitivity of NA neurons to sensory stimuli. These latter, via the stimulation of cortical α_1-adrenergic receptors, may then enable a functional DA subcortical transmission. The mesocortical DA pathway has been omitted for sake of clarity. Ra, raphe nuclei; LC, locus coeruleus; VTA, ventral tegmental area.

References

Aghajanian GK (1980) Mescaline and LSD facilitate the activation of locus coeruleus neurons by peripheral stimuli, *Brain Res* **186**:492–8.

Aghajanian GK (1985) Modulation of a transient outward current in serotonergic neurones by α_1-adrenoceptors, *Nature* **315**:501–3.

Artigas F, Romero L, de Montigny C, Blier P (1996) Acceleration of the effect of selected antidepressant drugs in major depression by 5-HT1A antagonists, *Trends Neurosci* **19**:378–83.

Ashby CR Jr, Tassin JP (1995) The modulation of dopaminergic neurons by norepinephrine. In: Asbhy CR Jr, ed., *Interactions of Neurotransmitters with Dopamine* (CRC Press: New York) 3–49.

Ashby CR Jr, Jiang LH, Kasser RJ, Wang RY (1990) Electrophysiological characterization of 5-hydroxytryptamine2 receptors in the rat medial prefrontal cortex, *J Pharmacol Exp Ther* **252:**171–8.

Aston-Jones G, Bloom F (1981) Norepinephrine-containing locus coeruleus neurons in behaving rats exhibit pronounced responses to the non-noxious environmental stimuli, *J Neurosci* **1:**887–900.

Blanc G, Trovero F, Vezina P et al (1994) Blockade of prefrontocortical α1-adrenergic receptors prevents locomotor hyperactivity induced by subcortical D-amphetamine injection, *Eur J Neurosci* **6:**293–8.

Blandina P, Goldfarb J, Walcott J, Green JP (1991) Serotonergic modulation of the release of endogenous norepinephrine from rat hypothalamic slices, *J Pharmacol Exp Ther* **256:**341–9.

Bolden-Watson C, Richelson E (1993) Blockade by newly-developed antidepressants of biogenic amine uptake into rat brain synaptosomes, *Life Sci* **52:**1023–9.

Chiang C, Aston-Jones G (1993) A 5-hydroxytryptamine2 agonist augments γ-aminobutyric acid and excitatory amino acid inputs to noradrenergic locus coeruleus neurons, *Neuroscience* **54:**409–20.

Dailey JW, Yan QS, Mishra PK, Burger RL, Jobe PC (1992) Effects of fluoxetine on convulsions and on brain serotonin as detected by microdialysis in genetically epilepsy-prone rats, *J Pharmacol Exp Ther* **260:**533–40.

Darracq L, Blanc G, Glowinski J, Tassin JP (1997) Importance of the noradrenaline/dopamine coupling in the locomotor activating effects of low doses of D-amphetamine, *J Neurosci* (submitted).

De Deuwaerdere P, Bonhomme N, Le Moal M, Spampinato U (1995) d-Fenfluramine increases striatal extracellular dopamine in vivo independently of serotonergic terminals or dopamine uptake sites, *J Neurochem* **65:**1100–8.

Garcia-Colunga J, Awad JN, Miledi R (1997) Blockage of muscle and neuronal nicotinic acetylcholine receptors by fluoxetine (Prozac), *Proc Natl Acad Sci USA* **94:**2041–4.

Gaspar P, Berger B, Alvarez C, Henry JP, Vigny A (1985) Catecholaminergic innervation of the septal area in man. Immunocytochemical study using TH and DBH antibodies, *J Comp Neurol* **241:**12–33.

Gaspar P, Stepniewska I, Kaas JH (1992) Topography and collateralization of the DA projections to motor and lateral prefrontal cortex in owl monkeys, *J Comp Neurol* **325:**1–21.

Gillibert C (1994) Libération des monoamines dans le cortex préfrontal du rat au cours du cycle veille-sommeil: analyse en microdialyse, DEA Thesis, University Paris VI.

Gorea E, Davenne D, Lanfumey L, Chastanet M, Adrien J (1991) Regulation of noradrenergic coerulean neuronal firing mediated by 5-HT2 receptors: hypoglossal nucleus, *Neuropharmacol* **30:**1309–18.

Grenhoff J, Svensson T (1993) Prazosin modulates the firing pattern of dopaminergic neurons in rat ventral segmental area. *Europ J Pharmacol* 233: 79–84.

Grenhoff J, Tung C, Ugedo L, Svensson T (1990) Effects of amperozide, a putative antipsychotic drug, on rat midbrain dopamine neurons recorded *in vivo*, *Pharmacol Toxicol* **60**(suppl 1): 29–33.

Haskins JT, Much EA, Andree TH (1987) Biochemical and electrophysiological studies of the psychotropic compound, Amperozide, *Brain Res Bull* **19:**465–71.

Hervé D, Blanc G, Glowinski J, Tassin JP (1982) Reduction of dopamine utilization in the prefrontal cortex but not in the nucleus accumbens after selective destruction of noradrenergic fibers innervating the ventral tegmental area in the rat, *Brain Res* **237:**510–16.

Hervé D, Pickel VM, Joh TH, Beaudet A (1987) Serotonin axon terminals in the ventral tegmental area of the rat: fine structure and synaptic input to dopamine neurons, *Brain Res* **435:**71–83.

Hughes ZA, Stanford SC (1996) Increased noradrenaline efflux induced by local infusion of fluoxetine in the rat frontal cortex, *Eur J Pharmacol* **317:**83–90.

Ichikawa J, Meltzer HY (1992) Amperozide, a novel antipsychotic drug, inhibits the ability of D-amphetamine to increase dopamine release in vivo in rat striatum and nucleus accumbens, *J Neurochem* **58:**2285–91.

Jordan S, Kramer GL, Zukas PK, Moeller M, Petty F (1994) In vivo biogenic amine efflux in medial prefrontal cortex with imipramine, fluoxetine and fluvoxamine, *Synapse* **18:**294–9.

Klimek V, Nielsen M (1987) Chronic treatment with antidepressants decreases the number of 3H-SCH 23390 binding sites in the rat striatum and limbic system, *Eur J Pharmacol* **139:**163–9.

Le Moal M, Stinus L, Simon H et al (1977) Behavioral effects of a lesion in the ventral mesencephalic tegmentum: evidence for involvement of A10 dopaminergic neurons, *Adv Biochem Psychopharmacol* **16:**237–45.

Lindvall O, Stenevi U (1978) Dopamine and noradrenaline neurons projecting to the septal area in the rat, *Cell Tissue Res* **190:**383–407.

Lisoprawski A, Jouvent R (1989) Agonistes dopaminergiques et émoussement affectif, *L'Encéphale* **XV:** 197–200.

Maj J, Rogoz Z, Skuza G, Sowinska H (1984) Repeated treatment with antidepressant drugs increases the behavioural responses to apomorphine, *J Neural Transm* **60:**273–82.

Ni YG, Miledi R (1997) Blockage of 5-HT2C serotonin receptors by fluoxetine (Prozac), *Proc Natl Acad Sci USA* **94:**2036–40.

Nomikos GG, Iurlo M, Andersson JL, Kimura K, Svensson TH (1994) Systemic administration of amperozide, a new atypical antipsychotic drug, preferentially increases dopamine release in the rat medial prefrontal cortex, *Psychopharmacol (Berl)* **115:**147–56.

Pan WHT, Sung JC, Fuh SMR (1996) Local application of amphetamine into the ventral tegmental area enhances dopamine release in the nucleus accumbens and the medial prefrontal cortex through noradrenergic neurotransmission, *J Pharmacol Exp Ther* **278:**725–31.

Pehek EA, Meltzer HY, Yamamoto BK (1993) The atypical antipsychotic drug amperozide enhances rat cortical and striatal dopamine efflux, *Eur J Pharmacol* **240:**107–9.

Peroutka SJ, Snyder SH (1980) Long-term antidepressant treatment decreases spiroperidol-labelled serotonin receptor binding, *Science* **210:**88–90.

Pessia M, Jiang ZG, North RA, Johnson SW (1994) Actions of 5-hydroxytryptamine on ventral tegmental area neurons of the rat in vitro, *Brain Res* **654:**324–30.

Phillipson OT (1979) Afferent projections to the ventral tegmental area of tsaï and interfascicular nucleus: a horse radish peroxidase study in the rat, *J Comp Neurol* **187:**117–44.

Randrup A, Braestrup C (1977) Uptake inhibition of biogenic amines by newer antidepressant drugs: relevance to the dopamine hypothesis of depression, *Psychopharmacology* **53:**309–14.

Randrup A, Munkvad I, Fog R et al (1975) Mania, depression and brain dopamine. *Curr Dev Psychopharmacol* **2:**207–48.

Room P, Postema F, Korf J (1981) Divergent axon collaterals of rat locus coeruleus neurons: a demonstration by a fluorescent double-labeling technique, *Brain Res* **221:**219–30.

Saavedra JM (1977) Distribution of 5-HT and synthetizing enzymes in discrete areas of the brain, *Fed Proc* **3:**2133–48.

Sadikot AF, Parent A (1990) The monoaminergic innervation of the amygdala in the squirrel monkey: an immunohistochemical study, *Neuroscience* **36:**431–47.

Schmidt CJ, Fadayel GM (1995) The selective 5-HT2A receptor antagonist, MDL 100,907, increases dopamine efflux in the prefrontal cortex of the rat, *Eur J Pharmacol* **273:**273–9.

Simon H, LeMoal M, Calas A (1979) Efferents and afferents of the ventral tegmental A10 region studied after local injections of 3H-leucine and horse radish peroxidase, *Brain Res* **178:**17–40.

Sorensen SM, Kehne JH, Fadayel GM et al (1993) Characterization of the 5-HT2 receptor antagonist MDL 100907 as a putative atypical antipsychotic: behavioural, electrophysiological and neurochemical studies, *J Pharmacol Exp Ther* **256:**684–91.

Steinbusch HWM (1981) Distribution of serotonin immunoreactivity in the central nervous system of the rat-cell-bodies and terminals, *Neuroscience* **6:**557–618.

Swanson LW, Hartman BK (1975) The central adrenergic system. An immunofluorescence study of the location of cell bodies and their efferent connections in the rat utilizing dopamine b-hydroxylase as a marker, *J Comp Neurol* **163:**467–506.

Taghzouti K, Simon H, Hervé D et al (1988) Behavioural deficits induced by an electrolytic lesion of the rat ventral mesencephalic tegmentum are corrected by a superimposed lesion of the dorsal noradrenergic system, *Brain Res* **440:**172–6.

Tassin JP (1994) Interrelation entre les neuromédiateurs impliqués dans la dépression et les antidépresseurs, *L'Encéphale* **20:**623–8.

Tassin JP (1995) A hypothesis on the sequential action of antidepressants on monoaminergic neurotransmitter systems. In: Fillion G, Briley M, eds, *Antidepressant Drugs for the 21st Century: How to Find and Develop Antidepressants* (Euro Conferences, Institut Pasteur: Paris) 43–71.

Tassin JP, Stinus L, Simon H et al (1978) Relationship between the locomotor hyperactivity induced by A10 lesions and the destruction of the fronto-cortical dopaminergic innervation in the rat, *Brain Res* **141:**267–81.

Tassin JP, Lavielle S, Hervé D et al (1979) Collateral sprouting and reduced activity of the rat mesocortical dopaminergic neurons after selective destruction of the ascending noradrenergic bundles, *Neuroscience* **4:**1569–82.

Tassin JP, Simon H, Glowinski J, Bockaërt J (1982) Modulations of the sensitivity of dopaminergic receptors in the prefrontal cortex and the nucleus accumbens. Relationship with locomotor activity. In: Collu R, Ducharme J, Barbeau A, Tolis G eds, *Brain Peptides and Hormones* (Raven Press: New York) 17–30.

Tassin JP, Studler JM, Hervé D, Blanc G, Glowinski J (1986) Contribution of noradrenergic neurons to the regulation of dopaminergic (D1) receptor denervation supersensitivity in rat prefrontal cortex, *J Neurochem* **46:**243–8.

Tassin JP, Trovero F, Vezina P, Blanc G, Glowinski J, Hervé D (1995) L'hetero-régulation des récepteurs ou la présence d'une relation fonctionnelle entre deux ensembles neuronaux, *Med Sci* **11:**829–36.

Trovero F, Hervé D, Blanc G, Glowinski J, Tassin JP (1992) *In vivo* partial inactivation of dopamine D1 receptors induces hypersensitivity of cortical dopamine-sensitive adenylate cyclase:

permissive role of α1-adrenergic receptors, *J Neurochem* **59:**331–7.

Trovero F, Marin P, Tassin JP, Premont J, Glowinski J (1994) Accelerated resensitization of the D1 dopamine receptor-mediated response in cultured cortical and striatal neurons from the rat: respective role of alpha1-adrenergic and N-methyl-D-aspartate receptors, *J Neurosci* **14:**6280–8.

Ugedo L, Grenhoff J, Svensson TH (1989) Ritanserin, a 5-HT2 receptor antagonist, activates midbrain dopamine neurons by blocking serotonergic inhibition, *Psychopharmacology* **98:**45–50.

Vetulani J, Sulser F (1975) Actions of various antidepressant treatments reduces reactivity of noradrenergic cyclic AMP generating system in limbic forebrain, *Nature* **257:**495–6.

Vezina P, Blanc G, Glowinski J, Tassin JP (1991) Opposed behavioural outputs of increased dopamine transmission in prefrontocortical and subcortical areas: a role for the cortical D1 dopaminergic receptor, *Eur J Neurosci* **3:**1001–7.

Wang RY (1981) Dopaminergic neurons in the rat ventral segmental area. II. Effects of D- and L-amphetamine, *Brain Res Rev* **3:**153–65.

Willner P (1983) Dopamine and depression: a review of recent evidence. I Empirical studies. II Theoretical approaches. III The effects of antidepressant treatments, *Brain Res Rev* **6:**211–46.

2

Electrophysiology of brain noradrenaline neurons and the mode of action of antidepressant drugs

Torgny H Svensson, Love Linnér and Lotta Arborelius

Introduction

Despite several decades of clinical research there exists no unequivocal evidence implicating brain noradrenaline (NA) neurons in the pathogenesis of depression (see Schatzberg and Schildkraut, 1995). At the same time, however, several sets of data strongly suggest that facilitation of brain noradrenergic neurotransmission represents one specific way by means of which an antidepressant effect can be achieved through pharmacological treatment of this disorder. Thus, in work by Delgado et al (1993), depressed patients in remission treated with NA reuptake inhibitors, such as desipramine or mazindol, developed a rapid increase in depression score during challenge with α-methylparatyrosine (AMPT), whereas only 1 of 9 patients treated with selective serotonin reuptake inhibitors (SSRIs) did. In contrast, 50% of patients having a therapeutic antidepressant response to an SSRI experienced a transient depressive relapse when plasma tryptophan was rapidly depleted, whereas only 1 of 13 patients treated with desipramine relapsed (Delgado et al, 1990). Consequently, in spite of numerous reports demonstrating extensive functional connections between brain NA- and 5-hydroxytryptamine (5-HT)-carrying neuronal systems, it appears that an antidepressant drug action can, indeed, be obtained via facilitation of brain noradrenergic neurotransmission alone, largely independent of an even impaired brain 5-HT availability. Conversely, the antidepressant effect of SSRIs can evidently also be obtained under conditions of reduced central catecholamine availability. Thus, there appear to exist several, largely independent pharmacological means to achieve a therapeutic effect in depression. At the same time, this phenomenon seems to provide the opportunity for synergistic interactions, when combining two or more pharmacological principles in depression. Clinical studies suggest, indeed, that drugs affecting both NA and 5-HT reuptake, e.g. tricyclic antidepressants (TCAs), display higher antidepressant efficacy than SSRIs alone (e.g. DUAG, 1986, 1990; Perry 1996). Also, several reports indicate an improved antidepressant effect of an SSRI when combined with a selective NA reuptake inhibitor (Nelson et al, 1991; Seth et al, 1992). Thus, although this chapter will focus on the electrophysiology of the NA system and antidepressant drug therapy, a brief commentary on the physiological interaction between central NA and 5-HT systems seems necessary. Since the AMPT challenge test actually involves deple-tion of both NA and dopamine (DA) in the brain, and mesolimbic DA is known to be critically involved with motivational behaviour, the functional interaction between brain NA and DA systems will also be discussed within this context. There are now numerous reviews discussing brain NA systems, depression and the mode of action of antidepressant drugs (e.g. Brady, 1994; Weiss et al, 1995/1996; Harro and Oreland, 1996). Consequently, this chapter will address a few specific issues, namely (1) mechanisms underlying the delay in onset of action of monoamine reup-take inhibitors and potential limitations to the efficacy of these drugs, (2) the significance of stress-induced activation of the locus coeruleus (LC) NA system for the function of the mesolimbic reward system and the effect of chronic antidepressant treatment within this context and (3) the interaction between brain NA and 5-HT systems and its significance for antidepressant drug action.

Feedback inhibition of brain NA and 5-HT systems and mechanisms of action of antidepressants

Early studies employing single cell recording techniques to analyse the effects of TCAs on the function of brain NA neurons within the LC revealed an acute, inhibitory action, which was particularly pronounced for secondary amines, such as desipramine (DMI), with a preferential action on NA reuptake mechanisms in brain. Moreover, this effect seemed to represent a so-called negative feedback mechanism, since it was antagonized by previous depletion of brain NA (Nybäck et al, 1975). Subsequent studies demonstrated that the feedback inhibition of LC neu-rons by TCAs such as DMI or imipramine (IMI) is caused by activation of somatodendritic α_2-autoreceptors and, moreover, that during chronic drug treatment this feedback inhibition becomes somewhat attenuated, probably related to functional desensitization of the α_2-autoreceptors within the LC (Svensson and Usdin, 1978). We also hypothesized that such chronic antidepressant drug treatment would cause stabilization against changes in LC activity, particularly reduction in neuronal activity. Since only some antidepressants caused functional desensitization of the somatodendritic α_2-autoreceptors within the LC, this phenomenon could not be ascribed any general significance in antidepressant therapy

(Scuvée-Moreau and Svensson, 1982). Numerous studies have subsequently confirmed and extended these initial findings, thus demonstrating that several TCAs and monoamine oxidase inhibitors administered chronically continue to cause some depression of LC neuronal firing rates, although the reduction is smaller than that seen after acute drug administration (see Brady, 1994). As discussed elsewhere in this book, chronic antidepressant therapies also frequently cause alterations in other central NA-related receptors, such as downregulation of β-receptors and upregulation of central α_1-adrenoceptors (e.g. Svensson, 1983; Baker and Greenshaw, 1989; Chapter 5). However, regardless of such long-term, adaptive changes in brain NA receptors, the recent clinical data by Delgado et al (1993) suggest that changes in the central availability of catecholamines alone can significantly influence the magnitude of the antidepressant effect. Also, the extracellular concentration of NA in brain, i.e. the cerebral cortex, has been shown to depend on the noradrenergic neuronal impulse flow in a frequency-dependent fashion (L'Heureux et al, 1986). Therefore, the initial, marked feedback inhibition of LC neuronal activity seen after acute administration of, for example, desipramine or maprotiline (Ceci and Borsini, 1996), as well as the remaining, partial inhibition of the NA cells during chronic drug treatment, might to some extent contribute both to the slow onset of action and to the limited, maximal efficacy of such antidepressant drugs.

In our original study (Svensson and Usdin, 1978), we observed that administration of antagonists at α_2-adrenoreceptors, but not α_1-adrenoreceptors, very effectively antagonized the feedback inhibition of LC neurons by, for example, DMI or IMI. Moreover, although both acute DMI and idazoxan have subsequently been found to increase central, cortical NA release, as assessed by microdialysis in awake, freely moving rats (Dennis et al, 1987), DMI potentiated the augmenting effect of systemically injected idazoxan on central NA release to a greater extent than it potentiated the effect of idazoxan locally infused into the cerebral cortex. The increase in brain NA output caused by idazoxan in normal animals seems to be executed largely via blockade of presynaptic α_2-adrenoreceptors located on the nerve terminals (Dennis et al, 1987). However, its effect in DMI-treated rats may, in contrast, to a significant extent also involve blockade of somatodendritic α_2-autoreceptors. One explanation may be that under physiological conditions these autoreceptors are not subjected to any major tone from the endogenous agonist, in contrast to the situation following acute DMI administration. Interestingly, also during chronic DMI treatment, basal levels of NA in central dialysis samples have been found to be considerably elevated (see Abercrombie and Finlay, 1991). A systematic study of the effects of α_2-adrenoceptor antagonists on brain NA systems in animals subjected to chronic antidepressant drug treatment seems, however, not to have been performed, as yet. The recent development in the serotonergic field concerning the combination of autoreceptor antagonists and antidepressant drugs (see below) makes this issue even more interesting.

Almost 20 years ago the first evidence was presented that the feedback inhibition of brain 5-HT systems caused by acute administration of a 5-HT reuptake-inhibiting antidepressant drug, IMI, is subjected to attenuation during chronic treatment (Svensson, 1978). Moreover, this phenomenon was suggested to be related to subsensitive serotonergic autoreceptors. Subsequently, this original and biochemically based notion was confirmed utilizing electrophysiological methods in studies of SSRIs (Blier and de Montigny, 1983; Chaput et al, 1986). Accordingly, central 5-HT release from serotonergic terminal areas, as revealed by assessment of extracellular concentrations of 5-HT in the frontal cortex and hypothalamus by means of microdialysis, was found to increase much more after chronic than after acute administration of fluvoxamine and fluoxetine, respectively (Bel and Artigas, 1993, Rutter et al, 1994). Evidence for desensitization of 5-HT_{1A} autoreceptors during chronic SSRI treatment was also obtained, in the sense that the effects of 5-HT_{1A} receptor agonists on both serotonergic neuronal activity and release were found to be attenuated (Chaput et al, 1986; Invernizzi et al, 1994; Rutter et al, 1994; Kreiss and Lucki, 1995). Clearly, since brain 5-HT availability seems to determine the magnitude of the clinical antidepressant effect obtained with SSRIs (see above), the delayed enhancement of brain serotonergic neurotransmission observed experimentally might have a bearing on the slow onset of action of clinical response to these drugs. Interestingly, administration of the selective 5-HT_{1A} receptor antagonist (S)-UH-301 was found to significantly augment the increase in hippocampal 5-HT concentration induced by acute citalopram administration (Hjorth, 1993) and, moreover, initial, open clinical experiments utilizing pindolol as a 5-HT_{1A} receptor antagonist seemed to indicate that the combination of an SSRI with a 5-HT_{1A} receptor antagonist might both shorten the onset of action and increase efficacy in the treatment of depression (Artigas et al, 1994). Subsequently, in our experiments with SSRIs and 5-HT_{1A} autoreceptor antagonists, we observed that the addition of a 5-HT_{1A} receptor antagonist markedly increased the activity of serotonergic cells in the dorsal raphe nucleus in not only rats treated acutely, but also, and even more potently, in animals treated chronically with citalopram (Arborelius et al, 1995). In parallel experiments, utilizing microdialysis in freely moving rats, the 5-HT_{1A} autoreceptor antagonist accordingly augmented the increased central 5-HT availability obtained not only with animals treated acutely but also, and even more potently, with animals treated chronically with citalopram (Arborelius et al, 1996). Thus, from an experimental standpoint a physiological substrate for an enhanced clinical efficacy of SSRIs through the addition of a 5-HT_{1A} autoreceptor antagonist could easily be envisaged.

Although the final confirmation of the initial clinical findings by Artigas et al (1994) remains to be seen, even a lack of effectiveness of pindolol may not necessarily allow the conclusion that the new therapeutic principle is invalid, because pindolol is an effective β-adrenoceptor blocking agent and such drugs can, clearly, precipitate depressive symptomatology in clinical practice. Most significantly, β-adrenoceptor antagonists also, especially during subchronic treatment, cause suppression of both LC NA activity and brain 5-HT synthesis (Dahlöf et al, 1981; Hallberg et al, 1982), and direct clinical evidence suggests that reduced synthesis of 5-HT in brain may rapidly reverse the antidepressant effects of both IMI and tranylcypromine (Shopsin et al, 1975, 1976) (see also above). Therefore, more selective $5\text{-}HT_{1A}$ receptor antagonists than pindolol, available for clinical use, are needed for a comprehensive analysis of this issue.

Against the background of the above findings and considerations, we have recently begun to analyse the effect of administration of an α_2-autoreceptor antagonist, idazoxan, on the firing rate of LC neurons in rats treated not only acutely, but also chronically, with TCAs such as DMI or IMI (Linnér et al, unpublished). Our preliminary results demonstrate that the α_2-autoreceptor antagonist not only effectively and rapidly reverses the feedback inhibition of LC neurons by acute IMI administration, in accordance with our previous results (see above), but also, and even more potently, activates the LC neurons in animals chronically treated with IMI (Figure 2.1); this is tentatively related, at least in part, to subsensitivity of the α_2-autoreceptors. Thus, the addition of an α_2-autoreceptor antagonist to an NA reuptake-inhibiting antidepressant drug should probably also significantly enhance brain NA availability during chronic antidepressant treatment. Consequently, combining an α_2-adrenoceptor antagonist with, for example, a TCA might, theoretically, both contribute to shortening the onset of antidepressant action and help to improve the efficacy during chronic treatment, although potential cardiovascular side-effects of such a drug combination must be considered. A previous study (Charney et al, 1986) observed, however, no enhanced clinical efficacy when yohimbine was combined with DMI early in treatment in a placebo-controlled study. Yet other studies document augmentation by yohimbine of both electroconvulsive therapy (ECT) (Sachs et al, 1986) and bupropion, a DA reuptake inhibitor (Pollack and Hammerness, 1993), in depression. Tentatively, the combined postsynaptic α_1-adrenoceptor-blocking actions of both antidepressant drugs and, to some extent, yohimbine might have reduced a putative synergistic effect of the combination of an α_2-autoreceptor antagonist and a TCA in depression (see below). Thus, further experiments with combinations of, for example, idazoxan and TCAs could still yield very interesting results. In fact, recent results suggest an antidepressant action of idazoxan alone (e.g. Grossman et al, 1994).

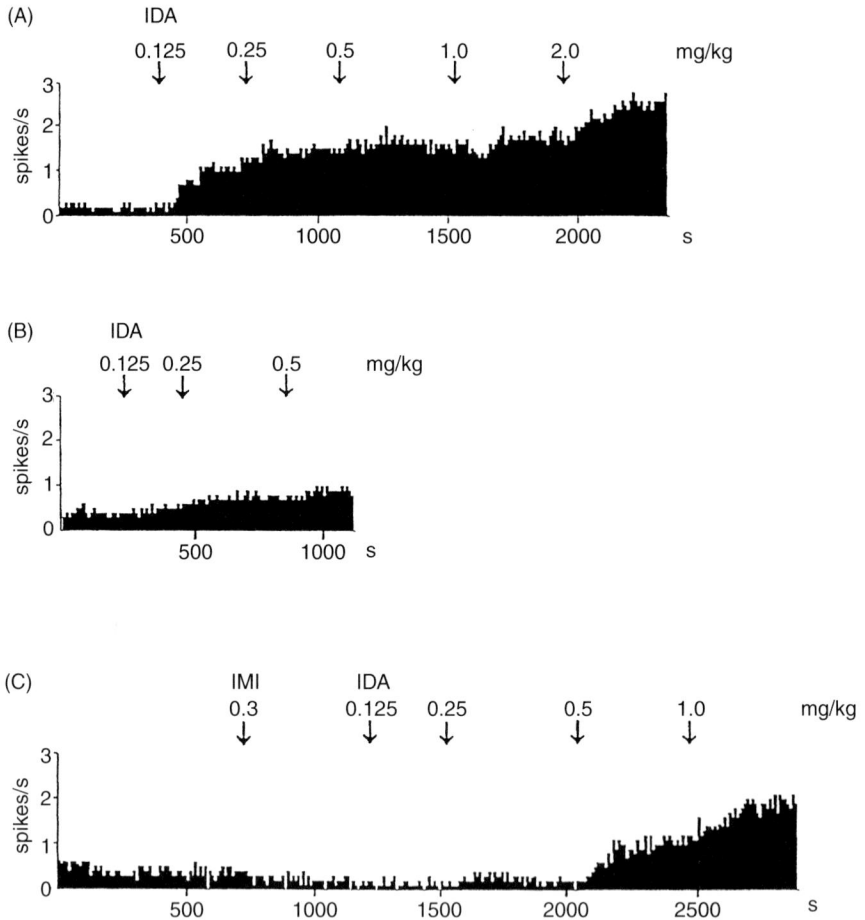

Figure 2.1

Effects on the firing rate of single NA neurons in the LC of incremental doses of the α_2-adrenoceptor antagonist idazoxan (IDA) administered intravenously to rats pretreated with: (A) chronic imipramine (IMI, 2×10 mg/kg per day for 14 days); (B) chronic saline (2×1 ml/kg per day for 14 days); (C) acute IMI (0.3 mg/kg intravenously). In (A) and (B), IDA was administered 12–16 h after the last injection of IMI or saline respectively.

Functional interaction between central NA and DA systems and mechanisms of action of antidepressants

The finding that catecholamine depletion can precipitate a depressive relapse in patients treated with some antidepressants can, admittedly, be interpreted to implicate, at least indirectly, brain DA in the antidepressant effect of drugs such as DMI or mazindol. Several experimental observations are, in fact, compatible with this notion, in particular some recent electrophysiological observations from our laboratory, which may have considerable interest from a pathophysiological perspective (Grenhoff et al, 1993). A number of studies provide biochemical, anatomical, behavioural and electrophysiological evidence for a stimulatory action of brain NA neurons on midbrain DA neurons (e.g. Andén and Grabowska, 1976; Donaldson et al, 1976; Tassin et al, 1979; Hervé et al, 1982; Grenhoff and Svensson, 1988, 1989; Lategan et al, 1990, 1992; Mavridis et al, 1991; Trovero et al, 1991). Subsequent pharmacological studies suggest, indeed, that brain NA neurons exert an excitatory, modulatory influence on the electrophysiological activity of DA neurons in the ventral tegmental area (VTA) via excitatory, postsynaptic α_1-adrenoceptors (Grenhoff and Svensson, 1993; Grenhoff, North and Johnson, 1995). For example, administration of prazosin caused regularization of the firing pattern of the VTA DA cells and reduced burst firing, but not firing rate; that is, phasic, but not tonic, activity in the mesolimbic DA system was suppressed. In other experiments we demonstrated that electrical stimulation of the LC profoundly affects the function of midbrain DA neurons (Grenhoff et al, 1993). The mainly excitatory effect of regular, single-pulse LC stimulation on the DA cells was antagonized both by pretreatment with a high dose of reserpine and by prazosin in a dose which effectively blocks central α_1-adrenoceptors. Such receptors may generally serve a modulatory function in brain, enhancing other excitatory afferent inputs to the cells. Thus, an enhanced central availability of brain NA, achieved, for example, by means of antidepressants such as DMI, may help to facilitate reward-related activation responses of the mesolimbic DA neurons, which, for example, may be elicited via activation of excitatory amino acid afferents to the VTA (Westerink et al, 1996).

Our experiments also showed, however, that more intense, burst-type LC stimulation, especially when repeated, instead causes a reserpine-resistant inhibition of the DA neurons, indicating that it could be due to a non-adrenergic mechanism, e.g. release of a neuropeptide such as galanin, which co-exists with NA in LC neurons (Holets et al, 1988) and inhibits central neurons via postsynaptic mechanisms (Seutin et al, 1989; Bartfai et al, 1991). A large body of experimental evidence demonstrates that brain NA neurons in the LC are profoundly activated by stress, particularly when of uncontrollable nature (e.g. Korf et al, 1973; Anisman and Sklar, 1979; Weiss et al, 1981; Svensson, 1987; Abercrombie and Jacobs, 1987; Abercrombie et al, 1988; Brady, 1994; Kitayama et al, 1994; Harro and Oreland, 1996), a phenomenon that seems to involve central release of corticotropin-releasing factor (CRF) (see Valentino et al, 1983, 1990; Owens and Nemeroff, 1991; Weiss et al, 1994). Such findings are of considerable interest, since both preclinical and clinical experience show that repeated, intense stress may contribute to depressive symptomatology (e.g. Katz et al, 1981; Anisman and Zacharko, 1990).

Thus, repeated stress exposures may, via profound activation of the LC, cause suppression of the mesolimbic DA reward system and, hence, contribute to anhedonia and reduced incentive behaviour, i.e. characteristic symptoms in melancholic depression (Anisman et al, 1980).

The above pathophysiological notion is, indeed, consistent with the hypothesis that mesolimbic DA neurons represent part of the central mechanisms that mediate the actions of at least some antidepressant drugs (e.g. Fibiger and Phillips, 1981; Borsini et al, 1985; Willner, 1985; Delini-Stula et al, 1988; Muscat, Sampson and Willner, 1990). The therapeutic effect of the atypical antidepressant drug bupropion, which seems to act largely via facilitation of mesolimbic DA function in brain (see Cooper et al, 1980; Nomikos et al, 1992), provides essential support for this contention. Such a mechanism may, in fact, be of particular significance in the treatment of severe, melancholic depression: whereas both repeated electroconvulsive treatment (see Modigh, 1975; Heal and Green, 1978; Nomikos et al, 1991a) and chronic TCA treatment have been found, in several ways, to facilitate brain DA neurotransmission, in particular the functional output of the mesolimbic DA system (e.g. Fibiger et al, 1990; Nomikos et al, 1991b), an effect that seems not to be shared by the SSRIs (Spyraki and Fibiger, 1981; Martin-Iverson et al, 1983), which also appear to possess less efficacy in severe depression. Recently, experiments utilizing intracellular recordings have provided further evidence for α_1-adrenoceptor-mediated control of midbrain DA neurons. Thus, the observation that rats are rewarded by intracranial self-stimulation not only of the VTA (Corbett and Wise, 1980; Fibiger et al, 1987), but also the noradrenergic locus coeruleus (Ritter and Stein, 1973; Segal and Bloom, 1976) may be related to NA-induced, α_1-adrenoceptor-mediated depolarization of the DA neurons. Given the large body of evidence linking physiological activation of the mesolimbic DA neurons to behavioural reward (e.g. Schultz and Romo, 1990; Le Moal and Simon, 1991; Ljungberg et al, 1992), this notion seems justified. Consequently, the physiological interaction between brain NA neurons, predominantly originating in the LC, and the DA neurons in the VTA, may represent a key substrate for the mediation of a full antidepressant effect, whether obtained by ECT or by antidepressants such as TCAs.

Functional interactions between brain NA and 5-HT neurons and mechanisms of action of antidepressants

A thorough discussion of the physiology of brain NA neurons and the mode of action of antidepressant drugs necessarily also has to include the functional interaction between NA and 5-HT neurons in brain. This interaction takes place at several sites in brain, one being the dorsal raphe nucleus (DRN). In fact, 20 years ago pharmacological experiments provided the first evidence for a tonic regulation of 5-HT neurons in the DRN by its noradrenergic input; an excitatory control mechanism, mediated via postsynaptic α_1-adrenoceptors (Svensson et al, 1975). Accordingly, the α_2-adrenoreceptor agonist clonidine was found to reduce not only brain NA neuronal activity, e.g. in the LC, but also, secondary to this effect, the firing rate of 5-HT neurons in the DRN, an indirect action that could be effectively reversed by administration of a high dose of clonidine, activating postsynaptic central α_1-adrenoceptors, or l-amphetamine, which potently releases NA in the central nervous system (Svensson, 1971; Bunney et al, 1975). Subsequent studies have confirmed and extended these original findings and conclusions (Baraban and Aghajanian, 1980, 1981), demonstrating inter alia the suppression of 5-HT cell-firing in the DRN by means of administration of α_1-adrenoceptor antagonists. In addition, systemic administration of prazosin was found to markedly reduce extracellular 5-HT levels in the hippocampus (Claustre et al, 1991). Conversely, administration of the α_2-adrenoceptor antagonist idazoxan was observed to enhance the firing activity of DRN 5-HT neurons (Freedman and Aghajanian, 1984; Garratt et al, 1991), probably via activation of NA release from noradrenergic terminals in the DRN. In addition, α_2-adrenergic heteroreceptors on serotonergic nerve terminals contribute to modulate nerve terminal, i.e. hippocampal, 5-HT release in vivo as assessed by means of microdialysis (Tao and Hjorth, 1992). Clearly, the noradrenergic interaction with serotonergic neurons in the DRN may serve as a significant site of action for several antidepressant drugs, such as the α_2-adrenergic receptor antagonist mirtazapine which, in addition, seems to facilitate nerve terminal release of 5-HT via blockade of α_2-heteroreceptors (see de Montigny et al, 1995; de Boer, 1996). The excitatory α_1-adrenoceptors within the DRN may also contribute to activate the 5-HT neurons indirectly following administration of selective NA and 5-HT reuptake inhibitors such as venlafaxine (Muth et al, 1991) or duloxetine (Kihara and Ikeda, 1995; Kasamo et al, 1996), which, in contrast to many TCAs, lack potent α_1-adrenoceptor blocking action: the feedback inhibition of brain 5-HT neurons in the DRN, secondary to the 5-HT reuptake inhibitory effect of such drugs, should, if anything, be attenuated by a concomitant facilitation of NA release in the DRN. Thus, the purported short latency of action and tentatively improved efficacy of this type of compound (Derivan et al, 1995) might in part be related to such a mechanism. Clearly, an antidepressant action appears possible to achieve through several, largely independent pharmacological principles, such as facilitation of brain NA or 5-HT neurotransmission, as mentioned previously. Yet the 5-HT–NA interactions described above may offer specific mechanisms to further improve the efficacy of SSRIs in depression. Indeed, addition of yohimbine to fluvoxamine in the treatment of refractory depression has been reported to enhance the antidepressant effect of the SSRI in a recent single-blind study (Cappiello et al, 1995).

Brain 5-HT–NA physiological interactions occur via several mechanisms and in different areas; another one is represented by the major central noradrenergic nucleus, the LC, itself. In fact, this interaction may have a bearing on the usefulness of SSRIs in the treatment of panic attack disorder, a well-established clinical effect of the 5-HT reuptake inhibitors that does not appear to be shared with the NA reuptake inhibitors. Previously, several experimental studies have demonstrated that the serotonergic input to the LC selectively suppresses glutamate-evoked responses of LC neurons, while leaving basal activity largely unaffected (Chouvet et al, 1988; Aston-Jones et al, 1991). Moreover, SSRIs such as fluoxetine, sertraline or citalopram were subsequently found to significantly suppress LC hyperactivity evoked by its excitatory amino acid inputs through pharmacological means (Engberg, 1992; Akaoka and Aston-Jones, 1993). Clearly, the intense arousal associated with panic attacks must also involve profound activation responses of brain NE neurons in the LC, a phenomenon that may well contribute to the symptomatology (see Svensson, 1987). Moreover, such evoked LC activations should in all probability involve some of its major, excitatory afferent inputs, which utilize excitatory amino acids as neuronal messengers (Aston-Jones et al, 1986). Accordingly, a continued treatment of panic attack disorder with SSRIs may help to suppress part of the most intense arousal reactions in brain through the 5-HT–NA interaction in the LC area. Such an effect may gradually, over time, contribute to extinguishing the overall neurobiological hyperreactivity.

Concluding remarks

A major conclusion from the above findings and considerations seems to be that a maximally effective antidepressant drug treatment should probably involve a synergistic interaction between two or more therapeutically significant, basic pharmacological principles, which by themselves may be effective in the treatment of affective disorder, but may have to be combined to achieve full efficacy in melancholic depression. Another, tentative conclusion is that drugs acting as antagonists at some of the central, postsynaptic monoaminergic receptors, such as α_1-adrenoceptors or β-receptors, may possess an intrinsic limitation to a rapid onset of action or, potentially, a less than optimal clinical efficacy. In addition, the relatively novel therapeutic principle of combining autoreceptor antagonists, acting at, for example, some α_2-adrenoceptors or 5-HT$_{1A}$-autoreceptors, with various monoamine reuptake inhibitors deserves further exploration both at the preclinical and clinical level of investigation. Finally, continued exploration of the interaction between brain NA systems and various neuropeptides such as CRF and galanin, for its potential significance in future antidepressant pharmacotherapies, seems warranted.

● Acknowledgements
This work was supported by the Swedish Medical Research Council (grant No 04646), the Karolinska Institute and Astra Arcus AB, Södertälje, Sweden.

References

Abercrombie ED, Finlay JM (1991) Monitoring extracellular norepinephrine in brain using in vivo microdialysis and HPLC-EC. In: Robinsson TE, Justice, JB Jr, eds, *Microdialysis in the Neurosciences* (Elsevier Science Publishers BV: Amsterdam) 253–74.

Abercrombie ED, Jacobs BL (1987) Single-unit response of noradrenergic neurons in the locus coeruleus of freely moving cats, I. Acutely presented stressful and nonstressful stimuli, *J Neurosci* **7:**2837–43.

Abercrombie ED, Keller RW, Zigmond MJ (1988) Characterization of hippocampal norepinephrine release as measured by microdialysis perfusion: pharmacological and behavioral studies, *Neuroscience* **27:**897–904.

Akaoka H, Aston-Jones G (1993) Indirect serotonergic agonists attenuate neuronal opiate withdrawal, *Neuroscience* **54:**561–5.

Andén NE, Grabowska M (1976) Pharmacological evidence for a stimulation of dopamine neurons by noradrenaline neurons in the brain, *Eur J Pharmacol* **39:**275–82.

Anisman H, Sklar LS (1979) Catecholamine depletion in mice upon reexposure to stress: mediation of the escape deficits produced by inescapable shock, *J Comp Physiol* **93:**610–25.

Anisman H, Zacharko RM (1990) Multiple neurochemical and behavioral consequences of stressors: implications for depression, *Pharmacol Ther* **46:**119–36.

Anisman H, Suissa A, Sklar L (1980) Escape deficits induced by uncontrollable stress: antagonism by dopamine and norepinephrine agonists, *Behav Neural Biol* **28:**34–47.

Arborelius L, Nomikos GG, Grillner P et al (1995) 5-HT$_{1A}$ receptor antagonists increase the activity of serotonergic cells in the dorsal raphe nucleus in rats treated acutely or chronically with citalopram, *Naunyn Schmiedeberg's Arch Pharmacol* **352:**157–65.

Arborelius L, Nomikos GG, Hertel P et al (1996) The 5-HT$_{1A}$ receptor antagonist (S)-UH-301 augments the increase in extracellular concentrations of 5-HT in the frontal cortex produced by both acute and chronic treatment with citalopram, *Naunyn Schmiedeberg's Arch Pharmacol* **353:**630–40.

Artigas F, Perez V, Alvarez F (1994) Pindolol induces a rapid improvement of depressed patients treated with serotonin reuptake inhibitors, *Arch Gen Psychiatry* **51:**248–51.

Aston-Jones G, Ennis M, Pieribone VA (1986) The brain nucleus locus coeruleus: restricted afferent control of a broad efferent network, *Science* **234:**734–7.

Aston-Jones G, Akaoka H, Charléty P et al (1991) Serotonin selectively attenuates glutamate-evoked activation of noradrenergic locus coeruleus neurons, *J Neurosci* **11:**760–9.

Baker GB, Greenshaw AJ (1989) Effects of long-term administration of antidepressants and neuroleptics on receptors in the central nervous system, *Cell Mol Neurobiol* **9:**1–44.

Baraban JM, Aghajanian GK (1980) Suppression of firing activity of 5-HT neurons in the dorsal raphe by α-adrenoceptor antagonists, *Neuropharmacology* **19:**355.

Baraban JM, Aghajanian GK (1981)

Noradrenergic innervation of serotonergic neurons in the dorsal raphe: demonstration by electron microscope autoradiography, *Brain Res* **204:**1.

Bartfai T, Bedecs K, Land T et al (1991) M-15: high-affinity chimeric peptide that blocks the neuronal actions of galanin in the hippocampus, locus coeruleus, and spinal cord, *Proc Natl Acad Sci USA* **88:**10961–5.

Bel N, Artigas F (1993) Chronic treatment with fluvoxamine increases extracellular serotonin in frontal cortex but not in raphe nuclei, *Synapse* **15:**243–5.

Blier P, de Montigny C (1983) Electrophysiological investigations on the effect of repeated zimelidine administration on serotonergic neurotransmission in the rat, *J Neurosci* **3:**1270–8.

Borsini F, Pulvirenti L, Samanin R (1985) Evidence of dopamine involvement in the effect of repeated treatment with various antidepressants in the behavioural 'despair' test in rats, *Eur J Pharmacol* **110:**253.

Brady LS (1994) Stress, antidepressant drugs, and the locus coeruleus, *Brain Res* **35:**545–6.

Bunney BS, Walters JR, Kuhar MJ et al (1975) D&L amphetamine stereoisomers: comparative potencies in affecting the firing of central dopaminergic and noradrenergic neurons, *Psychopharmacol Commun* **1:**177–90.

Cappiello A, McDougle CJ, Malison RT et al (1995) Yohimbine augmentation of fluvoxamine in refractory depression: a single-blind study, *Biol Psychiatry* **38:**765–7.

Ceci A, Borsini F (1996) Effects of desipramine and maprotiline on the coeruleus-cortical noradrenergic system in anaesthetized rats, *Eur J Pharmacol* **312:**189–93.

Chaput Y, de Montigny C, Blier P (1986) Effects of a selective 5-HT reuptake blocker, citalopram on the sensitivity of 5-HT autoreceptors: electrophysiological studies in the rat brain, *Naunyn Schmiedeberg's Arch*

Pharmacol **333:**342–8.

Charney DS, Price LH, Heninger GR (1986) Desipramine–yohimbine combination treatment of refractory depression: implications for the beta-adrenergic receptor hypothesis of antidepressant action, *Arch Gen Psychiatry* **43:**1156–61.

Chouvet G, Akaoka H, Aston-Jones G (1988) Serotonin selectively decreases glutamate-induced excitation of locus coeruleus neurons, *CR Acad Sci Paris* **306:**339–44.

Claustre Y, Rouquier L, Serrano A et al (1991) Effect of the putative 5-HT$_{1A}$ receptor antagonist NAN-190 on rat brain serotonergic transmission, *Eur J Pharmacol* **204:**71–7.

Cooper BR, Hester TJ, Maxwell RA (1980) Behavioral and biochemical effects of the antidepressant bupropion (Wellbutrin): evidence for selective blockade of dopamine uptake in vivo, *J Pharmacol Exp Ther* **215:**127–34.

Corbett D, Wise RA (1980) Intracranial self-stimulation in relation to the ascending dopaminergic systems of the midbrain: a moveable electrode mapping study, *Brain Res* **185:**1–15.

Dahlöf C, Engberg G, Svensson TH (1981) Effects of β-adrenoceptor antagonists on the firing rate of noradrenergic neurones in the locus coeruleus of the rat, *Naunyn Schmiedeberg's Arch Pharmacol* **317:**26–30.

de Boer TH (1996) The pharmacologic profile of mirtazapine, *J Clin Psychiatry* **57:**19–25.

de Montigny C, Haddjeri N, Mongeau R et al (1995) The effects of mirtazapine on the interactions between central noradrenergic and serotonergic systems, *CNS Drugs* **4:**13–17.

Delgado PL, Charney DS, Price LH et al (1990) Serotonin function and the mechanism of antidepressant action, *Arch Gen Psychiatry* **47:**411–18.

Delgado PL, Miller HL, Salomon RM et al (1993) Monoamines and the mechanism of antidepressant action: effects of catecholamine depletion on mood of patients treated with antidepressants, *Psychopharmacology* **29:**389–96.

Delini-Stula A, Radeke E, Van Riezen H (1988) Enhanced functional responsiveness of the dopaminergic system—the mechanism of antidepressant in the behavioural despair test in the rat, *Neuropsychopharmacology* **27:**943.

Dennis T, L'Heureux R, Carter C et al (1987) Presynaptic alpha$_2$ adrenoceptors play a major role in the effects of idazoxan on cortical noradrenaline release (as measured by in vivo dialysis) in the rat, *J Pharmacol Exp Ther* **241:**642–9.

Derivan A, Entsuah A, Kikta D (1995) Venlafaxine: measuring the onset of antidepressant action, *Psychopharmacology* **31:**439–47.

Donaldson IM, Dolphin A, Jenner P et al (1976) The roles of noradrenaline and dopamine in contraversive circling behaviour seen after unilateral electrolytic lesions of the locus coeruleus, *Eur J Pharmacol* **39:** 179–91.

DUAG (1986) Citalopram: clinical effect profile in comparison with clomipramine. A controlled multicenter study, *Psychopharmacology* **90:**131–8.

DUAG (1990) Paroxetine: a selective reuptake inhibitor showing better tolerance, but weaker antidepressant effect than clomipramine in a controlled multicenter study, *J Affect Disord* **18:**289–99.

Engberg G (1992) Citalopram and 8-OH-DPAT attenuate nicotine-induced excitation of central noradrenaline neurons, *J Neural Transm* **89:**149–54.

Fibiger HC, Phillips AG (1981) Increased intracranial selfstimulation in rats after long-term administration of desipramine, *Science* **214:**683.

Fibiger HC, LePiane FG, Jakubovic A et al (1987) The role of dopamine in intracranial self-stimulation of the ventral tegmental area, *J Neurosci* **7:**3888–96.

Fibiger HC, Phillips AG, Blaha CD (1990) Dopamine and the neural substrates of reward: implications for the mechanisms of action of antidepressant drugs, *Adv Biosci* **77:**51.

Freedman JE, Aghajanian GK (1984) Idazoxan (RX781094) selectively antagonizes α_2-adrenoceptors on rat central neurons, *Eur J Pharmacol* **105:**265.

Garratt JC, Crespi F, Mason R et al (1991) Effects of idazoxan on dorsal raphe 5-hydroxytryptamine neuronal function, *Eur J Pharmacol* **193:**87–93.

Grenhoff J, Svensson TH (1988) Clonidine regularizes substantia nigra dopamine cell firing, *Life Sci* **42:**2003–9.

Grenhoff J, Svensson TH (1989) Clonidine modulates cell firing in rat ventral tegmental area, *Eur J Pharmacol* **165:**11–18.

Grenhoff J, Svensson TH (1993) Prazosin modulates the firing pattern of dopamine neurons in rat ventral tegmental area, *Eur J Pharmacol* **233:**79–84.

Grenhoff J, Nisell M, Ferré S et al (1993) Noradrenergic modulation of midbrain dopamine cell firing elicited by stimulation of the locus coeruleus in the rat, *J Neural Transm* **93:**11–25.

Grenhoff J, North AR, Johnson SW (1995) Alpha$_1$-adrenergic effects on dopamine neurons recorded intracellularly in the rat midbrain slice, *Eur J Neurosci* **7:**1707–13.

Grossman F, Potter WZ, Brown E et al (1994) A double blind study comparing idazoxan to bupropion. In: *American Psychological Association Annual Meeting New Research* (Abstract NR600) 213.

Hallberg H, Almgren O, Svensson TH (1982) Reduced brain serotonergic activity after repeated treatment with β-adrenoceptor antagonists, *Psychopharmacology* **76:**114–17.

Harro J, Oreland L (1996) Depression as a spreading neuronal adjustment disorder, *Eur Neuropsychopharmacol* **6:**207–23.

Heal DJ, Green AR (1978) Repeated electroconvulsive shock increases the behavioural responses of rats to injection of both dopamine and dibutyryl cyclic AMP into the nucleus accumbens, *Neuropharmacology* **17:**1085–7.

Hervé D, Blanc G, Glowinski J et al (1982) Reduction of dopamine utilization in the prefrontal cortex but not in the nucleus accumbens after selective destruction of noradrenergic fibers innervating the ventral tegmental area in the rat, *Brain Res* **237:**510–16.

Hjorth S (1993) Serotonin 5-HT$_{1A}$ autoreceptor blockade potentiates the ability of the 5-HT reuptake inhibitor citalopram to increase nerve terminal output of 5-HT in vivo: a microdialysis study, *J Neurochem* **60:**776–9.

Holets VR, Hökfelt T, Rökaeus Å et al (1988) Locus coeruleus neurons in the rat containing neuropeptide Y, tyrosine hydroxylase or galanin and their efferent projections to the spinal cord, cerebral cortex and hypothalamus, *Neuroscience* **24:**893–906.

Invernizzi R, Bramante M, Samanin R (1994) Chronic treatment with citalopram facilitates the effect of a challenge dose on cortical serotonin output: role of presynaptic 5-HT$_{1A}$ receptors, *Eur J Pharmacol* **260:** 243–6.

Kasamo K, Blier P, de Montigny C (1996) Blockade of serotonin and norepinephrine uptake processes by duloxetine: in vitro and in vivo studies in the rat brain, *Am Soc Pharmacol Exp Ther* **277:**278–86.

Katz RJ, Roth KA, Carroll BJ (1981) Acute and chronic stress effects on open field activity in the rat: implications for a model of depression, *Neurosci Biobehav Rev* **5:**247–51.

Kihara T, Ikeda M (1995) Effects of duloxetine, a new serotonin and norepinephrine uptake inhibitor, on extracellular monoamine levels in rat frontal cortex, *J Pharmacol Exp Ther* **272:**177–83.

Kitayama I, Nakamura S, Yaga T et al (1994) Degeneration of locus coeruleus axons in stress-induced depression model, *Brain Res Bull* **35:**573–80.

Korf J, Aghajanian GK, Roth RH (1973) Increased turnover of norepinephrine in the rat cerebral cortex during stress: role of the locus coeruleus, *Neuropharmacology* **12:**933–8.

Kreiss DS, Lucki I (1995) Effects of acute and repeated administration of antidepressant drugs on extracellular levels of 5-hydroxytryptamine measured *in vivo*, *J Pharmacol Exp Ther* **274:**866–76.

Lategan AJ, Marien MR, Colpaert FC (1990) Effects of locus coeruleus lesions on the release of endogenous dopamine in the rat nucleus accumbens and caudate nucleus as determined by intracerebral microdialysis, *Brain Res* **523:**134–8.

Lategan AJ, Marien MR, Colpaert FC (1992) Suppression of nigrostriatal and mesolimbic dopamine release in vivo following noradrenaline depletion by DSP-4: a microdialysis study, *Life Sci* **50:**995–9.

Le Moal M, Simon H (1991) Mesocorticolimbic dopaminergic network: functional and regulatory roles, *Physiol Rev* **71:**155–234.

L'Heureux R, Dennis T, Curet O et al (1986) Measurement of endogenous noradrenaline release in the rat cerebral cortex in vivo by transcortical dialysis: effects of drugs affecting noradrenergic transmission, *J Neurochem* **46:**1794–801.

Ljungberg T, Apicella P, Schultz W (1992) Responses of monkey dopamine neurons during learning of behavioral reactions, *J Neurophysiol* **67:**145–63.

Martin-Iverson MT, Leclere JF, Fibiger HC (1983) Cholinergic–dopaminergic interactions and the mechanisms of action of antidepressants, *Eur J Phar-*

macol **94:**193–201.

Mavridis M, Colpaert FC, Millan MJ (1991) Differential modulation of (+)-amphetamine-induced rotation in unilateral substantia nigra-lesioned rats by α_1 as compared to α_2 agonists and antagonists, *Brain Res* **562:**216–24.

Modigh (1975) Electroconvulsive shock and postsynaptic catecholamine effects: increased psychomotor stimulant action of apomorphine and clonidine in reserpine pretreated mice by repeated ECS, *J Neural Transm* **36:**19–32.

Muscat R, Sampson D, Willner P (1990) Dopaminergic mechanism of imipramine action in an animal model of depression, *Biol Psychiatry* **28:**223.

Muth EA, Moyer JA, Haskins JT et al (1991) Biochemical, neurophysiological, and behavioral effects of Wy-45,233 and other identified metabolites of the antidepressant venlafaxine, *Drug Dev Res* **23:**191–9.

Nelson JC, Mazure CM, Bowers MB et al (1991) A preliminary open study of the combination of fluoxetine and desipramine for rapid treatment of major depression, *Arch Gen Psychiatry* **48:**303–7.

Nomikos GG, Athanasios, Zis P et al (1991a) Effects of chronic electroconvulsive shock on interstitial concentrations of dopamine in the nucleus accumbens, *Psychopharmacology* **105:**230–8.

Nomikos GG, Damsma G, Wenkstern D et al (1991b) Chronic desipramine enhances amphetamine-induced increases in interstitial concentrations of dopamine in the nucleus accumbens, *Eur J Pharmacol* **195:**63–73.

Nomikos GG, Damsma G, Wenkstern D et al (1992) Effects of chronic bupropion on interstitial concentrations of dopamine in rat nucleus accumbens and striatum, *Neuropsychopharmacology* **7:**7–14.

Nybäck HV, Walters JR, Aghajanian GK et al (1975) Tricyclic antidepressants: effects on the firing rates of brain noradrenergic neurons, *Eur J Pharmacol* **32:**302–12.

Owens MJ, Nemeroff CB (1991) Physiology and pharmacology of corticotropin-releasing factor, *Pharmacol Rev* **43:**425–73.

Perry PJ (1996) Pharmacotherapy for major depression with melancholic features: relative efficacy of tricyclic versus selective serotonin reuptake inhibitor antidepressants, *J Affect Disord* **39:**1–6.

Pollack MH, Hammerness P (1993) Adjunctive yohimbine for treatment in refractory depression, *Biol Psychiatry* **33:**220–1.

Ritter S, Stein L (1973) Self stimulation of noradrenergic cell group (A6) in locus coeruleus of rats, *J Comp Physiol Psychol* **85:**443–52.

Rutter JJ, Gundlah C, Auerbach SB (1994) Increase in extracellular serotonin produced by uptake inhibitors is enhanced after chronic treatment with fluoxetine, *Neurosci Lett* **171:**183–6.

Sachs GS, Pollack MH, Brotman AW et al (1986) Enhancement of ECT benefit by yohimbine, *J Clin Psychiatry* **47:**508–10.

Schatzberg AF, Schildkraut JJ (1995) Recent studies on norepinephrine systems in mood disorders. In: Bloom FE, Kupfer DJ, eds, *Psychopharmacology: The Fourth Generation of Progress* (Raven Press: New York) 911–20.

Schultz W, Romo R (1990) Dopamine neurons of the monkey midbrain: contingencies of responses to stimuli eliciting immediate behavioral reactions, *J Neurophysiol* **63:**607–24.

Scuvée-Moreau JJ, Svensson TH (1982) Sensitivity in vivo of central α_2- and opiate receptors after chronic treatment with various antidepressants, *J Neural Transm* **54:**51–63.

Segal M, Bloom FE (1976) The action of norepinephrine in the rat hippocampus. III. Hippocampal cellular responses to locus coeruleus stimulation in the awake rat, *Brain Res* **107:**499–511.

Seth R, Jennings AL, Bindman J et al (1992) Combination treatment with noradrenaline and serotonin reuptake inhibitors in resistant depression, *Br J Psychiatry* **161:**562–5.

Seutin V, Verbanck P, Massotte L et al (1989) Gelanin decreases the activity of locus coeruleus neurons in vitro, *Eur J Pharmacol* **164:**373–6.

Shopsin B, Gershon S, Goldstein M et al (1975) Use of synthesis inhibitors in defining a role for biogenic amines during imipramine treatment in depressed patients, *Psychopharmacol Commun* **1:**239–49.

Shopsin B, Friedman E, Gershon S (1976) Parachlorophenylaline reversal of tranylcypromine effects in depressed patients, *Arch Gen Psychiatry* **33:**811–91.

Spyraki C, Fibiger HC (1981) Behavioural evidence for supersensitivity of postsynaptic dopamine receptors in the mesolimbic system after chronic administration of desipramine, *Eur J Pharmacol* **74:**195–206.

Svensson TH (1971) Functional and biochemical effects of d- and l-amphetamine on central catecholamine neurons, *Naunyn Schmiedeberg's Arch Pharmacol* **271:**170–80.

Svensson TH (1978) Attenuated feedback inhibition of brain serotonin synthesis following chronic administration of imipramine, *Naunyn Schmiedeberg's Arch Pharmacol* **302:**115–18.

Svensson TH (1983) Mode of action of antidepressant agents and ECT—adaptive changes after subchronic treatment. In: Angst J, ed., *The Origins of Depression: Current Concepts and Approaches* (Springer Verlag: Berlin, Heidelberg, New York, Tokyo) 367–83.

Svensson TH (1987) Peripheral, autonomic regulation of locus coeruleus noradrenergic neurons in brain: putative implications for psychiatry and psychopharmacology, *Psychopharmacology* **92:**1–7.

Svensson TH, Usdin T (1978) Feedback inhibition of brain noradrenaline neurons by tricyclic antidepressants: α-receptor mediation, *Science* **202:**1089–91.

Svensson TH, Bunney BS, Aghajanian GK (1975) Inhibition of both noradrenergic and serotonergic neurons in brain by the α-adrenergic agonist clonidine, *Brain Res* **92:**291–306.

Tao R, Hjorth S (1992) α_2-Adrenoceptor modulation of rat ventral hippocampal 5-hydroxytryptamine release in vitro, *Naunyn Schmiedeberg's Arch Pharmacol* **345:**137.

Tassin JP, Lavielle S, Hervé D et al (1979) Collateral sprouting and reduced activity of the rat mesocortical dopaminergic neurons after selective destruction of the ascending noradrenergic bundles, *Neuroscience* **4:**1569–82.

Trovero F, Blanc G, Hervé D et al (1991) Contribution of an α_1-adrenergic receptor subtype to the expression of the 'ventral tegmental syndrome', *Neuroscience* **47:**69–76.

Valentino RJ, Foote SL, Aston-Jones G (1983) Corticotropin-releasing factor activates noradrenergic neurons of the locus coeruleus, *Brain Res* **270:**363–7.

Valentino RJ, Curtil AL, Parris DG et al (1990) Antidepressant actions on brain noradrenergic neurons, *J Pharmacol Exp Ther* **253:**833–40.

Weiss JM, Goodman PA, Losito BG et al (1981) Behavioral depression produced by an uncontrollable stressor: relationship to norepinephrine, dopamine, and serotonin levels in various regions of the rat brain, *Brain Res* **3:**167–205.

Weiss JM, Stout JC, Aaron MF et al (1994) Depression and anxiety: role of the locus coeruleus and corticotropin-releasing factor, *Brain Res Bull* **35:**561–72.

Weiss JM, Demetrikopoulos K, West CHK (1995/1996) Hypothesis linking the noradrenergic and dopaminergic systems in depression, *Depression* **3:**225–45.

Westerink BHC, Bouma M, Enrico P (1996) Stress- and reward-induced increase in extracellular dopamine in mesocortical and mesolimbic neurons: role of glutamatergic afferents to the VTA. In: Gonzáles-Mora JL, Borges R, Mas M, eds, *Monitoring Molecules in Neuroscience*, Proceedings of the 7th International Conference on *in vivo* Methods, University of La Laguna, Santa Cruz de Tenerife, Spain, 321–2.

Willner P (1985) *Depression: a Psychobiological Synthesis* (John Wiley & Sons: Chichester).

3

The possible role of 5-HT$_{1B}$ autoreceptors in the action of serotonergic antidepressant drugs

Mike Briley and Chantal Moret

The selective serotonin reuptake inhibitors (SSRI) fluoxetine, fluvoxamine, paroxetine, sertraline and citalopram are effective antidepressants (Boyer and Feighner, 1991). Their efficacy appears to be generally similar to that of tricyclic antidepressants (TCA), except in more severe depression, where they are probably somewhat less efficacious than the TCAs. From the fundamental point of view, the efficacy of such 'pharmacologically clean' drugs with a single acute pharmacological action makes them valuable tools for investigating the neurobiological mechanisms involved in antidepressant therapy and possibly the aetiology of depression.

The in vitro selectivity of SSRIs for the inhibition of serotonin uptake as compared to their inhibition of the uptake of noradrenaline varies from 20-fold (fluoxetine) to over 300-fold (paroxetine and citalopram) (Johnson, 1992). In addition, their metabolites are either inactive or less active at inhibiting monoamine uptake than the parent compound (Johnson, 1992). Binding studies have shown the absence of high-affinity interactions with a wide range of neurotransmitter receptors. Thus in vivo and certainly at clinical doses these compounds can be considered to have a single acute pharmacological action. In spite of the rapid onset of this effect in humans (in a few hours at most), the earliest signs of therapeutic improvement appear only after about two weeks in depression and longer in other disorders such as obsessive compulsive disorders (OCD).

Logically, one would expect that inhibition of serotonin reuptake would result in an immediate increase in the synaptic level of serotonin. SSRIs, however, when systemically administered acutely to animals, cause only modest or negligible increases in the levels of extracellular serotonin, as measured by in vivo microdialysis, in the cortex, or other brain areas inner-vated by the dorsal raphe, of freely moving rats or guinea pigs. The maximal increase in terminal regions is about 100%, whereas in the dorsal raphe nucleus extracellular levels of serotonin are increased by 4–6-fold (Adell and Artigas, 1991; Bel and Artigas, 1992; Invernizzi et al, 1992).

A possible exception is the systemic administration of fluoxetine, which results in increases of approximately four-fold in two terminal regions, the thalamus (Dailey et al, 1992) and the striatum (Perry and Fuller, 1992). Since studies comparing fluoxetine with other SSRIs have not been carried out in the same laboratory, these differences may result from methodological differences rather than a specific effect of fluoxetine. In addition, there are at present no data on the effect of fluoxetine on extracellular serotonin levels in the raphe.

The dorsal raphe nucleus is the richest region in serotonin and possesses a high density of serotonin reuptake sites (Palkovits et al, 1981). Nevertheless, it is equally sensitive to the inhibition of serotonin uptake by specific inhibitors as the various terminal regions. Thus the difference between the raphe and the terminal regions appears not to be due to different degrees of inhibition of serotonin reuptake.

Electrophysiological studies have shown that the firing rate of dorsal raphe neurons is under the control of 5-HT_{1A} receptors located on somatodendrites in the dorsal raphe nucleus (Sprouse and Aghajanian, 1987) and that stimulation of these receptors by systemic administration of 5-HT_{1A} agonists reduces the firing of these neurons. Increased levels of extracellular serotonin resulting from uptake inhibition activate these autoreceptors in the dorsal raphe nucleus, leading to a feedback inhibition of release in the terminal regions through decreased firing of the dorsal raphe serotonergic neurons. Thus systemic administration of the 5-HT_{1A} receptor antagonists, $S\text{-}(-)5\text{-fluoro-8-hydroxy-2-(di-}n\text{-propylamino)tetralin}$ HCl ((S)-UH-301) or $(-)$penbutolol (Hjorth, 1993), potentiates the increase in extracellular serotonin levels in the cortex or hippocampus produced by the systemic administration of citalopram (see Artigas et al, 1996).

A release-controlling serotonergic feedback mechanism in the terminal regions

This feedback control of the firing rate of the dorsal raphe appears, however, not to be the only negative feedback modulation of serotonergic neurotransmission. Studies from our group and elsewhere have shown that the release of serotonin from nerve terminals is under the control of inhibitory 5-HT autoreceptors (reviews: Moret, 1985; Middlemiss, 1988). These autoreceptors have been shown to be of the 5-HT_{1B} subtype (Engel et al, 1986; Hoyer and Middlemiss, 1989; Schlicker et al, 1989).

The genes encoding the 5-HT_{1B} receptor in rodents and in non-rodents, including humans (previously called the $5\text{-HT}_{1D\beta}$ receptor), are species homologues (Hoyer and Middlemiss, 1989; Hartig et al, 1992) with an overall homology of amino acid sequence of 92% (96% in the membrane-spanning domain). Although the pharmacological differences between these receptor subtypes are greater than usually seen between species homologues, they have similar regional distributions (Waeber et al, 1989) and functions. Both receptor subtypes are found in high densities in substantia nigra, globus pallidus, striatum and basal ganglia, where they function as 5-HT inhibitory autoreceptors on serotonergic nerve terminals (Moret, 1985; Engel et al, 1986; Middlemiss, 1988; Schlicker et al, 1989; Starke et al, 1989; Hoyer et al, 1990) regulating the release of 5-HT. Other 5-HT$_{1B}$ receptors are located, as heteroreceptors, on non-serotonergic terminals, while yet others may be situated postsynaptically on the target neurons of 5-HT projections (Vergé et al, 1986; Offord et al, 1988).

Several studies have suggested that more than one type of 5-HT autoreceptor may exist. Whereas 0.1 µM methiothepin was sufficient to shift the concentration–effect curve for the effect of lysergic acid diethylamide (LSD) on electrically evoked release of [^{3}H]5-HT from rat hypothalamic slices (Moret and Briley, 1986), 1 µM methiothepin was required to antagonize the inhibitory effect of dihydroergoscritine (DHEC), suggesting that LSD and DHEC might act on different subtypes of 5-HT autoreceptors, for which methiothepin had different affinities. A similar approach using guinea pig hippocampal slices (Wilkinson and Middlemiss, 1992) found that the ability of methiothepin to antagonize the inhibitory effect of sumatriptan or 5-carboxamidotryptamine (5-CT) was less marked than for 5-HT. These authors also suggested a possible heterogeneity in the receptor mediating the inhibition of [^{3}H]5-HT release in guinea pig hippocampus. More recently, in 5-HT$_{1B}$ 'knock-out' mice, in which the gene for the 5-HT$_{1B}$ receptor has been deleted, the relatively selective 5-HT$_{1B}$ receptor agonist CP 93129 (3-(1,2,5,6-tetrahydropyrid-4-yl)pyrolol[3,2,6]pyrid-5-one) was no longer able to reduce the release of 5-HT from brain slices in vitro. 5-CT, however, still inhibited the electrically evoked release of [^{3}H]5-HT in frontal cortex and hippocampal slices. Since 5-CT binds with high affinity to multiple 5-HT receptors, the authors suggested that the inhibition by 5-CT may involve receptors other than the 5-HT$_{1B}$ receptor (Pineyro et al, 1995).

In vitro, fast cyclic voltammetry has been used to measure the modulation by 5-HT$_{1D}$ receptors of the release of 5-HT in slices of the guinea pig dorsal raphe nucleus. These studies demonstrated that agonists decreased release, while antagonists by themselves had no effect, suggesting that although these receptors are functional they are not tonically activated (Starkey and Skingle, 1994; Hutson et al, 1995), at least in these in vitro preparations.

The direct, in vivo, study of 5-HT autoreceptor function has become more refined since the advent of intracerebral microdialysis, a technique which allows direct in vivo sampling and measurement of neurotransmitters and their metabolites in the extracellular fluid of the brain of anaesthetized or freely moving animals (Di Chiara, 1990).

The lack of compounds acting selectively at 5-HT$_{1B}$ receptors without an action at 5-HT$_{1A}$ receptors makes the study of release-controlling 5-HT autoreceptors in vivo particularly complex. Nevertheless, microdialysis in terminal regions such as guinea pig frontal cortex has shown that the local infusion of the relatively non-selective 5-HT$_{1B}$ agonist, 5-CT, through the microdialysis probe reduces the extracellular level of serotonin by a maximum of 40–50% (Lawrence and Marsden, 1992), while infusion of the non-selective 5-HT$_1$ receptor antagonist, methiothepin, into the guinea pig substantia nigra results in a large (as much as 10-fold) increase in the level of extracellular serotonin (Briley and Moret, 1993).

RU 24969 has been reported to decrease extracellular 5-HT levels in the hippocampus of anaesthetized rat when administered systemically (Sharp et al, 1989a,b; Martin et al, 1992). A similar reduction of dialysate 5-HT has also been obtained with this compound in the frontal cortex of anaesthetized rats (Brazell et al, 1985; Sleight et al, 1989) and in the diencephalon of awake rats (Auerbach et al, 1991) following systemic administration. Since RU 24969 has significant affinity for 5-HT$_{1A}$ receptors, and 5-HT$_{1A}$ receptor agonists, such as 8-hydroxy-2-(di-*n*-propylamino)-tetralin (8-OH-DPAT), gepirone, ipsapirone and buspirone (Sharp et al, 1989a,b), produce similar effects, it is difficult to determine whether the effects of RU 24969 are due to stimulation of somatodendritic 5-HT$_{1A}$ receptors controlling the firing of raphe neurons or terminal release-controlling 5-HT$_{1B}$ receptors. However, unlike 5-HT$_{1A}$ agonists, local administration of RU 24969 onto 5-HT$_{1A}$ receptor-rich cell bodies in the raphe nucleus did not decrease the extracellular levels of the serotonin metabolite, 5-hydroxyindole acetic acid (5-HIAA) (measured by voltammetry) (Martin and Marsden, 1987), suggesting that its effects on somatodendritic 5-HT$_{1A}$ receptors are weak. In addition, local administration of RU 24969 through the microdialysis probe via the perfusion medium directly into the terminal regions induced a decrease of extracellular 5-HT in the hippocampus of anaesthetized rat (Hjorth and Tao, 1991; Bosker et al, 1995) and in the diencephalon of awake rats. TFMPP applied locally into the diencephalon also decreased dialysate 5-HT levels (Auerbach et al, 1991). It is worth noting that the effects of local administration of RU 24969 and TFMPP are only obtained in the presence of a 5-HT uptake inhibitor in the perfusion medium (Auerbach et al, 1991; Hjorth and Tao, 1991). These compounds possess a non-negligible affinity for the 5-HT membrane carrier and are taken up into the nerve terminals, where, by displacement, they induce the release of 5-HT, thus masking their autoreceptor-mediated inhibitory effects. The effect of the local infusion of RU 24969 was attenuated by simultaneous infusion of the non-selective 5-HT autoreceptor antagonist, methiothepin, into the hippocampus (Martin et al, 1992).

Hjorth and Tao (1991) have shown that CP-93,129, a 5-HT$_{1B}$ receptor agonist with about 100-fold higher affinity for 5-HT$_{1B}$ than for 5-HT$_{1A}$ binding sites, when administered via the dialysis perfusion medium, caused a reduction of 5-HT output in the hippocampus of anaesthetized rats. This effect was significantly antagonized by co-infusion of methiothepin. In contrast to RU 24969 and TFMPP, CP-93,129 decreased dialysate 5-HT both in the presence and in the absence of a 5-HT uptake inhibitor, indicating that this compound is devoid of any action at the level of the 5-HT uptake site (Hjorth and Tao, 1991). Thus CP-93,129 is possibly the agonist of choice for studying 5-HT$_{1B}$ receptors controlling 5-HT release from serotonergic terminals in vivo. From the above results it would appear that 5-HT release in terminal areas in vivo is modulated by 5-HT$_{1B}$ autoreceptors in the rat.

In the rat hypothalamus, methiothepin, when applied locally via the microdialysis probe, increased the extracellular levels of 5-HT both in the absence and in the presence of the 5-HT uptake inhibitor citalopram, suggesting that in awake animals 5-HT autoreceptors in the terminal projection areas are tonically activated and exert a potent inhibitory effect on the release of 5-HT (Moret and Briley, 1996a).

Local (via microdialysis probe) administration of the 5-HT$_{1A/B}$ agonist 5-CT into the frontal cortex of the freely moving guinea pig decreased extracellular 5-HT levels (Lawrence and Marsden, 1992). Sumatriptan, when added to the perfusion medium, similarly reduced extracellular levels of 5-HT in the frontal cortex of anaesthetized guinea pigs (Sleight et al, 1990), presumably via an activation of 5-HT$_{1B}$ autoreceptors. In guinea pig hypothalamus, local, through the probe, administration of naratriptan, which is somewhat more selective for 5-HT$_{1B}$ compared to 5-HT$_{1A}$ receptors, also decreased the extracellular levels of 5-HT, an effect which was attenuated by the non-selective 5-HT$_1$ antagonist methiothepin at 1 μM, a concentration which did not modify by itself the outflow of 5-HT (Moret and Briley, 1996b).

In vitro methiothepin has been shown to increase, by itself, the electrically evoked release of [^{3}H]5-HT from slices of rat hypothalamus (Langer and Moret, 1982) and guinea pig hypothalamus and substantia nigra (Moret, unpublished data). In freely moving guinea pig, methiothepin increases, in a concentration-dependent (10–100 μM) manner, the extracellular levels of 5-HT when applied through the probe into the hypothalamus (Moret, unpublished data). This suggests that, as in the rat (see above), 5-HT autoreceptors in the hypothalamus are tonically activated in the freely moving guinea pig and exert a potent inhibitory effect on the release of 5-HT. When this inhibition is removed by an antagonist, such as methiothepin, there is a major increase in 5-HT release. A similar effect has been found with methiothepin in guinea pig substantia nigra (Briley and Moret, 1993).

A serotonergic feedback mechanism controlling serotonin synthesis

The activity of the rate-limiting enzyme of serotonin synthesis, tryptophan hydroxylase, is also under feedback control. Recently, Hjorth et al (1995) showed, in the rat, that the 5-HT$_{1B/2C}$ receptor agonist TFMPP suppresses 5-HT synthesis in vivo as estimated by the accumulation of 5-hydroxy-tryptophan (5-HTP) after the inhibition of the amino acid decarboxylase, i.e. an index of tryptophan hydroxylation (Carlsson et al, 1972). This suppression, which was evident in terminal projection areas such as the limbic forebrain and striatum, was also observed in axotomized animals, indicating that it was independent of neuronal firing. Furthermore, a similar inhibitory effect of TFMPP on 5-HT synthesis was found in vitro in slice preparations in the presence of depolarizing concentrations of potassium. In vitro, the effect of TFMPP was attenuated by the non-selective 5-HT receptor antagonist methiothepin, as well as the 5-HT$_{1B}$ receptor antagonists propranolol and cyanopindolol. By comparison, the decrease of 5-HT synthesis in forebrain regions induced in vivo by 8-OH-DPAT was prevented by transection of the brain. in addition, 8-OH-DPAT did not decrease 5-HT synthesis in vitro. These data thus suggest that the reduction of rat brain 5-HT synthesis by TFMPP is mediated by 5-HT autoreceptors located on the serotonergic axon terminals, and that this is a direct effect and independent of 5-HT neuronal firing.

This finding confirms a number of earlier suggestions. Using a similar ex vivo protocol, Moret and Briley (1993, 1997) found that methiothepin administered systemically increased the synthesis of 5-HT in rat brain, whereas the 5-HT$_{1A}$/5-HT$_2$ receptor antagonist spiperone had no effect, suggesting that 5-HT$_{1B}$ autoreceptors may be involved in the modulation of 5-HT synthesis.

In guinea pig brain, systemic administration of GR 127935 (N-[4-methoxy-3-(4-methyl-1-piperazinyl)phenyl]-2'-methyl-4'-(5-methyl-1,2,4-oxadiazol-3-yl) [1,1-biphenyl]-4-carboxamide), a reportedly selective 5-HT$_{1B}$ receptor antagonist (Roberts et al, 1994), increases 5-HT synthesis in the frontal cortex (maximum effect 233% of control). Smaller, but significant, increases (50–60%) in 5-HT synthesis have also been found in other regions, such as the hypothalamus, hippocampus and substantia nigra, following systemic administration of similar doses of GR 127935 (Moret and Briley, 1996b).

Taken together, these findings in both rat and guinea pig strongly suggest that the terminal 5-HT$_{1B}$ autoreceptors can play a role in the regulation of 5-HT synthesis. The future availability of specific agonists and antagonists for these receptors will help to clarify and characterize their involvement in the control of this key step of 5-HT neurotransmission.

The effect of chronic administration of SSRIs on the feedback mechanisms

Administration of citalopram (50 mg/kg PO) to rats for 21 days followed by a washout of 24 h resulted in an increased in vitro stimulation-induced release of 5-HT from hypothalamic slices preloaded with [^{3}H]5-HT (Moret and Briley, 1990). In addition, the concentration–effect curve of the agonist LSD was significantly shifted to the right compared with control animals, indicating a desensitization of the autoreceptor for the agonist. We suggested that repeated administration of the selective 5-HT reuptake inhibitor resulted in a decreased efficacy of the terminal autoreceptor, allowing an increased release of 5-HT (Moret and Briley, 1990).

By using fast cyclic voltammetry, O'Connor and Kruk (1994) have shown that repeated administration of the selective 5-HT reuptake inhibitor fluoxetine (5 mg/kg IP) for 21 days with a 24-h washout resulted in an enhancement of electrically stimulated 5-HT overflow from brain slices containing suprachiasmatic nucleus and a significant shift to the right in the concentration–response curve for the 5-HT$_{1B}$ receptor agonist RU 24969 in comparison to brain slices from control (vehicle-treated) animals, again demonstrating a downregulation of the terminal 5-HT$_{1B}$ autoreceptors in this brain region.

In guinea pigs, Blier and Bouchard (1994) have found that the electrically induced release of [^{3}H]5-HT was increased by a chronic treatment with paroxetine, a 5-HT reuptake inhibitor (14 days with 48 h withdrawal) in slices of hypothalamus, hippocampus and frontal cortex, and that the inhibitory effect of the non-selective 5-HT agonist 5-methoxytryptamine was attenuated in the hypothalamus and the hippocampus. Thus the terminal 5-HT$_{1B}$ autoreceptor also appears to be desensitized in the guinea pig after long-term blockade of 5-HT uptake.

The desensitization of the terminal release-controlling autoreceptor has also been deduced from indirect electrophysiological measurements (Chaput et al, 1986, 1991; Blier et al, 1988). Neurons in the CA$_3$ region of the hippocampus possess postsynaptic 5-HT$_{1A}$ receptors which, when stimulated by the serotonergic innervation from the raphe, induce a hyperpolarization of these cells. Thus by electrically stimulating the raphe neurons and measuring the hyperpolarization of cells in the hippocampus, it is possible to measure the overall efficiency of this serotonergic pathway. The intravenous administration of the autoreceptor antagonist methiothepin produces an increased hyperpolarization through an increased release resulting from the blockade of the terminal autoreceptors mediating the feedback inhibition of release. The extent of the effect of methiothepin can thus be used to deduce the sensitivity of the terminal autoreceptor.

Three weeks' administration of citalopram (20 mg/kg per day IP for 14 days) (Chaput et al, 1986), fluoxetine (10 mg/kg per day IP for 14 days)

(Blier et al, 1988) or paroxetine (5 mg/kg per day IP for 21 days) (Chaput et al, 1991) increases the efficiency of serotonergic neurotransmission by attenuation of the effect of the terminal autoreceptor. The increased efficacy of the stimulation of the raphe on the hyperpolarization of the CA_3 hippocampal cells induced by an intravenous injection of the autoreceptor antagonist methiothepin was abolished in SSRI-treated rats (Chaput et al, 1991).

Recently, Moret and Briley (1996a) attempted to demonstrate the increase in synaptic 5-HT using in vivo microdialysis on freely moving rats after a chronic administration of citalopram under exactly the same conditions as used in the previous in vitro study (Moret and Briley, 1990). Somewhat unexpectedly, no change was seen in the basal extracellular levels of endogenous 5-HT in chronic drug-treated animals. In addition, the enhancing effect of methiothepin, administered through the microdialysis probe, was similar in both control and chronically treated animals. These results suggest that, under the conditions of this study, repeated administration of citalopram followed by a washout of 24 h does not lead to a desensitization of the terminal 5-HT autoreceptor of sufficient magnitude for it to be measured in vivo, in contrast to the effects shown in vitro. At present, no clear explanation exists for the discrepancy between in vitro and in vivo findings. Methodological differences (slices preloaded with [^{3}H]5-HT in vitro compared to endogenous 5-HT in vivo; electrically stimulated release in vitro compared to basal release in vivo etc.) may be important. It is possible, however, that, in vivo, other regulatory mechanisms come into play, such as those controlling the firing rate of the raphe nucleus and the synthesis of 5-HT, both of which are under the control of the somatodendritic 5-HT$_{1A}$ autoreceptors. In the in vitro slice preparation where axon terminals have been physically separated from the cell bodies these latter influences are absent. Thus it may not be possible to distinguish a change in the sensitivity of the terminal autoreceptor by studying the levels of extracellular 5-HT if there are concomitant changes in other parts of the system.

In contrast, when studied without washout, extracellular levels of 5-HT were increased by both acute and repeated citalopram administration (Moret and Briley, 1996a). In rats treated chronically without washout, methiothepin (administered locally via the probe) had a greater maximal effect on 5-HT outflow than in rats receiving acute citalopram treatment. This study shows that a 5-HT uptake inhibitor and an autoreceptor antagonist are both capable of increasing extracellular levels of 5-HT. Furthermore, these two effects are additive or possibly synergistic, suggesting that a terminal 5-HT autoreceptor antagonist or a combination of such a drug with a 5-HT uptake inhibitor would produce a greater increase of extracellular levels of 5-HT in hyposerotonergic states and thus be potentially useful in the treatment of depressive disorders resistant to therapy by a single drug. Repeated administration of citalopram (50 mg/kg per day IP) for 21 days also modifies the synthesis of 5-HT. This treatment results in an increased basal rate of 5-HTP accumulation after inhibition of the aromatic amino acid decarboxylase with *m*-hydroxybenzylhydrazine (NSD 1015), indicating an increased activity of tryptophan hydroxylase. Interestingly, however, acute administration of citalopram still inhibits the synthesis with a dose–response curve which is approximately parallel to that of control animals (Moret and Briley, 1992). Thus the activity of tryptophan hydroxylase would appear to be under complex control. The chronic inhibition of serotonin synthesis produced by the repeated administration of an SSRI appears to result in an increased basal enzyme activity, probably as a result of increased enzyme concentration due to enzyme induction. Serotonin synthesis is, however, still responsive, with apparently little or no change in its sensitivity, to temporarily increased levels of serotonin produced by the acute administration of an SSRI. Since both the somatodendritic 5-HT$_{1A}$ autoreceptor and the terminal 5-HT$_{1B}$ autoreceptor are thought to be desensitized under these conditions (see above), the receptor mediating the attenuation of tryptophan hydroxylase activity (if it is indeed receptor mediated) would appear to be different from either of these two receptor subtypes. As shown above, there is no lack of other 5-HT receptor subtypes which could be implicated, and further studies are required in this area.

Thus by different indirect mechanisms, several different types of antidepressant therapy lead, after a few weeks, to a common effect, an increased serotonergic neurotransmission. An obvious consequence of this mechanism is that total or partial inactivation of one or more of the various serotonergic feedback systems should lead to a more rapid increase in serotonergic neurotransmission and consequently an alleviation of the symptoms of depression. Since 5-HT$_{1A}$ receptors exist both pre- and postsynaptically (Miquel et al, 1991, 1992), their blockade may be self-defeating. 5-HT$_{1B}$ receptors, however, appear to be localized mainly presynaptically, either as autoreceptors on serotonergic terminals (Moret, 1985; Engel et al, 1986) or as heteroreceptors on the terminals of other transmitters such as GABA (Hen, 1992), acetylcholine (Maura et al, 1989) etc. Thus selective 5-HT$_{1B}$ autoreceptor antagonists may represent an interesting new therapeutic class for the treatment of depression as well as other hyposerotonergic conditions, such as OCD. These findings are particularly interesting in the context of depressive illness. In spite of the rapid onset of uptake blockade in humans (within a few hours in platelets), the earliest signs of therapeutic improvement in depressive symptoms appear only after 2 weeks of treatment with selective 5-HT uptake inhibitors (for a general review of selective 5-HT uptake inhibitors, see Boyer and Feighner, 1991). The latency of the therapeutic effects has been attributed to the need for adaptive changes to be brought about by long-term treatment (review: see Briley and Moret, 1993). One of these adaptive changes may be the desensitization of the terminal

5-HT$_{1B}$ autoreceptor as described above, with the subsequent rise of synaptic levels of 5-HT and the stimulation of one or more postsynaptic receptors which is thought to be an essential long-term action of these antidepressants.

Evidence from functional studies in animals and humans

Animal studies

There is little information available on the behavioural effects of direct 5-HT$_{1B}$ autoreceptor stimulation. In the learned helplessness (LH) paradigm, rats that are exposed to uncontrollable footshocks fail to learn an escape response, such as a lever press in an operant cage or to move into another compartment in a shuttle box apparatus, whereas rats exposed to controllable shocks are able to acquire these escape responses. In this model, exposure to uncontrollable stress produces a number of signs seen in depressed patients, such as weight loss, changes in sleep pattern, decreased locomotion and performance deficits in learning tasks (Sherman et al, 1979). These symptoms, and specifically the performance deficits, are reduced by a variety of clinically effective antidepressant drugs (Martin et al, 1990). In addition, the density of serotonin uptake sites as measured by [^{3}H]imipramine or [^{3}H]paroxetine binding (Sherman and Petty, 1984; Edwards et al, 1991) are reduced in LH rats as compared to controls. This closely resembles the clinical situation, where there have been numerous reports (review: Briley, 1985) of decreases in serotonin uptake sites labelled by [^{3}H]imipramine (and other more selective ligands) in platelets of depressed patients (Briley et al, 1980) and in the postmortem brain of suicide victims (Stanley et al, 1982).

In LH rats, 5-HT$_{1B}$ receptors are upregulated (increased receptor binding) in the cortex, hippocampus and septum and downregulated in the hypothalamus (Edwards et al, 1991). These results suggest that a change in 5-HT$_{1B}$ receptor responsiveness might be related to the escape deficit. 5-HT release measured in vivo by microdialysis in the cortex of LH rats is decreased (Petty et al, 1992), which is compatible with 5-HT$_{1B}$ autoreceptors being upregulated.

The 5-HT$_{1B}$ receptor agonist CGS 12066B does not modify the escape deficit in the paradigm, but it does reduce the ability of the 5-HT reuptake blockers citalopram and fluvoxamine to reverse the behavioural deficit resulting from uncontrollable shocks (Martin and Puech, 1991), suggesting that 5-HT$_{1B}$ receptor agonists, by their inhibition of 5-HT release, might reduce the stimulation of 5-HT transmission induced by 5-HT reuptake blockers. Finally, a recent study has shown that methiothepin, a nonselective antagonist at the 5-HT$_{1B}$ autoreceptor (Moret, 1985), exhibits antidepressant-like activity in the olfactory bulbectomized rat model of depression (McNamara et al, 1995).

Human studies

Neuroendocrine and behavioural challenge studies of 5-HT$_{1B}$ receptors in humans have used sumatriptan. While this drug is relatively selective for the 5-HT$_{1B}$ receptor, it is reputed to penetrate the blood–brain barrier only to a limited extent. The most specific neuroendocrine response induced in humans by the administration of sumatriptan is a major (greater than five-fold) increase in plasma levels of growth hormone (Franceschini et al, 1994; Herdman et al, 1994). This effect, which is prevented by prior administration of the non-selective 5-HT$_1$ receptor antagonist cyprohepta-dine (Franceschini et al, 1994), has been suggested to result from an inhibition of the release of somatostatin via 5-HT$_{1B}$ heteroreceptors (Mota et al, 1995). As yet there have been no studies on depressed patients.

The administration of the non-selective 5-HT agonist *m*-chloro-phenylpiperazine (mCPP) to untreated patients suffering from OCD causes a marked and transient exacerbation of their symptoms (Zohar et al, 1987; Hollander et al, 1992), whereas the administration to healthy vol-unteers does not, in general, induce any symptomatology. This effect, which can be prevented by pretreatment with the non-selective 5-HT receptor antagonist metergoline (Pigott et al, 1991), has been suggested to result from stimulation of 5-HT receptors that are supersensitive in OCD patients. This idea has found support in the observation that the effects of mCPP are blunted in patients whose OCD has been success-fully treated with clomipramine (Zohar et al, 1988), which presumably normalizes these supersensitive receptors. mCPP has high affinity for 5-HT$_{1A}$, 5-HT$_{1B}$ and 5-HT$_{2C}$ receptors. Since more selective serotonergic agonists, such as ipsapirone (5-HT$_{1A}$) and MK-212 (2-chloro-6-(1-piper-azinyl) pyrazine) (5-HT$_{2C}$), do not produce the exacerbation of OCD symptoms (Bastani et al, 1990), it would appear that the receptors involved are probably of the 5-HT$_{1B}$ subtype. In addition, since OCD symptoms are unaltered by modification of synaptic 5-HT levels through tryptophan depletion (Barr et al, 1994), the receptors involved are probably not 5-HT autoreceptors but more likely 5-HT$_{1B}$ heteroreceptors. The putative role of 5-HT$_{1B}$ receptors has been recently tested by admin-istering sumatriptan to OCD patients, who reacted with a marked and transient aggravation of their OCD symptomatology (Dolberg et al, 1995). These studies suggest that supersensitive 5-HT$_{1B}$ receptors may indeed be involved in the pathophysiology of OCD and may represent a potential target for its treatment.

Conclusion

5-HT autoreceptors are capable of modulating 5-HT neurotransmission via the control of the release and synthesis of 5-HT. The induction of the depressive-like state of LH induces 5-HT_{1B} receptor supersensitivity (Edwards et al, 1991) in various brain regions. An increase in 5-HT_{1B} autoreceptor sensitivity is consistent with the decreased release of 5-HT from LH rats observed by microdialysis in the cortex (Petty et al, 1992). Increased serotonergic neurotransmission appears to be associated with an increased level of anxiety (Chopin and Briley, 1987; Briley and Chopin, 1994). The frequent co-existence of high levels of anxiety with depression, a supposedly hyposerotonergic state, is, nevertheless, difficult to explain. In the case, however, of supersensitivity of 5-HT_{1B} auto- and heteroreceptors, a decreased release of 5-HT resulting from an increased autoinhibition and an increased level of anxiety resulting from activation of supersensitive 5-HT_{1B} heteroreceptors, decreasing GABA release, for example, could be expected. This corresponds to the situation found in the LH model of depression, where 5-HT_{1B} auto- and heteroreceptors both appear to be supersensitive. Interestingly, rats exposed to repeated inescapable shocks, such as the 'LH rats', not only show a number of 'depressive' signs (Sherman et al, 1979), but also exhibit behaviour associated with high levels of anxiety (Vandijken et al, 1992a,b). To date there is no indication as to whether 5-HT_{1B} receptors are supersensitive in anxious or depressed patients, but the above animal data make this an attractive working hypothesis. Repeated administration of 5-HT uptake-blocking antidepressants would be expected to desensitize both pre- and postsynaptic 5-HT_{1B} receptors. Desensitization of presynaptic 5-HT_{1B} autoreceptors has already been demonstrated in vitro in rats following chronic treatment with citalopram (Moret and Briley, 1990). If 5-HT_{1B} auto- and heteroreceptors are supersensitive in depression and anxiety, direct antagonism of 5-HT_{1B} receptors may well produce both antidepressant and anxiolytic effects more rapidly than with selective 5-HT uptake-blocking agents.

As mentioned above, a totally independent line of reasoning has led Zohar and coworkers (Dolberg et al, 1995) to a similar conclusion in OCD where 5-HT_{1B} receptors appear to be supersensitive and their desensitization through long-term administration of 5-HT reuptake inhibitors is possibly responsible for their therapeutic effect. As in depression, a significant gain in the delay of onset of action can be envisaged by the use of specific 5-HT_{1B} receptor antagonists to treat OCD.

In conclusion, several lines of evidence suggest that changes in the sensitivity of 5-HT_{1B} auto- and heteroreceptors may be fundamental to several psychiatric disorders. Further investigation into 5-HT_{1B} receptor function in psychopathology would appear to be potentially rewarding. In addition, the development of new selective agonists and antagonists could be important in both research and therapy.

References

Adell A, Artigas F (1991) Differential effects of clomipramine given locally or systemically on extracellular 5-hydroxytryptamine in raphe nuclei and frontal cortex—an in vivo brain microdialysis study, *Naunyn Schmiedebergs Arch Pharmacol* **343:**237–44.

Artigas F, Romero L, De Montigny C, Blier P (1996) Acceleration of the effect of selected antidepressant drugs in major depression by 5-HT$_{1A}$ antagonists, *Trends in Neuroscience* **19:**378–83.

Auerbach SB, Rutter JJ, Juliano PJ (1991) Substituted piperazine and indole compounds increase extracellular serotonin in rat diencephalon as determined by in vivo microdialysis, *Neuropharmacology* **30:**307–11.

Barr LC, Goodman WK, McDougle CJ et al (1994). Tryptophan depletion in patients with obsessive-compulsive disorder who respond to serotonin reuptake inhibitors, *Arch Gen Psychiatry* **51:**309–17.

Bastani B, Nash F, Meltzer H (1990) Prolactin and cortisol responses to MK-212, a serotonin agonist, in obsessive-compulsive disorder, *Arch Gen Psychiatry* **47:**946–51.

Bel N, Artigas F (1992) Fluvoxamine preferentially increases extracellular 5-hydroxytryptamine in the raphe nuclei: an in vivo microdialysis study, *Eur J Pharmacol* **229:**101–3.

Blier P, Bouchard C (1994) Modulation of 5-HT release in the guinea pig brain following long-term administration of antidepressant drugs, *Br J Pharmacol* **113:**485–95.

Blier P, Chaput Y, De Montigny C (1988) Long-term 5-HT reuptake blockade, but not monoamine oxidase inhibition, reduces the function of the terminal 5-HT autoreceptor: an elecrophysiological study in the rat brain, *Naunyn Schmiedebergs Arch Pharmacol* **337:**246–54.

Bosker FJ, Van Esseveldt KE, Klompmakers AA, Westenberg HGM (1995) Chronic treatment with fluvoxamine by osmotic minipumps fails to induce persistent functional changes in central 5-HT$_{1A}$ and 5-HT$_{1B}$ receptors, as measured by in vivo microdialysis in dorsal hippocampus of conscious rats, *Psychopharmacology* **117:**358–63.

Boyer WF, Feighner JP (1991) The efficacy of selective serotonin reuptake inhibitors in depression. In: Feighner JP, Boyer WF, eds, *Selective Serotonin Reuptake Inhibitors* (Wiley: Chichester) 89–108.

Brazell MP, Marsden CA, Nisbet AP, Routledge C (1985) The 5-HT$_1$ receptor agonist RU-24969 decreases 5-hydroxytryptamine (5-HT) release and metabolism in the rat frontal cortex in vitro and in vivo, *Br J Pharmacol* **86:**209–16.

Briley M (1985) Imipramine binding: its relationship with serotonin uptake and depression. In: Green AR, ed., *Neuropharmacology of Serotonin* (Oxford University Press: Oxford) 50–78.

Briley M, Chopin P (1994) Is anxiety associated with a hyper- or hyposerotonergic state? In: Palomo T, Archer T, eds, *Strategies for Studying Brain Disorders*, Vol. 1, *Depression, Anxiety and Drug Abuse Disorders* (Editorial Complutence: Donoso Cortés, Madrid) 197–209.

Briley M, Moret C (1993) Neurobiological mechanisms involved in antidepressant therapies, *Clin Neuropharmacol* **16:**387–400.

Briley M, Langer SZ, Raisman R, Sechter D, Zarifian E (1980) 3H-Imipramine binding sites are decreased in platelets of untreated depressed patients, *Science* **209:**303–5.

Carlsson A, Davis JN, Kehr W, Lindqvist M, Atack CV (1972) Simultaneous measurement of tyrosine and tryptophan hydroxylase activities in brain in vivo using an inhibitor of the aromatic amino acid decarboxylase, *Naunyn Schmiedebergs Arch Pharmacol* **275:**153–68.

Chaput Y, De Montigny C, Blier P (1986) Effects of a selective 5-HT reuptake blocker, citalopram, on the sensitivity of 5-HT autoreceptors: electrophysiological studies in rat brain, *Naunyn Schmiedebergs Arch Pharmacol* **333:**342–8.

Chaput Y, De Montigny C, Blier P (1991) Presynaptic and postsynaptic modifications of the serotonin system by long-term administration of antidepressant treatments—an in vivo electrophysiologic study in the rat, *Neuropsychopharmacology* **5:**219–29.

Chopin P, Briley M (1987) Animal models of anxiety: the effect of compounds that modify 5-HT neurotransmission, *Trends Pharmacol Sci* **8:** 383–8.

Dailey JW, Yan QS, Mishra PK, Burger RL, Jobe PC (1992) Effects of fluoxetine on convulsions and on brain serotonin as detected by microdialysis in genetically epilepsy-prone rats, *J Pharmacol Exp Ther* **260:**533–40.

Di Chiara G (1990) In vivo brain dialysis of neurotransmitters, *Trends Pharmacol Sci* **11:**116–21.

Dolberg OT, Sasson Y, Cohen R, Zohar J (1995) The relevance of behavioral probes in obsessive-compulsive disorder, *Eur Neuropsychopharmacol* **5:**161–2.

Edwards E, Harkins K, Wright G, Henn FA (1991) 5-HT$_{1B}$ receptors in an animal model of depression, *Neuropharmacology* **30:**101–5.

Engel G, Göthert M, Hoyer D, Schlicker E, Hillenbrand K (1986) Identity of inhibitory presynaptic 5-hydroxytryptamine (5-HT) autoreceptors in the rat brain cortex with 5-HT$_{1B}$ binding sites, *Naunyn Schmiedebergs Arch Pharmacol* **332:**1–7.

Franceschini R, Cataldi A, Garibaldi A et al (1994) The effects of sumatriptan on pituitary secretion in man, *Neuropharmacology* **33:**235–9.

Hartig PR, Branchek TA, Weinshank RL (1992) A subfamily of 5-HT$_{1D}$ receptor genes, *Trends Pharmacol Sci* **13:**152–9.

Hen R (1992) Of mice and flies—commonalities among 5-HT receptors, *Trends Pharmacol Sci* **13:**160–5.

Herdman JRE, Delva NJ, Hockney RE, Campling GM, Cowen PJ (1994) Neuroendocrine effects of sumatriptan, *Psychopharmacology* **113:**561–4.

Hjorth S (1993) Serotonin 5-HT$_{1A}$ autoreceptor blockade potentiates the ability of the 5-HT reuptake inhibitor citalopram to increase nerve terminal output of 5-HT in vivo: a microdialysis study, *J Neurochem* **60:**776–9.

Hjorth S, Tao R (1991) The putative 5-HT$_{1B}$ receptor agonist CP-93,129 suppresses rat hippocampal 5-HT release in vivo—comparison with RU 24969, *Eur J Pharmacol* **209:**249–52.

Hjorth S, Suchowski CS, Galloway MP (1995) Evidence for 5-HT autoreceptor-mediated, nerve impulse-independent, control of 5-HT synthesis in the rat brain, *Synapse* **19:**170–6.

Hollander E, DeCaria CM, Nitescu A (1992) Serotonergic function in obsessive-compulsive disorder, *Arch Gen Psychiatry* **49:**21–8.

Hoyer D, Middlemiss DN (1989) Species differences in the pharmacology of terminal 5-HT autoreceptors in mammalian brain, *Trends Pharmacol Sci* **10:**130–2.

Hoyer D, Schoeffter P, Waeber C, Palacios JM (1990) Serotonin 5-HT$_{1D}$ receptors, *Ann NY Acad Sci* **600:**168–82.

Hutson PH, Bristow LJ, Cunningham JR et al (1995) The effects of GR127935, a putative 5-HT$_{1D}$ receptor antagonist, on brain 5-HT metabolism, extracellular 5-HT concentration and behaviour in the guinea pig, *Neuropharmacology* **34:**383–92.

Invernizzi R, Belli S, Samanin R (1992) Citalopram's ability to increase the extracellular concentrations of serotonin in the dorsal raphe prevents the drug's effect in the frontal cortex, *Brain Res* **584:**322–4.

Johnson AM (1992) Paroxetine—a pharmacological review, *Int Clin Psychopharmacol* **6:**15–24.

Langer SZ, Moret C (1982) Citalopram antagonizes the stimulation by lysergic acid diethylamide of presynaptic inhibitory serotonin autoreceptors in the rat hypothalamus, *J Pharmacol Exp Ther* **222:**220–6.

Lawrence AJ, Marsden CA (1992) Terminal autoreceptor control of 5-hydroxytryptamine release as measured by in vivo microdialysis in the conscious guinea pig, *J Neurochem* **58:**142–6.

Martin KF, Marsden CA (1987) In vivo voltammetry in the suprachiasmatic nucleus of the rat: effects of RU 24969, methiothepin and ketanserin, *Eur J Pharmacol* **121:**135–9.

Martin KF, Hannon S, Phillips I, Heal DJ (1992) Opposing roles for 5-HT$_{1B}$ and 5-HT$_3$ receptors in the control of 5-HT release in rat hippocampus in vivo, *Br J Pharmacol* **106:**139–42.

Martin P, Puech AJ (1991) Is there a relationship between 5-HT$_{1B}$ receptors and the mechanisms of action of antidepressant drugs in the learned helplessness paradigm in rats? *Eur J Pharmacol* **192:**193–6.

Martin P, Beninger RJ, Hamon M, Puech AJ (1990) Antidepressant-like action of 8-OH-DPAT, a 5-HT$_{1A}$ agonist, in the learned helplessness paradigm: evidence for a postsynaptic mechanism, *Behav Brain Res* **38:**135–44.

Maura G, Fedele E, Raiteri M (1989) Acetylcholine release from rat hippocampal slices is modulated by 5-hydroxytryptamine, *Eur J Pharmacol* **165:**173–9.

McNamara MG, Kelly JP, Leonard BE (1995) Some behavioural effects of methiothepin in the olfactory bulbectomised rat model of depression, *Med Sci Res* **23:**583–5.

Middlemiss DN (1988) Autoreceptors regulating serotonin release. In: Sanders-Bush E, ed., *The Serotonin Receptors* (Humana Press: Clifton, NJ) 210–24.

Miquel MC, Doucet E, Boni C et al (1991) Central serotonin-1A receptors—respective distributions of encoding messenger RNA, receptor protein and binding sites by in situ hybridization histochemistry, radioimmunohistochemistry and autoradiographic mapping in the rat brain, *Neurochem Int* **19:**453–65.

Miquel MC, Doucet E, Riad M, Adrien J, Verge D, Hamon M (1992) Effect of the selective lesion of serotoninergic neurons on the regional distribution of 5-HT1A receptor messenger RNA in the rat brain, *Mol Brain Res* **14:**357–62.

Moret C (1985) Pharmacology of the serotonin autoreceptor. In: Green AR, ed., *Neuropharmacology of Serotonin* (Oxford University Press: Oxford) 21–49.

Moret C, Briley M (1986) Dihydroergocristine-induced stimulation of the 5-HT autoreceptor in the hypothalamus of the rat, *Neuropharmacology* **25:**169–74.

Moret C, Briley M (1990) Serotonin autoreceptor subsensitivity and antidepressant activity, *Eur J Pharmacol* **180:**351–6.

Moret C, Briley M (1992) Effect of antidepressant drugs on monoamine synthesis in brain in vivo, *Neuropharmacology* **31:**679–84.

Moret C, Briley M (1993) Which 5-HT receptors are involved in the modulation of 5-HT synthesis by the 5-HT uptake blocker, citalopram? *Br J Pharmacol* **108:**95P.

Moret C, Briley M (1996a) Effects of acute and repeated administration of citalopram on extracellular levels of serotonin in rat brain, *Eur J Pharmacol* **295:**189–97.

Moret C, Briley M (1996b) Effects of GR 127935 on terminal 5-HT1D autoreceptors and 5-HT synthesis in guinea pig brain, *Soc Neurosci Abstr* **22:**528.17.

Moret C, Briley M (1997) Ex vivo inhibitory effect of the 5-HT uptake blocker citalopram on 5-HT synthesis, *J Neural Transm* **104:**147–60.

Mota A, Bento A, Peñalva A, Pombo M, Dieguez C (1995) Role of the serotonin receptor subtype $5-HT_{1D}$ on basal and stimulated growth hormone secretion, *J Clin Endocrinol Metab* **80:**1973–7.

O'Connor JJ, Kruk ZL (1994) Effects of 21 days treatment with fluoxetine on stimulated endogenous 5-hydroxytryptamine overflow in the rat dorsal raphe and suprachiasmatic nucleus studied using fast cyclic voltammetry in vitro, *Brain Res* **640:**328–35.

Offord SJ, Ordway GA, Frazer A (1988) Application of $[^{125}I]$iodocyanopindolol to measure 5-hydroxytryptamine (1B) receptors in the brain of the rat, *J Pharmacol Exp Ther* **244:**144–53.

Palkovits M, Raisman R, Briley M, Langer SZ (1981) Regional distribution of [3H]-imipramine binding in the brain, *Brain Res* **210:**493–8.

Perry KW, Fuller RW (1992) Effect of fluoxetine on serotonin and dopamine concentration in microdialysis fluid from rat striatum, *Life Sci* **50:**1683–90.

Petty F, Kramer G, Wilson L (1992) Prevention of learned helplessness— in vivo correlation with cortical serotonin, *Pharmacol Biochem Behav* **43:**361–7.

Pigott TA, Zohar J, Hill JL (1991) Metergoline blocks the behavioural and neuroendocrine effects of orally administered m-chlorophenylpiperazine in patients with obsessive-compulsive disorder, *Biol Psychiatry* **29:**418–26.

Pineyro G, Castanon N, Hen R, Blier P (1995) Regulation of 5-HT release in 5-HT_{1B} knock-out mice: experiments in hippocampal, frontal cortex and midbrain raphe slices, *Soc Neurosci Abst* **21:**1368.

Roberts C, Thorn L, Price GW, Middlemiss DN, Jones BJ (1994) Effect of the selective $5-HT_{1D}$ receptor antagonist, GR 127935, on in vivo 5-HT release, synthesis and turnover in the guinea pig frontal cortex, *Br J Pharmacol* **112:**488P.

Schlicker E, Fink K, Göthert et al (1989) The pharmacological properties of the presynaptic serotonin autoreceptor in the pig brain cortex conform to the $5-HT_{1D}$ receptor subtype, *Naunyn Schmiedebergs Arch Pharmacol* **340:**45–51.

Sharp T, Bramwell SR, Hjorth S, Grahame-Smith DG (1989a) Pharmacological characterization of 8-OH-DPAT-induced inhibition of rat hippocampal 5-HT release in vivo as measured by microdialysis, *Br J Pharmacol* **98:**989–97.

Sharp T, Bramwell ST, Grahame-Smith DG (1989b) $5-HT_1$ agonists reduce 5-hydroxytryptamine release in rat hippocampus in vivo as determined by brain microdialysis, *Br J Pharmacol* **96:**283–90.

Sherman AD, Petty F (1984) Learned helplessness decreases 3H-imipramine binding in rat cortex, *J Affect Disord* **6:**25–32.

Sherman AD, Allers GL, Petty F, Henn FA (1979) A neuropharmacologically relevant animal model of depression, *Neuropharmacology* **18:**891–4.

Sleight AJ, Smith RJ, Marsden CA, Palfreyman MG (1989) The effects of chronic treatment with amitriptyline and MDL 72394 on the control of 5-HT release in vivo, *Neuropharmacology* **28:**477–80.

Sleight AJ, Cervenka A, Peroutka SJ (1990) In vivo effects of sumatriptan (GR-43175) on extracellular levels of 5-HT in the guinea pig, *Neuropharmacology* **29:**511–13.

Sprouse JS, Aghajanian GK (1987) Electrophysiological responses of serotonergic dorsal raphe neurons to 5-HT1A and 5-HT1B agonists, *Synapse* **1:**3–9.

Stanley M, Vigilio J, Gershon S (1982) Tritiated imipramine binding sites are decreased in the frontal cortex of suicides, *Science* **216:**1337–9.

Starke K, Göthert M, Kilbinger H (1989) Modulation of neurotransmitter release by presynaptic autoreceptors, *Physiol Rev* **69:**864–989.

Starkey SJ, Skingle M (1994) 5-HT$_{1D}$ as well as 5-HT$_{1A}$ autoreceptors modulate 5-HT release in the guinea pig dorsal raphé nucleus, *Neuropharmacology* **33:**393–402.

Vandijken HH, Mos J, van der Heyden JAM, Tilders FJH (1992a) Characterization of stress-induced long-term behavioural changes in rats—evidence in favor of anxiety, *Physiol Behav* **52:**945–51.

Vandijken HH, van der Heyden JAM, Mos J, Tilders FJH (1992b) Inescapable footshocks induce progressive and long-lasting behavioural changes in male rats, *Physiol Behav* **51:**787–94.

Vergé D, Daval G, Marcinkiewicz M et al (1986) Quantitative autoradiography of multiple 5-HT$_1$ receptor subtypes in the brain of control or 5,7-dihydroxytryptamine-treated rats, *J Neurosci* **6:**3474–82.

Waeber C, Dietl MM, Hoyer D, Palacios JM (1989) 5-HT$_1$ receptors in the vertebrate brain: regional distribution examined by autoradiography, *Naunyn Schmiedebergs Arch Pharmacol* **340:**486–94.

Wilkinson LO, Middlemiss DN (1992) Metitepine distinguishes two receptors mediating inhibition of [^{3}H]-5-hydroxytryptamine release in guinea pig hippocampus, *Naunyn Schmiedebergs Arch Pharmacol* **345:**696–9.

Zohar J, Mueller EA, Insel TR (1987) Serotonin responsivity in obsessive compulsive disorder, *Arch Gen Psychiatry* **44:**946–51.

Zohar J, Insel TR, Zohar-Kadoush RC, Hill JL, Murphy DL (1988) Serotonergic responsivity in obsessive-compulsive disorder: effects of clomipramine treatment, *Arch Gen Psychiatry* **45:**167–72.

4

Modulation of the serotonergic system by 5-HT-moduline

Gilles Fillion, Brigitte Grimaldi, Isabelle Cloëz-Tayarani, Alexandre Bonnin, Marie-Paule Fillion, Olivier Massot, Jean-Claude Rousselle, Laure Seguin and Jean-Christophe Seznec

Serotonergic neurotransmission and its neuromodulatory role

Neuroanatomy of the serotonergic system

Serotonin (5-hydroxytryptamine, 5-HT) is at the present time largely accepted as an important neurotransmitter which essentially has a role as a neuromodulator in the central nervous system (CNS).

The anatomic structure of the system is rather well adapted to that role, as it is very centralized: all the 5-HT cellular bodies are located in a single area, the raphe region. It projects to a vast majority of the brain areas (see Jacobs and Azmitia, 1992; Baumgarten and Grozdanovic, 1994). Thus, the centralization of the system may favor the function of control and modulation by the serotonergic system on other neurotransmissions.

However, since the number of serotonergic cells in the brain is quite limited, i.e. close to 11 500 in rat and 24 000 in cat raphe dorsalis (Wiklund et al, 1981), it is surprising that the serotonergic system may have a significant modulatory function on brain activity, as on the basis of the classical schematic representation of a neuron it could be expected that each 5-HT neuron would interact with only a few other neurons. A particular property of the serotonergic system confers on it a large enhancement of its capacity to interact with other neurons. Indeed, the system developed a large arborescence of the axonal projections, particularly well demonstrated in rodents (Kosofsky and Molliver, 1987) and monkeys (Takeuchi, 1988). Moreover, these fibers exhibit an extremely high number of varicosities (equivalent of neuron terminals) which contain serotonergic vesicles which are probably releasable outside the terminal. It was estimated that a single axon projecting from the raphe to the cortex in human brain could contain up to 500 000 varicosities and that in the rat brain the density of the terminals in the cortex could reach 6×10^6 per mm^3 of the tissue (Audet et al, 1989).

The ascending serotonergic projections originating from the dorsal and from the ventral raphe areas appear to have different targeting and different structural morphologies, the dorsal system being more collateralized than the ventral one (see Baumgarten and Grozdanovic, 1994). The very high capacity for interaction in the serotonergic system conferred by the very high number of varicosities is further enhanced by the fact that the major proportion of these varicosities are non-junctional, i.e. they do not form true synapses (Descarries et al, 1990). The corresponding transmission, also called volumic transmission (Fuxe et al, 1989), favors a further enhancement of the capacity for interaction of a single serotonergic fiber with other neurons.

The serotonergic system functions as an oscillator

Various experimental studies (Jacobs et al, 1990) have indicated that the serotonergic system exerts a tonic effect on CNS activity. The serotonergic neurons of the raphe discharge in a regular firing rate ranging from zero during paradoxical sleep to 5–7 Hz during active waking, intermediate values being observed during quiet waking (Jacobs and Fornal, 1993). Thus, the action potential progressing along the axonal branches of the 5-HT neuron may induce the release of the amine at each of its numerous varicosities. Therefore, this system appears to function as an oscillator, i.e. a regulatory device used in physics which releases a signal characterized by its amplitude and its frequency. The signal amplitude corresponds to the amount of 5-HT released from the varicosity, and the frequency is that of the neuronal discharge. The tight control of these two parameters confers on the oscillator its ability to finely regulate other functions. The frequency and amplitude of the serotonergic 'oscillator' are actually tightly controlled: the frequency of discharge of the 5-HT neurons is regulated by the various neuronal afferents to the raphe and also by the $5-HT_{1A}$ autoreceptors located in this area; the amplitude of the signal, the amount of 5-HT released from a single varicosity at each neuronal discharge, is controlled by neuronal afferents and by $5-HT_{1B}$ autoreceptors located on the neuronal varicosities. Therefore, it can be expected that a pharmacologic interaction at $5-HT_{1A}$ and $5-HT_{1B}$ autoreceptors should affect the serotonergic activity.

Neurophysiology and pathology

The anatomy and the widespread tonic activity of the system is in good agreement with the observation that the serotonergic activity is implicated in a large number of physiologic events: temperature regulation, sleep, learning and memory, behavior, nociception, feeding, sexual functions, hormonal secretions, locomotion, cardiovascular tonicity and also immune activity (see Zifa and Fillion, 1992). Thus, dysfunctions of the serotonergic interactions with other systems may also be involved in a number of pathologic disorders and particularly in depression (see Zifa and Fillion, 1992).

Role of 5-HT$_{1B}$ receptors in serotonergic activity

It is known that at least 14 different types of 5-HT-specific receptors are involved in the function of the serotonergic system. The facts that some of these receptors were only recently identified and that there is a lack of selective ligands to activate or antagonize these receptors have resulted in a poor pharmacologic characterization of the role of the different 5-HT receptors in serotonergic activity. This is also the case for the 5-HT$_{1B}$ receptors. Indeed, the clear identification of the various 5-HT$_{1B/1D}$ receptor subtypes is relatively recent and did not allow the development of numerous specific ligands.

Nevertheless, at the present time, the 5-HT$_{1B}$ receptor subtypes correspond to the r5-HT$_{1B}$ and h5-HT$_{1B}$ receptors, previously called 5-HT$_{1B}$ and 5-HT$_{1D\beta}$ respectively; these receptors have more than 90–95% structural identity in various mammalian species, although the pharmacologic properties of the two subtypes are different; for example, the r5-HT$_{1B}$ receptor recognizes β-adrenergic antagonists such as propranolol and cyanopindolol, while the h5-HT$_{1B}$ receptor does not. Site-directed mutagenesis showed that the difference originated from a single amino acid modification in the transmembrane domain 7: the rat amino acid asparagine-351 is changed to threonine-355 in humans (Metcalf et al, 1992; Oksenberg et al, 1992; Parker et al, 1993).

An additional receptor subtype called 5-HT$_{1D}$ (Hartig et al, 1996) (formerly 5-HT$_{1D\alpha}$) was initially identified in the dog (Libert et al, 1988) as an orphan receptor, and its existence was confirmed in humans and the rat (Hamblin et al, 1992; Weinshank et al, 1992); this receptor is clearly distinct from the 5-HT$_{1B}$ receptor (61% identity in humans), although its pharmacologic properties are similar. Indeed, the serotonin derivative 5-O-carboxymethylglycyl-([125I])-tyrosinamide ([125I]-GTI), which was presented as a good selective ligand for the 5-HT$_{1B}$ receptor (Hoyer et al, 1994), has a similar affinity for the 5-HT$_{1D}$ receptor subtype. Only recently, it was shown that ketanserin and ritanserin may discriminate between the two subtypes 5-HT$_{1B}$ and 5-HT$_{1D}$ (Zgombick et al, 1995).

Functional studies have indicated that 5-HT$_{1B}$ receptors can be separated into two categories. Autoreceptors are located on 5-HT varicosities, where they inhibit the evoked release of 5-HT (Middlemiss, 1984; Engel et al, 1986; Fink et al, 1995) and its biosynthesis (Hjorth et al, 1995); these autoreceptors are also present on somatodendritic fibers of the serotonergic system in the raphe (Piñeyro et al, 1995; Piñeyro and Blier, 1996). Postsynaptic 5-HT$_{1B}$ receptors are located on non-serotonergic terminals, where they inhibit the release of the transmitter contained in the corresponding neurons, i.e. acetylcholine (Harel-Dupas et al, 1991) and γ-aminobutyric acid (Feuerstein et al, 1996).

The distribution of 5-HT_{1B} receptors is wide and heterogeneous within the brain: the highest levels are found in brain areas involved in motor function, such as globus pallidus and ventral pallidum, entopeduncular nucleus and subtantia nigra (reticulata). They are also observed with a relatively high density in dorsal subiculum, subthalamic nucleus, superior colliculus, hypothalamic nuclei, central gray matter and substantia nigra (compacta). Lower densities are observed in olfactory tubercles and optic tracts, nucleus accumbens, amygdaloid nucleus, septum, dorsal raphe interpeduncular nucleus, ventral tegmental area, and frontal and parietal cortices (Bruinvels et al, 1993).

In situ hybridization studies have shown that 5-HT_{1B} mRNA is present in a number of regions which also exhibit 5-HT_{1B} receptors (Bruinvels et al, 1994) and have also demonstrated that some areas (globus pallidus and substantia nigra) which are very rich in 5-HT_{1B} receptors, did not show any corresponding mRNA. This observation confirms that 5-HT_{1B} receptors are transported to the nerve terminal in serotonergic (or non-serotonergic) neurons.

In sum, 5-HT_{1B} receptors may play an important role in the activity of the serotonergic system. Thus, any interaction affecting their regulatory function might have important functional consequences.

5-HT-moduline: characterization and properties

Isolation, purification and biochemical characterization

The existence of endogenous ligands interacting with 5-HT_1 receptor subtypes was previously postulated as a potential explanation of the observed direct and non-competitive interactions of antidepressant drugs with 5-HT_1 receptor subtypes (Fillion and Fillion, 1981). Horse, bovine and rat brains were submitted to extraction procedures involving acidic and organic treatments; the resulting extracts were tested for their capacity to interact with the binding of $[^3H]5\text{-HT}$ to 5-HT_{1B} receptors in rat brain membrane preparations. The active fractions were further purified by HPLC chromatography using different matrices and various mobile phases (Rousselle et al, 1996). Sequential purification steps allowed the isolation of a single fraction up to homogeneity; the corresponding endogenous compound was able to specifically interact with the binding of $[^3H]5\text{-HT}$ to 5-HT_{1B} receptors without affecting the binding of specific ligands to receptors for other neurotransmitters (muscarinic, dopaminergic, α- and β-adrenergic, histaminergic, opiate and benzodiazepine receptors).

Amino acid analysis, microsequencing and mass spectrometry analysis allowed the characterization of the endogenous compound as being a short peptide corresponding to leucine–serine–alanine–leucine (LSAL). This peptidic sequence was synthetized and its activity determined. As the endogenous peptide, the synthetic compound interacted specifically with the 5-HT$_{1B}$ receptor and not with any of the other tested receptors, strongly suggesting the identity of the synthetic peptide with the purified endogenous active compound (Rousselle et al, 1996).

Biochemical and pharmacologic properties

A first series of experiments was carried out to study the molecular mechanism of interaction of the peptide with the receptor. It was shown that LSAL interacted in a non-competitive way with the binding of [^{3}H]5-HT to 5-HT$_{1B}$ receptor, indicating that the site of action of the peptide, although it was located on the 5-HT$_{1B}$ receptor protein, was probably not identical to that able to recognize the amine. It was also observed that the apparent affinity of the interaction was particularly high, as the corresponding EC$_{50}$ was close to 10^{-10} M. The fact that LSAL did not show any activity at low temperature suggests that the interaction might involve conformational changes of the receptor protein. Interestingly, the specificity of interaction was further established by the demonstration that LSAL did not interact with any other serotonergic receptors, including 5-HT$_{1A}$, 5-HT$_{1E}$, 5-HT$_{1F}$, 5-HT$_{2A}$, 5-HT$_{2B}$, 5-HT$_{2C}$, 5-HT$_3$, 5-HT$_6$ and 5-HT$_7$ receptor subtypes. These results demonstrated that LSAL interacted solely with 5-HT$_{1B}$ receptors. Interestingly, the peptide was not able to interact with any of the transporters tested in our studies, namely 5-HT, noradrenaline, dopamine, choline and γ-aminobutyric acid, up to concentrations (10^{-5} M) 100 000 times higher than those active on 5-HT$_{1B}$ receptors. The specificity of the activity of LSAL was restricted to the actual sequence of the peptide: the peptide ALLS, the same amino acid composition as LSAL in a different sequence (scrambled peptide), is totally devoid of action up to concentrations 50 000 times higher than that of the active concentration of LSAL. The two dipeptides AL and LS resulting from the metabolism of the initial compound are also very poorly effective, being 10 000–100 000 times less active than LSAL respectively (Rousselle et al, 1996).

The interaction of LSAL with the 5-HT$_{1B}$ receptor protein is in good agreement with the functional results observed at the cellular level and in in vivo situations. Indeed, it was shown that LSAL at low concentrations (in the nanomolar range) markedly reversed the inhibitory effect of a 5-HT$_{1B}$-specific agonist (CGS 12066 B, CP 93129) on the synaptosomally evoked release of [^{3}H]5-HT (Massot et al, 1996). This antagonistic effect also appeared to involve a non-competitive interaction. Furthermore, intracerebroventricular administration of the peptide in mouse showed an antagonistic action on the effect of a selective $5\text{-}HT_{1B}$ agonist in an in vivo model of social interaction (Massot et al, 1996).

Thus, the pharmacologic studies of LSAL indicated that the peptide specifically interacted with $5\text{-}HT_{1B}$ receptors, inducing an antagonistic non-competitive interaction in binding experiments as well as in functional in vitro and in vivo studies. Therefore, the function of $5\text{-}HT_{1B}$ receptor being related to the serotonergic control of the release of various neurotransmitters and particularly that of 5-HT itself, the peptide LSAL, being responsible for a direct antagonistic activity at these receptors, was called 5-HT-moduline.

Binding of [³H]5-HT-moduline and autoradiographic studies

In order to study the binding of 5-HT-moduline itself, the peptide was radiolabeled using tritium. It was shown that [³H]5-HT-moduline bound to rat or guinea pig brain membrane preparation on binding sites able to recognize the peptide with a very high affinity corresponding to a dissociation constant close to 10^{-10} M; the similarity of the binding affinity with the EC_{50} of LSAL in preventing the binding of [³H]5-HT to $5\text{-}HT_{1B}$ receptors strongly suggested that the binding site corresponded well to that interacting with the $5\text{-}HT_{1B}$ receptor.

It was also shown that the binding of the tritiated peptide was prevented by the non-radiolabeled peptide itself (LSAL); in contrast, it was affected neither by the scrambled peptide (ALLS) nor by the metabolites AL or LS. Furthermore, no other tested peptides (TRH, galanin, bacitracin) had any displacing effect. These results indicated that the observed site binding [³H]5-HT-moduline was quite specific for the LSAL chemical structure. Moreover, the fact that cells transfected with the $5\text{-}HT_{1B}$ receptor gene expressing the corresponding receptor were able to bind [³H]5-HT-moduline, whereas the corresponding wild cells did not, demonstrated that the binding of 5-HT-moduline actually affected the receptor protein itself.

Autoradiographic studies were carried out (Massot et al, 1996, Cloëz-Tayarani et al, unpublished) and showed that the binding of [³H]5-HT-moduline very closely resembled that of [¹²⁵I]cyanopindolol labeling $5\text{-}HT_{1B}$ receptors in rat brain coronal sections. The distribution was seemingly the same, strongly suggesting that $5\text{-}HT_{1B}$ receptors were actually labeled by the peptide; this result was expected, since 5-HT-moduline was shown to specifically interact with $5\text{-}HT_{1B}$ receptors. Furthermore, this result demonstrates that all $5\text{-}HT_{1B}$ receptors are able to bind [³H]5-HT-moduline independently of their regional distribution or cellular localization.

The autoradiographic analysis of the binding of [³H]5-HT-moduline in $5\text{-}HT_{1B}$ knock-out mice in which $5\text{-}HT_{1B}$ receptors are not expressed

(Saudou et al, 1994) shows a total disappearance of the binding of [^{125}I]cyanopindolol and also that of [^{3}H]5-HT-moduline. This result demonstrates that the peptide binds to 5-HT$_{1B}$ receptor and not to any other protein (Cloëz-Tayarani et al, submitted).

5-HT-moduline distribution in the brain—immunocytochemistry

The target of 5-HT-moduline having been identified as the 5-HT$_{1B}$ receptor, it was of interest to know the localization of the peptide itself. First of all, a first series of experiments was carried out in vitro to determine whether or not the peptide could be released from an excitable tissue. Rat brain cortex synaptosomes were prepared and submitted to a potassium shock and centrifuged; then, the peptide was measured in the resulting supernatant, using its capacity to prevent the binding of [^{3}H]5-HT-moduline to 5-HT$_{1B}$ receptors. It was shown that 5-HT-moduline was released in K^{+}/Ca^{2+}-dependent manner, indicating that, in this respect, 5-HT-moduline behaves like other neurotransmitters and might be one (Massot et al, 1996).

In a second study, the technique of immunochemistry was used to obtain an efficient tool to detect and quantify 5-HT-moduline. Polyclonal antibodies were prepared in rabbit and raised against a complex established between LSAL and keyhole limpet hemocyanin (KLH), a known efficient antigen in mammals. The obtained polyclonal antibodies are clearly specific to the LSAL structure, since they bind LSAL and recognize neither the scrambled peptide (ALLS) nor the dipeptide AL or LS (Grimaldi et al, in press). Using this tool, immunocytochemistry was carried out on coronal sections of mouse brain. 5-HT-moduline immunoreactivity was observed in the cerebral cortex, including cingulate, retrosplenial, parietal and pyriform cortical regions; the basal ganglia was also labeled, namely the globus pallidus and substantia nigra, whereas the striatum did not seem to contain the peptide to a significant extent. The superior colliculi, subthalamic nuclei and hypothalamic areas were heavily labeled. The labeling appears to correspond to cellular profiles showing arborizations or axonal-like projections, suggesting that a neuronal system containing 5-HT-moduline is present in the brain and heterogeneously distributed (Figure 4.1).

The labeled cellular profiles are located throughout the brain according to a distribution different from that corresponding to the serotonergic cellular bodies (all located in the raphe). Thus, co-localization of 5-HT-moduline with 5-HT is unlikely; however, this conclusion has to await new results to be totally established. At the present time, it could be hypothesized that 5-HT-moduline is released from a neuronal system, probably distinct from the serotonergic system but closely interacting with it via 5-HT$_{1B}$ receptors.

Regulation of 5-HT$_{1B}$ receptors—potential role of 5-HT-moduline

Acute stress in rat and sensitivity of 5-HT$_{1B}$ receptors

The increase in 5-HT release in reaction to stress situations was proposed by Briley et al (1990), and the use of microdialysis techniques allowed the demonstration of the marked enhancement of the 5-HT release after physical or psychic stress (Shimizu et al, 1992; Kahawara et al, 1993).

The hypothesis that the increase in 5-HT release occurring immediately after stress could originate from regulation mechanisms affecting the 5-HT$_{1B}$ receptors was used as the basis of our experiments. Rats were submitted to a brief restraint stress (15–40 min), immobilized in a glass cylinder. The function of the 5-HT$_{1B}$ receptors was tested immediately after the restraint period by the analysis of the efficacy of a specific 5-HT$_{1B}$ agonist in inhibiting forskolin-stimulated adenylyl cyclase activation; this test was carried out using membranal preparations obtained from substantia nigra. It was shown that the sensitivity of the 5-HT$_{1B}$ receptors was clearly decreased in stressed rats compared to normal rats, since the dose–effect curve of the 5-HT$_{1B}$ agonist was shifted to the right in a very significant manner. This effect was highly reproducible and indicated that an acute restraint stress induced the desensitization of the 5-HT$_{1B}$ receptors. The functional consequence presumably corresponded to the enhancement of the release of 5-HT previously described (Kahawara et al, 1993) and possibly related to induced anxious states (Briley and Chopin, 1994).

The intracerebroventricular administration of 5-HT-moduline had an effect similar to that of the acute stress, as it also induced a significant shift to the right of the dose–response curve of a 5-HT$_{1B}$ agonist on the activity of the receptor (Seguin et al, 1997). Furthermore, this effect was clearly specific for 5-HT-moduline, since the scrambled peptide ALLS administered under the same experimental conditions did not produce any significant desensitization of the receptor.

These observations suggest that, during acute stress, a desensitization of 5-HT$_{1B}$ receptors occurs at least in substantia nigra, and may be the result of the interaction of 5-HT-moduline with these receptors.

Potential role of 5-HT-moduline in psychiatry and particularly in depression

The modulatory role of the 5-HT system is presumably complementary to those of other aminergic systems which also have modulatory activities in the CNS. The 5-HT system may affect the anterior brain, regulating

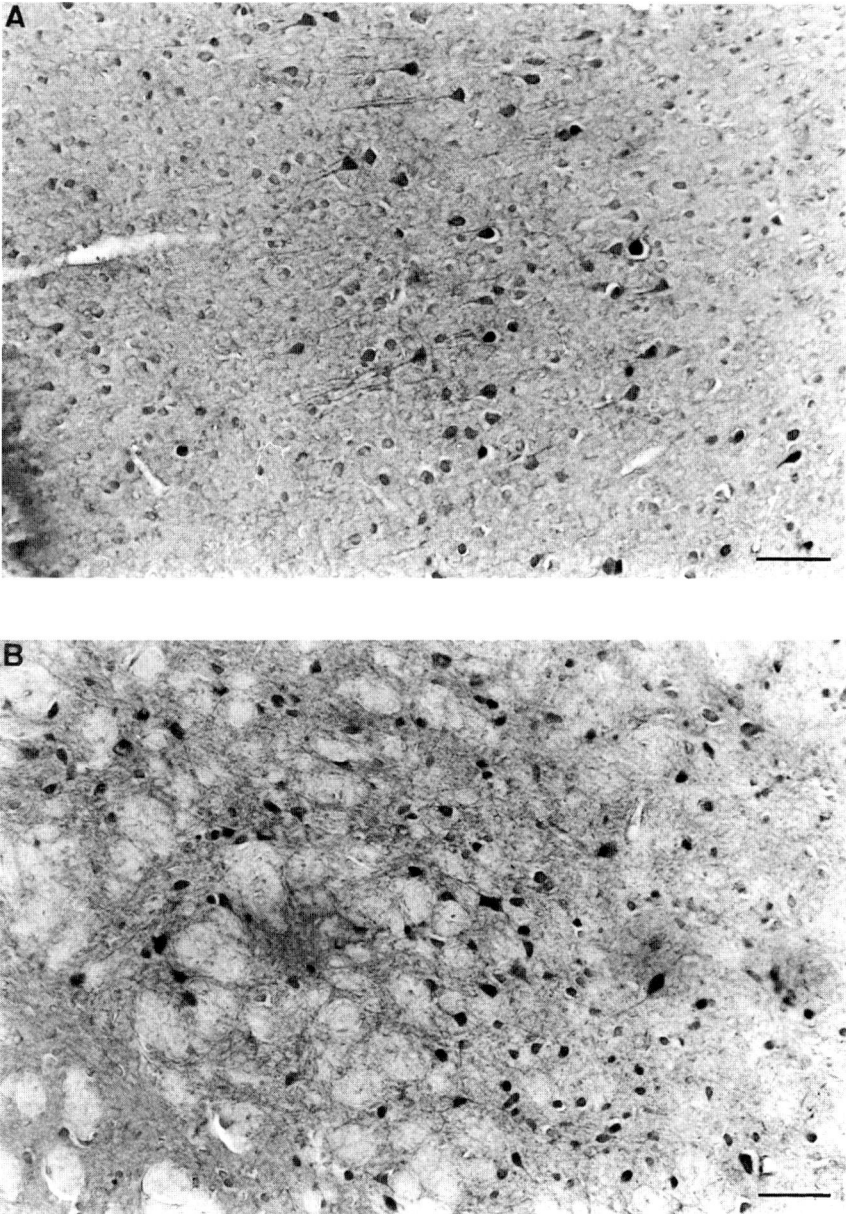

Figure 4.1

(A) 5-HT-moduline immunoreactivity in parietal cortex of mouse brain. The intensively immunolabeled cells are medium-sized and polygonal and exhibit long, labeled processes. These pyramidal neurons are generally vertically oriented. Scale bar = 50 µm. (B) 5-HT-moduline immunoreactivity in the globus pallidus. A dense distribution of intensively immunolabeled cells is observed; some of them are organized in clusters. Scale bar = 50 µm.

various transmissions linked to specific functions related to strategy, creativity, voluntary movements etc. It may also regulate the functions related to the activity of the lower brain: respiration, circulation, hormone secretions, impulsive behavior etc. 5-HT$_{1B}$ receptors are potentially involved in those mechanisms, since they are directly regulating the control of the 5-HT activity either as autoreceptors (modulation of the release of 5-HT) or as postsynaptic receptors directly mediating the effect of 5-HT on the release of other neurotransmitters.

The fact that 5-HT-moduline interacts with 5-HT$_{1B}$ receptors in in vitro assays using cultured cells indicates that the peptide may alter the functions of the two categories of receptors. An important question which has still to be answered is whether all 5-HT$_{1B}$ receptors in the brain are under the physiologic control of 5-HT-moduline; in other words, whether or not 5-HT-moduline is released in brain tissue and able to reach 5-HT$_{1B}$ autoreceptors as well as heteroreceptors. Nevertheless, the wide distribution of the 5-HT-moduline immunoreactivity within the brain tends to suggest that in the majority of brain areas the 5-HT$_{1B}$ receptors may indeed constitute a target for 5-HT-moduline used in physiologic events. Accordingly, the action of 5-HT-moduline as a regulator of 5-HT$_{1B}$ receptors may be a very efficient mechanism which finely tunes the activity of the serotonergic system; this mechanism may participate in the processes which maintain the homeostasis of the CNS and (or) in those which are involved in the adaptation of the response of the CNS to novel external stimuli.

The potential effect of 5-HT-moduline is indicated by the results obtained in the model of acute stress. Indeed, under those experimental conditions, 5-HT-moduline appears to be released and to induce the desensitization of 5-HT$_{1B}$ receptors, thus enhancing 5-HT release. This mechanism potentially represents an adaptive process in which the animal modifies various functions to elaborate an adequate response to the applied stimulus via changes in the serotonergic activity.

Thus, the presence or absence of 5-HT-moduline leads to a rapid induction of hypo/hypersensitization of the 5-HT$_{1B}$ receptor and appears to participate in the control of the serotonergic regulatory activity. The hypo/hypersensitivity of the receptor may represent a mechanism which finely tunes the adaptive processes elaborated in response to a given stimulus. A dysfunction affecting the mechanism of control of the sensitivity of the receptors potentially leads to pathologic situations, as previously proposed by Briley and Chopin (1994). Therefore, it could be speculated that a reduced or increased level of 5-HT-moduline may induce hyper/hyposensitization of the 5-HT$_{1B}$ autoreceptors and a decrease or increase in 5-HT synthesis and release. In particular, the hypersensitization of the 5-HT$_{1B}$ receptor possibly may be involved in certain depressive states, suicidal behavior and impulsivity. Current research is needed to specify the potential role of 5-HT-moduline in psychiatric disorders and especially depression.

References

Audet MA, Descarries L, Doucet G (1989) Quantified regional and laminar distribution of the serotonin innervation in the anterior half of the adult cerebral cortex, *J Chem Neuroanat* **2:**29–44.

Baumgarten HG, Grozdanovic Z (1994) Neuroanatomy and neurophysiology of central serotonergic systems, *J Serotonin Res* **3:**171–9.

Briley M, Chopin P (1994) Is anxiety associated with a hyper- or hyposerotonergic state? In: Palomo T, Archer T, eds, *Strategies for Studying Brain Disorders*, Vol. 1, *Depressive, Anxiety and Drug Abuse Disorders* (Complutense: Madrid, Farrand Press: London) 197–209.

Briley M, Chopin P, Moret C (1990) Effect of serotonin lesion on 'anxious' behaviour measured in the elevated plus-maze test in the rat, *Psychopharmacology* **101:**187–9.

Bruinvels AT, Palacios JM, Hoyer D (1993) Autoradiographic characterization and localisation of serotonin 5-HT$_{1B}$ compared to 5-HT$_{1D}$ binding sites in rat brain, *Naunyn Schmiedebergs Arch Pharmacol* **347:**569–82.

Bruinvels AT, Landwehrmeyer B, Gustafson EL et al (1994) Localization of 5-HT$_{1B}$, 5-HT$_{1D\alpha}$, 5-HT$_{1E}$ and 5-HT$_{1F}$ receptor messenger RNA in rodent and primate brain, *Neuropharmacology* **33:**367–86.

Descarries L, Audet MA, Doucet G et al (1990) Morphology of central serotonin neurons, *Ann NY Acad Sci* **600:**81–92.

Engel G, Göthert M, Hoyer D, Schlicker E, Hillenbrand K (1986) Identity of inhibitory presynaptic 5-hydroxytryptamine (5-HT) autoreceptors in the rat brain cortex with 5-HT$_{1B}$ binding sites, *Naunyn Schmiedebergs Arch Pharmacol* **332:**1–7.

Feuerstein TJ, Hüring H, van Velthoven V, Lücking CH, Landwehrmeyer GB (1996) 5-HT$_{1D}$-like receptors inhibit the release of endogenously formed [³H]GABA in human, but not in rabbit, neocortex, *Neurosci Lett* **209:**210–14.

Fillion G, Fillion M-P (1981) Modulation of affinity of postsynaptic serotonin receptors by antidepressant drugs, *Nature* **292:**349–51.

Fink K, Zenter J, Göthert M (1995) Subclassification of presynaptic 5-HT autoreceptors in the human cerebral cortex as 5-HT$_{1D\beta}$ receptors, *Naunyn Schmiedebergs Arch Pharmacol* **352:**451–4.

Fuxe K, Agnati LF, Zoli M, Bjelke B, Zini I (1989) Some aspects of the communicational and computational organization of the brain, *Acta Physiol Scand* **135:**203–16.

Hamblin MW, Metcalf MA, McGuffin RW, Karpelis S (1992) Molecular cloning and functional characterization of a human 5-HT$_{1B}$ serotonin receptor: a homologue of the rat 5-HT$_{1B}$ receptor with 5-HT$_{1D}$-like pharmacological specificity, *Biochem Biophys Res Commun* **184:**752–9.

Harel-Dupas C, Cloëz I, Fillion G (1991) The inhibitory effect of TFMPP on [³H]acetylcholine release in guinea-pig hippocampal synaptosomes is mediated by a 5-HT$_1$ receptor distinct from 1A-subtype, 1B-subtype, and 1C-subtype, *J Neurochem* **56:**221–7.

Hartig PR, Hoyer D, Humphrey PPA, Martin G (1996) Alignment of receptor nomenclature with the human genome: classification of 5-HT$_{1B}$ and 5-HT$_{1D}$ receptor subtypes, *Trends Pharmacol Sci* **17:**103–5.

Hjorth S, Suchowski SS, Galloway MP (1995) Evidence for 5-HT autoreceptor-mediated, nerve impulse-independent, control of 5-HT synthesis in the rat brain, *Synapse* **19:**170–6.

Hoyer D, Clarke DE, Fozard JR et al (1994) VII International union of pharmacology classification of receptors for 5-hydroxytryptamine (Serotonin), *Pharmacol Rev* **46:**158–203.

Jacobs BL, Azmitia EC (1992) Structure and function of the brain serotonin system, *Physiol Rev* **72:**165–229.

Jacobs BL, Fornal CA (1993) 5-HT and motor control: a hypothesis, *Trends Neurosci* **16:**346–52.

Jacobs BL, Wilkinson LO, Fornal CA (1990) The role of brain serotonin, a neurophysiologic perspective, *Neuropsychopharmacology* **3:**473–9.

Kahawara H, Yoshida M, Yokoo H, Nishi M, Tanaka M (1993) Psychological stress increases serotonin release in the rat amygdala and prefrontal cortex assessed by in vivo microdialysis, *Neurosci Lett* **162:**81.

Kosofsky BE, Molliver ME (1987) The serotonergic innervation of cerebral cortex: different classes of axon terminals arise from dorsal and median raphe nuclei, *Synapse* **1:**153–68.

Libert F, Parmentier M, Lefort A et al (1988) Selective amplification and cloning of four new members of the G-protein coupled receptor family, *Science* **244:**569–72.

Massot O, Rousselle JC, Fillion MP et al (1996) 5-Hydroxytryptamine-moduline, a new endogenous cerebral peptide, controls the serotoninergic activity via its specific interaction with 5-hydroxytryptamine$_{1B/1D}$ receptors, *Mol Pharmacol* **50:**752–62.

Metcalf MA, McGuffin RW, Hamblin MW (1992) Conversion of the human 5-HT$_{1D\beta}$ serotonin receptor to the rat-5-HT$_{1B}$ ligand-binding phenotype by Thr[335] Asn site directed mutagenesis, *Biochem Pharmacol* **44:**1917–20.

Middlemiss DN (1984) Stereoselective blockade at [3H]5HT binding sites and at the 5-HT autoreceptor by (−)propranolol, *Eur J Pharmacol* **101:**289–93.

Oksenberg J, Marsters SA, O'Dowd BF et al (1992) A single amino-acid difference confers major pharmacological variation between human and rodent 5-HT$_{1B}$ receptors, *Nature* **360:**161–3.

Parker EM, Grisel DA, Iben LG,

Shapiro RA (1993) A single amino acid difference accounts for the pharmacological distinction between the rat and human 5-hydroxytryptamine$_{1B}$ receptor, *J Neurochem* **60:**380–3.

Piñeyro G, Blier P (1996) Regulation of 5-hydroxytryptamine release from rat midbrain raphe nuclei by 5-hydroxytryptamine$_{1D}$ receptors: effect of tetrodotoxin, G protein inactivation and long-term antidepressant administration, *J Pharmacol Exp Ther* **276:**697–707.

Piñeyro G, Castanon N, Hen R, Blier P (1995) Regulation of [^{3}H]5-HT release in raphe, frontal cortex and hippocampus of 5-HT$_{1B}$ knock-out mice, *NeuroReport* **7:**353–9.

Rousselle JC, Massot O, Delepierre M, Zifa E, Rousseau B, Fillion G (1996) Isolation and characterization of an endogenous peptide from rat brain interacting specifically with the serotonergic$_{1B}$ receptor subtypes, *J Biol Chem* **271:**726–35.

Saudou F, Amara DA, Dierich A et al (1994) Enhanced aggressive behavior in mice lacking 5-HT$_{1B}$ receptor, *Science* **265:**1875–8.

Seguin L, Seznec J-C, Fillion G (1997) The endogenous cerebral tetrapeptide 5-HT-moduline reduces in vivo the functional activity of central 5-HT$_{1B}$ receptors in the rat, *Neurosci Res* **27:**277–80.

Shimizu N, Take S, Hori T, Oomura Y (1992) In vivo measurement of hypothalamic serotonin release by intracerebral microdialysis: significant enhancement by immobilization stress in rats, *Brain Res Bull* **28:**727–34.

Takeuchi Y (1988) Distribution of serotonin neurons in the mammalian brain. In: Osborne NN, Hamon M, eds, *Neuronal Serotonin* (John Wiley & Sons: London) 25–56.

Weinshank RJ, Zgombick JM, Macchi MJ, Branchek TA, Hartig PR (1992) Human serotonin$_{1D}$ receptor is encoded by a subfamily of two distinct genes: 5-HT$_{1D\alpha}$ and 5-HT$_{1D\beta}$, *Proc Natl Acad Sci USA* **89:**3630–4.

Wiklund L, Leger L, Persson M (1981) Monoamine cell distribution in the cat brain. A fluorescence histochemical study with quantification of indolaminergic and locus coeruleus cell groups, *J Comp Neurol* **203:**613–47.

Zgombick JM, Schechter LE, Kucharewicz SA, Weinshank RL, Branchek TA (1995) Ketanserin and ritanserin discriminate between recombinant human 5-HT$_{1D\alpha}$ and 5-HT$_{1D\beta}$ receptor subtypes, *Eur J Pharmacol* **291:**9–15.

Zifa E, Fillion G (1992) 5-Hydroxytryptamine receptors, *Pharmacol Rev* **44:**401–58.

5

Antidepressants and post-receptor events: the 'serotonin/norepinephrine link' revisited

S Paul Rossby and Fridolin Sulser

Introduction

A functional link between noradrenergic and serotonergic neuronal systems was first suggested by Dahlstrôm and Fuxe (1964), based on their anatomic mapping of cell bodies and terminals containing norepinephrine (NE) and serotonin (5-HT) in brain. Psychopharmacologic and electrophysiologic studies have since generated robust support for this link and have thus contributed substantially to the evolution of the heuristic monoamine hypotheses of depression (see, for example, review by Pryor and Sulser, 1991). Additionally, since stressful life events and vulnerability to stress are believed to be predisposing factors in the precipitation of depression (Paykel, 1979; Akiskal, 1985), and glucocorticoids are central to the stress response, the discovery that circulating glucocorticoids alter aminergic receptor sensitivity in brain (Mobley and Sulser, 1980; Mobley et al, 1983; Roberts et al, 1984; Harrelson et al, 1987) made it imperative to integrate the glucocorticoid system into any meaningful amine hypothesis of affective disorders. Thus the 'serotonin–norepinephrine–glucocorticoid link' hypothesis of affective disorders was formulated, emphasizing the role of adaptation at the receptor level in the mechanisms of antidepressant drug effects. Previously the emphasis had shifted from acute presynaptic events to delayed postsynaptic changes in receptor sensitivities (Vetulani and Sulser, 1975), and it has shifted again more recently to the convergence of aminergic signals beyond the receptors—leading ultimately to changes in programs of gene expression.

From research in C6 glioma cells to research in the mammalian brain

A link between aminergic (NE–5-HT) and endocrine (glucocorticoid) signals beyond the receptors was first demonstrated in C6 glioma cells at the level of gene expression. C6 glioma cells contain β-adrenoceptors positively linked to adenylate cyclase, and 5-HT receptors positively linked to phospholipase C, and are thus a useful model for the study of receptor-mediated signal–transcription coupling. In accordance with previously published results (Yoshikawa and Sabol, 1986), NE caused a 3–5-fold increase in the steady-state level of preproenkephalin (PPE) mRNA in C6 cells, and this rise was markedly enhanced by glucocorticoids. The NE-induced increase in steady-state PPE mRNA levels was mediated via the β-adrenoceptor-coupled adenylate cyclase system (Eiring et al, 1992). Whereas 5-HT alone did not alter the PPE mRNA level, co-incubation with isoproterenol significantly attenuated the increase in the PPE message (Figure 5.1). Although 5-HT did not alter either the density of β-adrenoceptors or their downregulation by isoproterenol (Eiring et al, 1992), it significantly diminished the isoproterenol-induced increase in endogenous and cyclic AMP-stimulated protein kinase A (PKA) activity (Table 5.1). Extrapolation of these findings to the central nervous system suggests that the nature of the aminergic link involves a connection between β-adrenoceptor desensitization and 5-HT receptor stimulation in the regulation of gene expression. It is noteworthy that in addition to

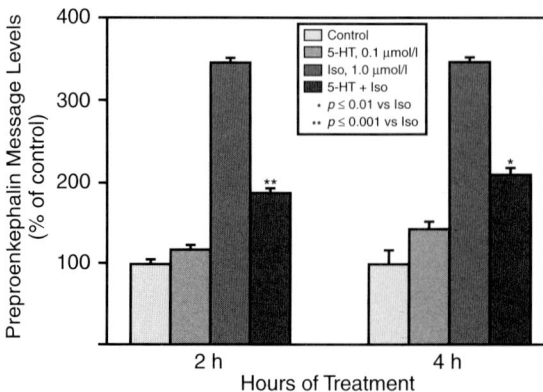

Figure 5.1

The effect of serotonin (5-HT) and isoproterenol on preproenkephalin message levels in rat C6 glioma cells. Confluent cultures were incubated, after the medium was changed, for 2 or 4 h with 5-HT, (−)-isoproterenol (Iso), both agents, or sterile water (controls). Using dot blot hybridization, 3.0 μg total cellular RNA per sample was analyzed for PPE message content and compared to control levels. Each bar represents the average of three separate experiments. From Eiring et al (1992).

Table 5.1   cAMP-dependent protein kinase activity in rat C6 glioma cells (soluble fraction).

	−cAMP (pmol/min per mg protein ± SEM)	+cAMP pmol/min per mg protein ± SEM)
Control	1155 ± 37	4479 ± 163
Isoproterenol (Iso) (1 μM)	6535 ± 302*	5868 ± 248
Serotonin (5-HT) (0.1 μM)	410 ± 86	4828 ± 209
Iso + 5-HT	5567 ± 266**	4935 ± 237***

*$p < 0.001$ versus control; **$p < 0.05$ versus Iso; ***$p < 0.02$ versus Iso. (Adapted from Manier et al, 1994).

demonstrating the convergence of aminergic signals beyond the β-adrenoceptor, the PKA results obtained in C6 glioma cells provided the first evidence of 'cross-talk' between aminergic receptor systems at the protein kinase level. Accordingly, the convergent regulation of voltage-gated sodium channels in mammalian brain by protein kinase A- and C-mediated phosphorylation (Li et al, 1993) provides an electrophysiologic correlate to the molecular data. They concluded that this regulation has the potential to serve as an integrative mechanism, because two inputs linked to different second messenger systems in the same neuron can induce a greater response than activation of either input alone.

Electrophysiologic and behavioral experiments involving antidepressant drugs continue to provide evidence for cross-talk between neuronal aminergic systems. For example, chronic administration of clinically effective antidepressants has been shown to increase the inhibitory response of forebrain neurons to microiontophoretically applied 5-HT (de Montigny and Aghajanian, 1978), and to increase behavioral responses to 5-HT and dopamine (Green and Deakin, 1980). The demonstration that these effects can be abolished by lesioning noradrenergic neurons (Green and Deakin, 1980; Gravel and de Montigny, 1987), strongly indicates functional interconnections (cross-talk) between serotonergic and noradrenergic signal transduction pathways. Cross-talk between these systems is also supported by clinical experience, and is discussed in Chapters 1, 8 and 16.

Pharmacologic studies with the dual reuptake inhibitor venlafaxine have recently increased our knowledge of the 'serotonin–norepinephrine link' in brain in vivo. Chronic administration of venlafaxine failed to alter either the density of β-adrenoceptors or the sensitivity of the β-adreno-ceptor-coupled adenylate cyclase system to NE in normal rats. However, it significantly decreased the cyclic AMP response to NE following 5-HT depletion (Table 5.2), i.e. in the absence of venlafaxine's strong 5-HT effect the NE component of its mechanism in brain was 'unmasked'. This is consistent with reports that venlafaxine rapidly desensitizes the

Table 5.2   The role of the 5-HT component of venlafaxine in the desensitization of the β-adrenoceptor-coupled adenylate cyclase (frontal cortex).

	Cyclic AMP response (pmol/mg protein ± SEM)
Controls (saline) (16)	55 ± 6
DMI (11)	27 ± 2***
Venlafaxine (15)	48 ± 3
PCPA (16)	47 ± 4
Venlafaxine (PCPA) (15)	37 ± 3**
DMI (PCPA) (8)	36 ± 5*

Rats were treated for 10 days with either desmethyl imipramine (DMI) (10 mg/kg per day IP) or venlafaxine (20 mg/kg IP b.i.d.). *p*-Chlorophenylalanine (PCPA) was administered at a dose of 200 mg/kg IP for 3 days, then 200 mg/kg IP every second day up to day 13. Drug treatments started at day 4. The animals were killed at day 14 and the cyclic AMP response to 100 μM NE determined in slices of the cortex. ***$p < 0.001$; **$p < 0.01$; *$p < 0.05$. Numbers in parentheses indicate the number of animals. Data from Nalepa et al (1997).

adenylate cyclase system to isoproterenol in the pineal gland (Moyer et al, 1984; Muth et al, 1991), which is richly innervated by noradrenergic neurons but is lacking serotonergic innervation (Wurtman et al, 1968).

As a step towards understanding the significance of these observations, we have hypothesized that since NE desensitizes β-adrenoceptors via PKA-mediated phosphorylation, the activation of protein kinase C (PKC) via 5-HT receptor cascades must somehow inhibit the activity of PKA (Nalepa et al, 1997). Though it has been difficult to unravel the precise mechanism of this cross-talk in brain in vivo, PKA/PKC counter-regulation of agonist-induced β-adrenoceptor desensitization has been demonstrated in various cell lines (Shih and Malbon, 1994). Accordingly, these studies demonstrated that antisense mRNA oliogodeoxynucleotides to PKA and the second messenger-independent/G-protein-coupled receptor kinase BARK1 nearly abolished agonist/receptor-mediated desensitization of the β-adrenoceptor-coupled adenylate cyclase system, whereas antisense PKC mRNA oligonucleotides enhanced the desensitization. More recently, Döbbeling and Berchtold (1996) have provided evidence in a fibroblast cell line that activation of the calcium and PKC pathways downregulates the PKA pathway. As pointed out earlier, cross-talk between 5-HT and NE at the PKA level has been demonstrated in C6 glioma cells (Manier et al, 1994). Though an extrapolation to the CNS in vivo is clearly premature at this time, these results are instrumental in formulating working hypotheses on the mode of action of venlafaxine (and antidepressants in general) beyond the monoaminergic receptors.

The mode of action of antidepressant drugs—a unified hypothesis

All clinically effective antidepressants alter noradrenergic and/or serotonergic neuronal systems at various levels of the aminergic signal transduction cascade or are converted in vivo to metabolites which, in concert with the parent drug, alter the synaptic availability of NE or 5-HT or both. Whereas the emphasis on the mode of action of antidepressants shifted in the mid-1970s from acute presynaptic to delayed postsynaptic receptor-mediated adaptive processes (Vetulani and Sulser, 1975), recent in vivo and in vitro studies (see above) now require a further conceptual shift of attention to 5-HT and NE receptor-coupled intracellular signal transduction processes that ultimately affect gene expression. Figure 5.2 depicts three representative second messenger signal transduction pathways affected by antidepressants and their convergence at the level of protein kinases (third messengers) which in turn control gene expression via phosphorylation of transcription factors (fourth messengers). It follows that selective NE reuptake inhibitors, selective 5-HT uptake inhibitors, monoamine oxidase (MAO) inhibitors and dual uptake inhibitors such as venlafaxine (and perhaps milnacipran) share a final common mechanism of action beyond the aminergic receptors.

Figure 5.2 also implies that PKA-mediated phosphorylation can be attenuated by either predominantly noradrenergic antidepressants (e.g. DMI) via desensitization of β-adrenoceptor-coupled adenylate cyclase or by selective 5-HT reuptake inhibitors (SSRIs) which do not affect the

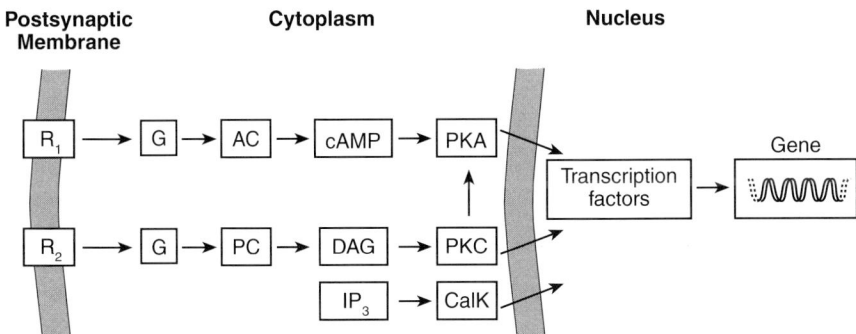

Figure 5.2

Hypothetical convergence of signal transduction cascades at the level of protein kinase-mediated phosphorylation of transcription factors. The cross-talk between PKA and PKC is also indicated: R_1, receptors linked to the cyclic AMP–PKA pathway (e.g. β); R_2, receptors linked to the DAG–PKC pathway and via IP_3 to the calcium/calmodulin-dependent protein kinase pathways (e.g. 5-HT$_{2A}$–5-HT$_{2C}$); G, G proteins; AC, adenylate cyclase; PC, phospholipase C; cAMP, cyclic AMP; DAG, diacyglycerol; IP_3, inositol triphosphate; PKA, protein kinase A; PKC, protein kinase C; CalK, Ca^{2+}/calmodulin-dependent protein kinase.

β-adrenergic system but instead activate PKC via diacylglycerol (DAG), which in turn downregulates PKA. Consequently, antidepressants which activate both signal transduction pathways (MAO inhibitors and dual amine uptake inhibitors) would be expected to be more potent in regulating the final link of the transduction cascade. Experiments are in progress in our laboratory to test this assumption. Whether or not this will translate into enhanced clinical efficacy or efficacy in therapy-resistant depression remains to be seen.

Finally, with regard to the pharmacology of antidepressant drugs, an important conclusion evidenced above is that β-adrenoceptor downregulation and/or desensitization of the β-adrenoceptor-coupled adenylate cyclase system is not a prerequisite for antidepressant activity, since an increased 5-HT signal can affect the final link of the aminergic transduction cascade without altering β-adrenoceptor density or sensitivity. The β-adrenoceptor changes are now viewed as being the consequence of an increased β-adrenoceptor/cyclic AMP–PKA-mediated information flow following chronic treatment with antidepressants that persistently increase the synaptic availability of NE (i.e. DMI-like drugs, MAO inhibitors). The results discussed in this section lend support to a unified mechanism of action of all antidepressants beyond the receptors at the level of protein kinase-mediated phosphorylation processes (revised 5-HT–NE link hypothesis).

Since PKA-mediated phosphorylation represents a highly efficient kinetic amplification mechanism (Walsh and Ashby, 1973; Cohen, 1982), small changes in the activity of this enzyme will have profound effects on the *net* signal transduction cascade. While studies using the pineal gland as a model system demonstrated long ago that the *net* noradrenergic signal transfer is deamplified following chronic treatment with tricyclic antidepressants (dark-induced *N*-acetyltransferase activity and melatonin formation) despite the persistent blockade of neuronal reuptake of NE (Heydorn et al, 1982; Friedman et al, 1984), studies on PKA-mediated phosphorylation of endogenous protein substrates in brain after chronic administration of antidepressants are now being pursued in many laboratories.

Antidepressants and programs of gene expression

Hoeffler et al (1989) presented evidence that cellular signal transduction pathways involving PKA and PKC coordinately modulate gene transcription via interactions between common as well as distinct *cis*-acting elements and DNA-binding proteins such as CREB, Fos, Jun, etc. Since antidepressant drugs change the activities of PKA and PKC, it is not surprising that this class of drugs affects gene transcription (Nestler et al, 1990; Brady et al, 1991; Peiffer et al, 1991; Rossby et al, 1995, 1996; Nibuya et al, 1995, 1996; Schwaninger et al, 1995). The translocation of

PKA from the cytosol to the nucleus following chronic treatment with anti-depressant drugs and electroconvulsive therapy (ECT) (Nestler et al, 1989) could provide the link between agonist receptor occupancy, PKA activation by cyclic AMP, and transcriptional activation by the phosphory-lation of DNA-binding proteins in the nucleus. This report is noteworthy because nuclear translocation of PKA (or its catalytic subunit) is appar-ently the rate-limiting step in CREB phosphorylation (at Ser-133), which in turn leads to the transcriptional activation of genes containing the palin-dromic CRE sequence 5'-TGACGTCA-3' (Hagiwara et al, 1993). Interest-ingly, although this probably represents the key phosphorylation event, it is not sufficient to generate the transactivation functions of CREB and therefore the phosphorylation of additional serines by other kinases has been postulated.

Phosphorylation of the kinase-inducible domain of CREB is believed to allosterically change the conformation of its transactivation domain, allowing interaction with the TATA box complex involved in the initiation of transcription (Meyer and Habener, 1993). It follows that since antide-pressant drug-induced changes in the activities of transcription factors (e.g. CREB) affect large numbers of eukaryotic genes (e.g. genes con-taining CRE elements in their promoter regions), antidepressant drugs alter programs of gene expression. We have advanced the view that the delay experienced clinically in therapeutic responses to antidepressants is the consequence of changes in programs of gene expression that determine the intensities of incoming signals, the sensitivities of neuronal systems to those signals, and the nature, amplitude and duration of cen-tral nervous system responses (Rossby et al, 1996).

An interesting view on the role of neurotrophins in the mode of action of antidepressants and in the psychopathology of depression was recently advanced by Duman et al (1997). It is based on the finding that acute and chronic ECT and chronic treatment with several different antidepres-sants increase the levels of mRNAs encoding brain-derived neurotrophic factor (BDNF) and its receptor, trkB (Nibuya et al, 1995). Since direct administration of BDNF into the midbrain has been reported to exert anti-depressant activity in animal models of depression (Siuciak et al, 1994), BDNF and trkB genes may be specifically targeted in programs of gene expression altered by antidepressant drugs. Whether or not an upregula-tion of the cyclic AMP–PKA–CREB cascade underlies the increased levels of BDNF and trkB mRNAs remains to be determined.

Results from our laboratory demonstrate that changes in gene expres-sion in response to antidepressant drug treatment occur via two funda-mentally different mechanisms: (1) via agonist receptor-mediated transduction cascades (Rossby et al, 1996) and (2) via a mechanism that is independent of agonist receptor-mediated signal transduction processes (Rossby et al, 1995). An example of the first mechanism is depicted in Figure 5.3. Chronic treatment of rats with fluoxetine approximately doubled steady-state levels of PPE mRNA in the amygdala. This increase was abolished in brains depleted of 5-HT by PCPA (5-HT levels were selectively reduced to less than 5% of control values), thus demonstrating that the action of this SSRI is dependent on the synaptic availability of 5-HT. An example of the second mechanism (agonist receptor cascade independent) is illustrated in Figure 5.4. In accord with studies by previous investigators (Peiffer et al, 1991; Seckl and Fink, 1992), the chronic administration of the noradrenergic antidepressant desipramine (DMI) significantly increased GRII mRNA in the rat hippocampus. Surprisingly, the increase following DMI was identical in the virtual absence of NE (DSP4 induced selective lesions of noradrenergic neurons which reduced NE levels to less than 5% of control values). Since DSP4-induced neurotoxic lesions can produce an increase in the density of β-adrenoceptors, thereby enhancing postsynaptic receptor

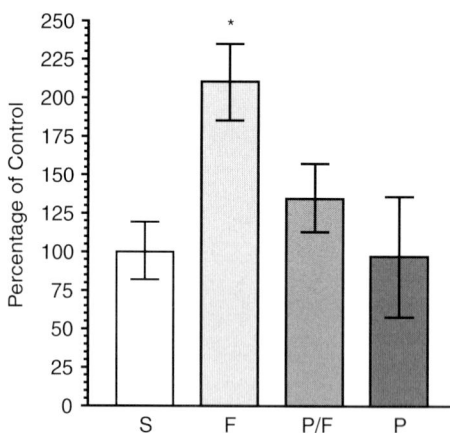

Figure 5.3

Steady-state levels of PPE mRNA in rat amygdala determined by northern blot hybridization analysis. Rats were treated for 13 days with saline (S, $n = 9$), fluoxetine (F, $n = 8$), PCPA plus fluoxetine (P/F, $n = 5$) or PCPA (P, $n = 6$). Values are expressed as percentage of control ± SEM. $*p = 0.0027$ versus saline. From Rossby et al (1996).

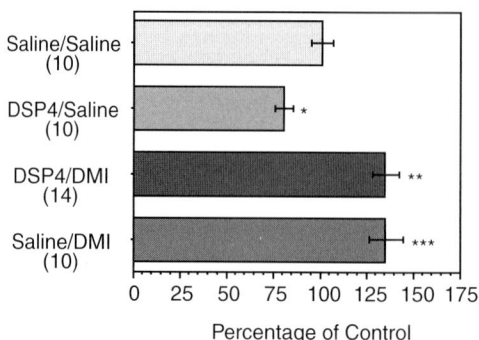

Figure 5.4

Steady-state levels of glucocorticoid type II receptor mRNA in total hippocampal RNA from rats treated with DSP4/saline ($n = 10$), DSP4/DMI ($n = 14$), and saline/DMI ($n = 10$), expressed as a percentage of controls treated with saline/saline. Significance was determined by ordinary ANOVA followed by a Newman–Keuls test. $*p < 0.05$ (DSP4/saline versus saline/saline); $**p < 0.001$ (DSP4/DMI versus DSP4/saline); $***p < 0.01$ (saline/DMI versus saline/saline). From Rossby et al (1995).

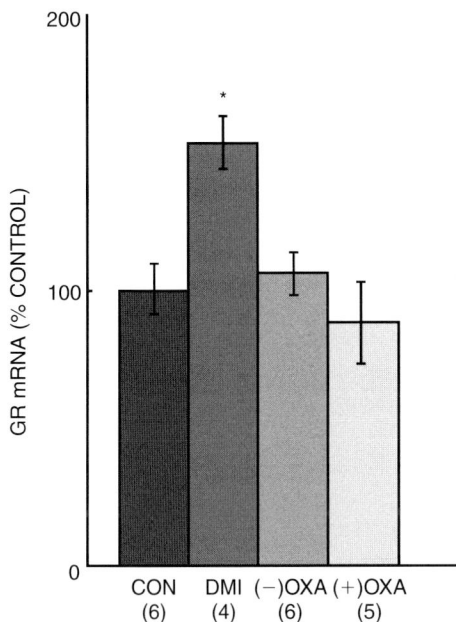

Figure 5.5

Steady-state levels of hippocampal GRII mRNA. Male Sprague–Dawley rats were treated for 7 days with saline (CON); 15 mg/kg IP desipramine (DMI); 20 mg/kg IP, b.i.d. of $(-)$-oxaprotiline $((-)OXA)$ or $(+)$-oxaprotiline $((+)OXA)$. Each bar represents the steady-state level of GRII mRNA $\pm$ SEM, expressed as percentage of control levels. Numbers in parentheses indicate number of animals. $*p < 0.01$ (versus control). From Eiring and Sulser (1997).

sensitivity to NE (Nalepa et al, 1997), it might have been argued that increased receptor sensitivity effectively compensated for the reduced synaptic availability of NE after DMI in DSP4-treated animals. However, subsequent results obtained with the two enantiomers of oxaprotiline have nullified this argument and support the previously reached conclusion concerning DMI (Rossby et al, 1995), i.e. that the synaptic availability of NE is not a prerequisite for the effect of DMI on GRII gene expression. Specifically, chronic treatment with neither $(+)$-oxaprotiline nor $(-)$-oxaprotiline increased the steady-state levels of GRII mRNA in rat hippocampus (Figure 5.5), and although one would not have expected $(-)$-oxaprotiline to alter hippocampal GRII mRNA (no blockade of NE uptake), the $(+)$ enantiomer, which produces NE uptake-blocking effects equal to those of DMI (Mishra et al, 1982), should have mimicked the activity of DMI. Finally, our results are consistent with previous in vitro studies which demonstrated that DMI significantly increases GRII promoter activity in CAT reporter gene constructs in the absence of NE (Pepin et al, 1992; Figure 5.6).

The direct effect of DMI (independent of the synaptic availability of the neurotransmitter NE) on gene expression is quite surprising, since other known effects of chronic administration of this tricyclic antidepressant are completely dependent on the synaptic availability of NE, e.g. β-adrenoceptor downregulation and desensitization of the β-adrenoceptor-coupled adenylate cyclase system (Wolffe et al, 1978; Schweitzer et al,

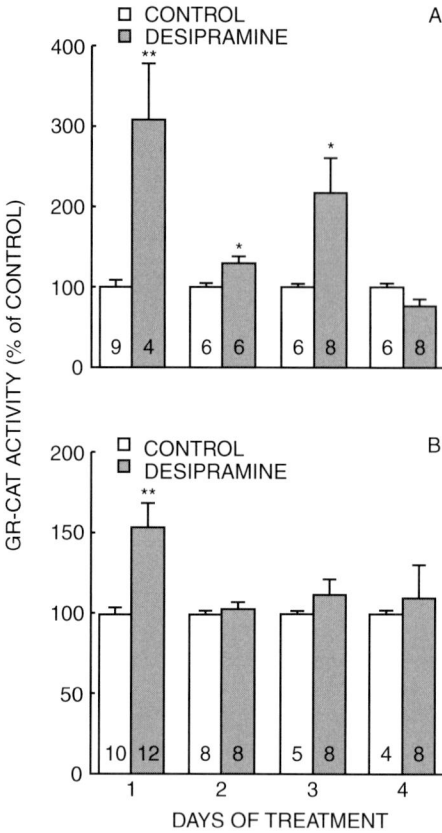

Figure 5.6

Promoter activity of the reporter plasmid pH GR2.7 CAT when stably transfected in LTK$^-$ (A) or Neuro 2A (B) cells incubated with 10^{-6} M DMI. $**p < 0.01$; $*p < 0.05$. From Pepin et al (1992).

1979; Janowsky et al, 1982). However, a previous report (rarely mentioned in the literature) demonstrated that DMI is taken up into cells in a dose- and time-dependent manner (Honegger et al, 1983), reaching intracellular concentrations high enough presumably to affect actions beyond the receptors. Since gene-specific transcription factors are composed of functionally distinct domains predisposing them to the effects of pharmaceutical agents (Peterson and Tupy, 1994), it is conceivable that the DMI effect on GRII gene expression could be mediated via modulation of transcription factors associated with GRII expression. The agonist receptor cascade-independent regulation of gene expression by the antidepressant DMI illustrates the potential of drugs to affect programs of gene expression by interacting directly with targets beyond the level of agonist receptor occupancy.

The concepts of plasticity and loss of plasticity in the central nervous system

We have stated (Rossby and Sulser, 1997) that the concept of 'plasticity' in the central nervous system (CNS) implies that the healthy CNS can adapt to conditions which threaten the physical and psychic/emotional well-being of the organism by altering programs of gene expression in specific neuronal and glial cell populations (Goelet et al, 1986; Comb et al, 1987; Morgan and Curran, 1988), and furthermore that research focusing on the nature and pathogenesis of affective disorders has identified what appear to be aberrant programs of gene expression (Sachar et al, 1973; Vetulani and Sulser, 1975), suggesting that the CNS of the person suffering from depression may be 'locked' into programs which no longer respond appropriately to changing external circumstances. Thus we have postulated that affective disorders involve loss of plasticity in specific programs of gene expression and that the currently available antidepressants do not restore plasticity in the CNS; they compensate for its loss.

Our assertion that CNS plasticity involves changes in programs of gene expression is supported by considerable evidence, including the following: (1) the redundancy of promoter sequences (e.g. CRE, AP-1, etc.) in the genome strongly suggests that transcription factors activated by intracellular signal transduction pathways can regulate the expression of sets of genes (Duman, 1995); (2) the activation of immediate early gene (IEG) expression (e.g. c-*fos* and c-*jun*) by pharmacologic (and environmental) stimuli results in the production of transcription factors which apparently orchestrate long-term adaptations of neuronal function by controlling the expression of late response genes (Sheng and Greenberg, 1990); and (3) steroid hormones modify the transcription rates of cell-specific gene networks (Yamamoto, 1985).

Glucocorticoid hypersecretion in major depression indicates a loss of plasticity in the hypothalamic–pituitary–adrenal system (HPA axis) and, consequently, in programs of gene expression which have evolved to protect the organism from over-reactions to stress. These programs are orchestrated at the genomic level by glucocorticoid–receptor complexes, which bind to specific DNA sequences (glucocorticoid response elements or GREs) and enhance (or decrease) the transcription of cell-type-specific 'networks' of genes (Yamamoto, 1985). The functional utility of the HPA axis, which regulates both the circadian and phasic release of adrenal glucocorticoids, depends upon its capacity for autoregulation, i.e. its sensitivity to feedback control. It should be emphasized that loss of plasticity in this system is extensively pathogenic because of the wide distribution of glucocorticoid receptors throughout the CNS (including glial cells) and, by implication, the large number of genes involved. Interestingly, it has been suggested that the DMI-induced increase in GRII receptor density (see above) could restore feedback inhibition in the HPA system and thus be responsible for its normalization during successful antidepressant pharmacotherapy (Barden et al, 1995). If this is indeed the case, it represents an important example of pharmacologic compensation for a loss of plasticity.

Finally, it should be noted that the delayed desensitization of the NE β-adrenoceptor-coupled adenylate cyclase system by virtually all clinically effective noradrenergic antidepressant treatments, including ECT (Vetulani and Sulser, 1975), was perhaps the first indication that antidepressants compensate for loss of plasticity at the level of gene expression. Implicit in this finding were the notions that at some time in the patient's history the amplitude of β-adrenergic receptor synthesis was increased in order to compensate for insufficient catecholamine levels, and that the CNS somehow lost the capacity to restore normal plasticity to this system, resulting in perpetual hypersensitivity.

Chronobiology of the CNS

In order to ultimately gain a complete understanding of the nature and etiopathology of depression, we cannot afford to ignore the rhythmic nature of gene expression as reflected by the circadian oscillations of: (1) α- and β-adrenergic, serotonergic, cholinergic, dopaminergic, opiate and benzodiazepine receptor numbers (Goodwin et al, 1982); (2) urinary metabolites of serotonin (5-hydroxyindole acetic acid, 5-HIAA), dopamine 3-methoxy-4-hydroxy-mandelic acid (VMA) and norepinephrine homovanillic acid (HVA) (Goodwin et al, 1982); (3) plasma levels of melatonin, NE, thyroid-stimulating hormone, adrenocorticotrophic hormone (ACTH), cortisol, corticosterone, growth hormone and prolactin (Nicholson et al, 1985; Goetz and Tolle, 1987; Linkowski et al, 1987; Mendlewicz, 1991); (4) region-specific levels of 5-HT and dopamine (Ozaki et al, 1993); and (5) messenger RNAs encoding tryptophan hydroxylase (Green et al, 1995), CRH (Kwak et al, 1993), glucocorticoid, mineralocorticoid and serotonin (5-HT$_{2C}$) receptors (Holmes et al, 1995), and immediate early genes (IEGs) c-*fos*, NGFI-A, NGFI-B, c-*jun*, *junB* and *junD* (Rusak et al, 1992). The waveforms of these circadian oscillations are characterized by amplitude, i.e. the extent of rhythmic change measured from peak to trough, and period, i.e. the duration of one complete cycle (Halberg et al, 1977).

The hypothesis linking affective disorders with disturbances in circadian rhythms was originally based on four clinical symptoms of depression, i.e. early morning awakening, diurnal variation in symptom severity, seasonality, and cyclicity of the illness (Kripke et al, 1978). The hypothesis states (in part) that 'long-term cycles of relapse and remission could occur if affective episodes resulted from an abnormal internal phase relationship between two circadian rhythms and if at least one of those rhythms escaped from entrainment to the day–night cycle and was free-running in and out of phase with the other rhythm'.

In support of this hypothesis, the peak amplitude of cortisol secretion has been shown to occur earlier in its circadian rhythm (a phase advance) in depressed patients compared with normal controls (Doig et al, 1966). This shift in timing was accompanied by a change in waveform and was confirmed by three independent studies involving reasonably large numbers of patients (Conroy et al, 1968; Fullerton et al, 1968). In one of these studies (Fullerton et al, 1968), the degree of phase advance was correlated with the severity of the depression. Phase advances in depressed patients have also been reported for circadian temperature rhythm, the onset of REM sleep, and urinary metabolites of 5-HT, dopamine and NE (Riederer et al, 1974; Wehr et al, 1980).

Finally, Linkowski et al (1987) have reported the effects of antidepressant treatment on the circadian rhythms of plasma ACTH and cortisol and the timing of REM sleep in patients suffering from major depressive illness. During the acute phase of the illness the patients presented with early onset of REM sleep, phase-advanced ACTH/cortisol rhythms, hypercortisolism, and shortened periods of quiescent nocturnal cortisol secretion. Following treatment with ECT or amytriptyline, the timing of the circadian rhythms of ACTH and cortisol and the duration of the quiescent period of cortisol secretion were normalized. REM latencies were increased and cortisol levels returned to normal due to a change in the amplitude of episodic pulses. The authors concluded that a disorder of circadian rhythmicity characterizes acute episodes of major depressive illness and that this chronobiological abnormality, as well as the hyper-secretion of ACTH and cortisol, are state rather than trait dependent.

Epilogue

The inclusion of chronobiological phenomena in the conceptual framework of our research requires another shift, i.e. we now hypothesize that the state of the CNS and thus the state of consciousness of an individual at each moment in time is determined by synchronicity at the level of gene expression (Jung, 1972). This concept is diametrically opposed to that of causality. Causality, based on the linear progressions of gene expression, is a matter of statistical probabilities ($p < 0.05$) and is thus not absolute, whereas synchronicity takes the actual coincidence of events in space and time as meaning something more than mere chance. Accordingly, when we can compare programs of gene expression in normal versus dysfunctional central nervous systems, we should be able to determine which genes are involved in the pathogenesis of psychiatric disorders and how they are involved. From a clinical perspective this should (hopefully) enable us to formulate therapies designed to restore plasticity in the CNS by altering not only the levels of gene expression but also the rhythms (waveforms and phase positions).

● Acknowledgments
Original research from our laboratories has been supported by USPHS grant MH-29228. We thank Mrs Doris Head for the expert typing of the manuscript.

References

Akiskal HS (1985) Interaction of biologic and psychologic factors in the origin of depressive disorders, *Acta Psychiatr Scand* **71**(suppl 319):131–9.

Barden N, Reul JMHM, Holsboer F (1995) Do antidepressants stabilize mood through actions on the hypothalamic–pituitary–adrenocortical system? *TINS* **18**:6–11.

Brady LS, Whitfield HJ Jr, Fox RJ et al (1991) Long-term antidepressant administration alters corticotropin releasing hormone, tyrosine hydroxylase and mineralocorticoid receptor gene expression in rat brain, *J Clin Invest* **87**:831–7.

Cohen P (1982) The role of protein phosphorylation in neuronal and hormonal control of cellular activity, *Nature* **296**:613–20.

Comb M, Hyman SE, Goodman HM (1987) Mechanisms of trans-synaptic regulation of gene expression, *Trends Neurosci* **10**:473–8.

Conroy RTWL, Hughes BD, Mills JN (1968) Circadian rhythms of plasma 11-hydroxycorticosteroids in psychiatric disorders, *Br J Med* **3**:405–7.

Dahlström A, Fuxe K (1964) Evidence for the existence of monoamine containing neurons in the central nervous system. I. Demonstration of monoamines in the cell bodies of brain stem neurons, *Acta Physiol Scand* **62**:1–5.

de Montigny C, Aghajanian GK (1978) Tricyclic antidepressants: long-term treatment increases responsivity of rat forebrain neurons to serotonin, *Science* **202**:1303–6.

Döbbeling U, Berchtold MW (1996) Down-regulation of the protein kinase A pathway by activators of protein kinase C and intracellular Ca^{2+} in fibroblast cells, *FEBS Lett* **391**:131–3.

Doig RJ, Mummery RV, Wills MR et al (1966) Plasma cortisol levels in depression, *Br J Psychiatry* **112**:1263–7.

Duman RS (1995) Regulation of intracellular signal transduction and gene expression by stress. In: Friedman MJ, Charney DS, Deutch AY, eds, *Neurobiological and Clinical Consequences of Stress: From Normal Adaptation to PTSD* (Lippincott-Raven: Philadelphia) 27–44.

Duman RS, Heninger GR, Nestler EJ (1997) A molecular and cellular theory of depression, *Arch Gen Psychiatry* (in press).

Eiring A, Sulser F (1997) An increased synaptic availability of norepinephrine is *not* essential for antidepressant induced increases in hippocampal GRII mRNA, *Neuropsychopharmacology* (submitted).

Eiring A, Manier DH, Bieck PR, Howells RD, Sulser F (1992) The 'serotonin/norepinephrine/glucocorticoid link' beyond the beta adrenoceptor, *Mol Brain Res* **16**:211–14.

Friedman E, Yocca FD, Cooper TD (1984) Antidepressant drugs with varying pharmacological profiles alter rat pineal beta adrenergic mediated function, *J Pharmacol Exp Ther* **228**:545–50.

Fullerton DT, Wenzel FJ, Ohrenz FN et al (1968) Circadian rhythm of adrenal cortical activity in depression, *Arch*

Gen Psychiatry **19:**674–88.

Goelet P, Castellucci VF, Schacher S et al (1986) The long and the short of long-term memory–a molecular framework, *Nature* **322:**419–22.

Goetz U, Tolle R (1987) Circadian rhythm of free urinary cortisol, temperature and heart rate in endogenous depressives and under antidepressant therapy, *Neuropsychobiology* **18:** 175–84.

Goodwin FK, Wirz-Justice A, Wehr TA (1982) Evidence that the pathophysiology of depression and the mechanism of action of antidepressant drugs both involve alterations in circadian rhythms. In: Costa E, Racagni G, eds, *Typical and Atypical Antidepressants: Clinical Practice* (Raven Press: New York) 1–12.

Gravel P, de Montigny C (1987) Noradrenergic denervation prevents sensitization of rat forebrain neurons to serotonin by tricyclic antidepressant treatment, *Synapse* **1:**233–9.

Green AR, Deakin JFW (1980) Brain noradrenaline depletion prevents ECS-induced enhancement of serotonin and dopamine mediated behavior, *Nature* **285:**232–3.

Green CB, Cahill GM, Bexharse JC (1995) Regulation of tryptophan hydroxylase expression by retinal circadian oscillator in vitro, *Brain Res* **677:**283–90.

Hagiwara M, Brindle P, Harootunian A et al (1993) Coupling of hormonal stimulation and transcription via the cyclic AMP-responsive factor CREB is rate limited by nuclear entry of protein kinase A, *Mol Cell Biol* **13:**4852–9.

Halberg F, Carandente F, Cornelissen G et al (1977) Glossary of chronobiology, *Chronobiologia* **4**(suppl 1):1–189.

Harrelson AL, Rosterre W, McEwen BS (1987) Adrenocortical steroids modify neurotransmitter stimulated cyclic AMP accumulation in the hippocampus and limbic brain of the rat, *J Neurochem* **48:**1648–55.

Heydorn WE, Brunswick DJ, Frazer A (1982) Effect of treatment of rats with antidepressants on melatonin concentrations in the pineal gland and serum, *J Pharmacol Exp Ther* **222:**534–43.

Hoeffler JP, Deutsch PJ, Lin J et al (1989) Cyclic adenosine monophosphate and phorbol esters—responsive signal transduction pathways converge at the level of transcriptional activation by the interactions of DNA-binding proteins, *Mol Endocrinol* **3:** 868–80.

Holmes MC, French KL, Seckl JR (1995) Modulation of serotonin and corticosteroid receptor gene expression in the rat hippocampus with circadian rhythm and stress, *Brain Res Mol Brain Res* **28:**186–92.

Honegger UE, Roscher AA, Wiesmann UN (1983) Evidence for lysosomotropic action of desipramine in cultured human fibroblasts, *J Pharmacol Exp Ther* **225:**436–41.

Janowsky AJ, Steranka LR, Gillespie DD et al (1982) Role of neuronal signal input in the down-regulation of central noradrenergic receptor function by antidepressant drugs, *J Neurochem* **39:**290–2.

Jung, CG (1972) Synchronicity: an acausal connecting principle. In: Jung CG, ed., *Collected Works of CG Jung*, Vol. 8 (Princeton University Press: Princeton, NJ) 417–531.

Kripke DF, Mullaney DJ, Atkinson M et al (1978) Circadian rhythm disorders in manic-depressives, *Biol Psychiatry* **13:**335–50.

Kwak SP, Morano MI, Young EA, Watson SJ, Akil H (1993) Diurnal CRH mRNA rhythm in the hypothalamus: decreased expression in the evening is not dependent on endogenous glucocorticoids, *Neuroendocrinology* **57:** 96–105.

Li M, West JW, Numan R et al (1993) Convergent regulation of sodium channels by protein kinase C and cyclic AMP-dependent protein kinase, *Science* **261:**1439–42.

Linkowski P, Mendlewicz J, Kerkofs M et al (1987) 24-hour profiles of adreno-corticotropin, cortisol, and growth hormone in major depressive illness: effect of antidepressant treatment, *J Clin Endocrinol Metab* **65:**141–52.

Manier DH, Eiring A, Sulser F (1994) The serotonin (5HT)/noradrenaline link beyond the beta adrenoceptors: is the 5HT effect mediated via 5HT1B receptors? *J Serotonin Res* **1:**113–18.

Mendlewicz J (1991) Sleep-related chronobiological markers of affective illness, *Int J Psychophysiol* **10:**245–52.

Meyer TE, Habener JF (1993) Cyclic adenosine 3'5'-monophosphate response element binding protein (CREB) and related transcription activating deoxyribonucleic acid binding proteins, *Endocrine Rev* **14:**269–90.

Mishra R, Gillespie DD, Lovell R (1982) Oxaprotiline: induction of central noradrenergic subsensitivity by its (+)-enantiomer, *Life Sci* **30:**1747–55.

Mobley PL, Sulser F (1980) Adrenal corticoids regulate sensitivity of noradrenaline receptor coupled adenylate cyclase in brain, *Nature* **286:**608–9.

Mobley PL, Manier DH, Sulser F (1983) Norepinephrine sensitive adenylate cyclase system in rat brain; role of adrenal corticosteroids, *J Pharmacol Exp Ther* **226:**71–7.

Morgan JI, Curran T (1988) Calcium as a modulator of the immediate-early gene cascade in neurons, *Cell Calcium* **9:**303–11.

Morgan JI, Curran T (1991) Stimulus-transcription coupling in the nervous system: involvement of the inducible proto-oncogenes fos and jun, *Annu Rev Neurosci* **14:**421–51.

Moyer JA, Muth EA, Haskins JT et al (1984) In vivo antidepressant profiles of the novel bicyclic compounds Wy-45030 and Wy-45881, *Soc Neurosci* **10:**26.

Muth EA, Moyer JA, Haskins JT et al (1991) Biochemical, neuropathophysiological and behavioral effects of Wy-45233 and other identified metabolites of the antidepressant venlafaxine, *Drug Dev Res* **23:**191–9.

Nalepa I, Manier DH, Gillespie DG et al (1997) Dual signaling by venlafaxine: I. The beta adrenoceptor desensitization hypothesis revisited, *Eur Neuropsychopharmacol* (submitted).

Nestler EJ, Terwilliger RZ, Duman RS (1989) Chronic antidepressant administration alters the subcellular distribution of cyclic AMP-dependent protein kinase in rat frontal cortex, *J Neurochem* **53:**1644–7.

Nestler EJ, McMahon A, Sabban EL et al (1990) Chronic antidepressant administration decreases the expression of tyrosine hydroxylase in the rat locus coeruleus, *Proc Natl Acad Sci USA* **87:**7522–6.

Nibuya M, Morinobu S, Duman RS (1995) Regulation of BDNF and trkB mRNA in rat brain by chronic electroconvulsive seizure and antidepressant drug treatment, *J Neurosci* **15:** 7539–47.

Nibuya M, Nestler EJ, Duman RS (1996) Chronic antidepressant administration increases the expression of CREB in rat hippocampus, *J Neurosci* **16:**2365–72.

Nicholson S, Lin J-H et al (1985) Diurnal variations in responsiveness of the hypothalamo–pituitary–adrenal axis in the rat, *Neuroendocrinology* **40:** 217–24.

Ozaki N, Duncan WC Jr, Johnson KA et al (1993) Diurnal variations in serotonin and dopamine levels in discrete brain regions of Syrian hamsters and their modification by chronic clorgyline treatment, *Brain Res* **627:**41–8.

Paykel ES (1979) In: Depue RA, ed., *The Psychobiology of the Depressive Disorders: Implications for the Effects of Stress* (Academic Press: New York) 245–62.

Peiffer A, Veilleaux S, Barden N (1991) Antidepressant and other centrally acting drugs regulate glucocorticoid receptor messenger RNA levels in rat brain, *Psychoneuroendocrinology* **16:** 505–15.

Pepin MC, Govindan MV, Barden N (1992) Increased glucocorticoid receptor gene promoter activity after antidepressant treatment, *Mol Pharmacol* **41:**1016–22.

Peterson MG, Tupy JL (1994) Transcriptional factors: a new frontier in pharmaceutical development, *Biochem Pharmacol* **47:**127–8.

Pryor JC, Sulser F (1991) Evolution of monoamine hypotheses of depression. In: Horton RW, Katona C, eds, *Biological Aspects of Affectiv Disorders* (Academic Press: London) 77–94.

Riederer P, Birkmayer W, Neumeyer E et al (1974) The daily rhythm of HVA, VMA (VA) and 5-HIAA in depression syndrome, *J Neural Transm* **35:**23–45.

Roberts VJ, Singhal RL, Roberts DCS (1984) Corticosterone prevents the increase in noradrenaline stimulated adenyl cyclase activity in rat hippocampus following adrenalectomy or metopirone, *Eur J Pharmacol* **103:** 235–40.

Rossby SP, Sulser F (1997) Events beyond the synapse. In: Skolnick P, ed., *Antidepressants: Current Trends and Future Directions* (Humana Press Inc: Totowa, NY) 195–212.

Rossby SP, Nalepa I, Huang M et al (1995) Norepinephrine-independent regulation of GRII mRNA *in vivo* by a tricyclic antidepressant, *Brain Res* **687:**79–82.

Rossby SP, Perrin C, Burt A et al (1996) Fluoxetine increases steady-state levels of preproenkephalin mRNA in rat amygdala by a serotonin dependent mechanism, *J Serotonin Res* **3:**69–74.

Rusak B, McNaughton L, Robertson HA et al (1992) Circadian variation in photic regulation of immediate-early gene mRNAs in rat suprachiasmatic nucleus cells, *Brain Res Mol Brain Res* **14:**124–30.

Sachar EJ, Hellman L, Roffwarg HP et al (1973) Disrupted 24-hour patterns of cortisol secretion in psychotic depression, *Arch Gen Psychiatry* **28:**19–24.

Schwaninger M, Schöfl C, Blume R et al (1995) Inhibition by antidepressant drugs of cyclic AMP response element-directed gene transcription, *Mol Pharmacol* **47:**1112–18.

Schweitzer JW, Schwartz R, Friedhoff AJ (1979) Intact presynaptic terminals required for beta-adrenergic receptor regulation by desipramine, *J Neurochem* **33:**377–9.

Seckl JR, Fink G (1992) Antidepressants increase glucocorticoid and mineralocorticoid receptor mRNA expression in rat hippocampus in vivo, *Neuroendocrinology* **55:**621–6.

Sheng M, Greenberg ME (1990) The regulation and function of c-fos and other immediate early genes in the nervous system, *Neuron* **4:**477–85.

Shih M, Malbon CC (1994) Oligodeoxynucleotides antisense to mRNA encoding protein kinase A, protein kinase C and β-adrenergic receptor kinase reveal distinctive cell-type specific roles in agonist-induced desensitization, *Proc Natl Acad Sci USA* **91:**12 193–7.

Siuciak JA, Lewis D, Wiegand SJ et al (1994) Brain derived neurotrophic factor (BDNF) produces an antidepressant-like effect in two animal models of depression, *Soc Neurosci* **20:**1106.

Vetulani J, Sulser F (1975) Action of various antidepressant treatments reduces reactivity of noradrenergic cyclic AMP generating system in limbic forebrain, *Nature* **257:**495–6.

Walsh DA, Ashby CS (1973) Protein kinases: aspects of their regulation and diversity, *Recent Prog Horm Res* **29:**329–59.

Wehr TA, Muscettola G, Goodwin FK (1980) Urinary 3-methoxy-4-hydroxy-phenylglycol circadian rhythm, *Arch Gen Psychiatry* **37:**254–63.

Wolffe BB, Harden TK, Sporn JR et al (1978) Presynaptic modulation of beta adrenergic receptors in rat cerebral cortex after treatment with antidepressants, *J Pharmacol Exp Ther* **207:** 446–57.

Wurtman RJ, Axelrod J, Kelly DE (1968) *The Pineal* (Academic Press: New York and London).

Yamamoto KR (1985) Steroid receptor regulated transcription of specific genes and gene networks, *Annu Rev Genet* **19:**209–52.

Yoshikawa K, Sabol SL (1986) Expression of the enkephalin precursor gene in C6 rat glioma cells: regulation by β adrenergic agonists and glucocorticoids, *Mol Brain Res* **1:**75–83.

6
Animal models of depression

Brian E Leonard

Introduction

Although the neuroanatomical and neurochemical composition of the human and sub-human brain is basically similar, there is no convincing evidence to suggest that even the most developed non-human primate suffers from an identifiable mental illness. To paraphrase Roth and Kerr (1970), the depressive state is probably peculiar to *Homo sapiens*. Thus the state of the mood and cognitive function, as exemplified by feelings of guilt, worthlessness and pessimism, are unlikely to be present in an animal species that does not have a well-defined concept of self-esteem or of the future. Other features of the depression syndrome such as apathy, loss of appetite and libido, and impaired attention and memory, might be simulated in animals following the appropriate behavioural manipulation. This has led several investigators to study changes in behaviour and brain neurotransmission that may be linked to reward and punishment.

Despite the advances which have been made in the development of animal models of depression in recent years, most of those routinely used by research laboratories in the pharmaceutical industry have remained surprisingly inept at accurately predicting clinically effective antidepressants, and in the generation of new hypotheses of the pathophysiology of depression. Thus, almost every significant advance in antidepressant drug treatment, from the discovery of iproniazid and imipramine to the second-generation antidepressants such as mianserin, has resulted either from astute clinical observation or serendipity.

Hitherto, most animal models which have been used for the selection of putative antidepressants have been based on the simple amine deficiency theory, which postulates that depression arises as a result of a deficiency in biogenic amine neurotransmitters in the synaptic cleft. Thus it has been assumed that antidepressants 'work' by blocking the reuptake of products of the intraneuronal metabolism of biogenic amine neurotransmitters, generally assumed to be noradrenaline and serotonin. As the ability of monoamine oxidase inhibitors and tricyclic antidepressants to antagonize the hypothermia and behavioural depression caused by acute reserpine treatment provided a useful model for the detection of imipramine and iproniazid-like drugs, a plethora of antidepressants has been developed which have similar pharmacological and toxicological profiles to the parent compounds. Sulser et al (1978) were the first investigators to report changes in the sensitivity of β-adrenoceptors following chronic antidepressant treatment or electroconvulsive shock (ECS); others later showed that changes occurred in the sensitivity of $5-HT_2$ receptors and α_2-adrenoceptors following chronic antidepressant treatment (Peroutka and Snyder, 1980; Smith et al, 1983), which led to the amine theory being modified to take into account the adaptation of receptors which appear to correlate with the onset of the antidepressant response. Whether such changes in receptor density are causally related to the therapeutic action of the antidepressants is unproven.

The purpose of this chapter is to describe some of the animal models of depression which have been developed. A valid animal model of depression should fulfil the following criteria:

1. It should show behavioural changes that simulate those occurring in the depressed patient, e.g. memory loss, motor retardation, deficits in cognition, irritability, anorexia, loss of libido.
2. It should show a normalization of these symptoms when antidepressant drugs are administered.
3. As the effective control of depression only occurs following chronic drug treatment, the animal model should only respond optimally to antidepressants that are chronically administered.

McKinney (1977) has succinctly summarized the criteria necessary for the establishment of an animal model of depression as: comparable symptomatology, comparable aetiology, comparable neurophysiological basis and the concordant effect of antidepressants. Willner (1995) has also summarized the criteria necessary for an animal model of depression under the headings of *predictive validity* (i.e. the extent to which the model only responds to clinically effective antidepressants), *face validity* (i.e. the similarity between the behaviour of the animal model and the symptoms of depression) and *construct validity* (i.e. the similarity between the underlying cause of depression and the cause of the abnormal behavioural changes in the animal model). Whereas it has been possible to develop rodent models of depression that satisfy the predictive validity, and to some extent the face validity, it has not been possible to reliably develop models of construct validity. This is because of the paucity of data relating to the biochemical changes that are causally related to depression, even though there is some evidence that changes in the function of the biogenic amine neurotransmitters may play a crucial role.

Many of the animal models of depression are based on the effects of stress, the changes resulting from the exposure of animals (usually rodents) to stress being reversed by antidepressant treatments. The stressors used vary from mild to severe stress, as exemplified by foot-shock, restraint stress and immersion in water. Chronic mild unavoidable stress has also been used to produce a model of depression (Willner, 1987) which has the advantage over many of the stress models in that the behavioural deficits can be corrected by chronic, but not acute, anti-depressant treatment. Other models are based on ethnological methods whereby the effects of social defeat are monitored. Most of these proce-dures are associated with a decrease in motor activity and/or reward behaviour (e.g. sucrose consumption) which may be reversed by acute and/or chronic antidepressant treatment, depending on the model stud-ied.

A second group of models is based on the effects of social isolation. Such studies have been mainly made on non-human primates, but more recently behavioural changes following the social isolation of rats have been shown to be useful. The first and second groups of model were largely developed 15–20 years ago and have undergone little change since their introduction.

The third group of models involves the reversal of changes that follows discrete lesions of the limbic system. Thus lesions of the amygdala, sep-tum and olfactory bulbs produce behavioural changes that can be reversed by the chronic administration of antidepressants.

A number of comprehensive reviews have been published in the last 10 years (see Henn and McKinney, 1987; Overstreet et al, 1988; Willner, 1990; Van Riezen and Leonard, 1991) and therefore this chapter merely gives an overview of some of the more popular models that are used for the development of novel antidepressants. In addition, an assessment will be made of the olfactory bulbectomized rat model which appears to offer a major advantage over most animal models in that many of the changes in the endocrine, immune and neurotransmitter systems are qualitatively similar to those occurring in depressed patients.

Developmental models of depression

Bowlby (1968) observed that the removal of children from their mothers induced depressive symptoms that were characterized by hyperactivity followed by despair and withdrawal. Harlow (1958) has shown that a sim-ilar behaviour could be elicited by the removal of the infant monkey from its mother. Despite the promising nature of the earlier studies, Kaufman (1974) has shown that far greater changes in infant behaviour occur in monkeys reared by their mothers in relative isolation from other monkeys than occurs in response to separation from the natural mother. The rela-tionship between such events as isolation from the mother in childhood and the onset of depression in the adult is still an unresolved question, and the behaviour of the monkey following prolonged isolation from its mother probably bears a closer resemblance to psychotic behaviour than depression (McKinney et al, 1973).

There is experimental evidence to suggest that social isolation is associated with a reduction in brain serotonin turnover (Garattini et al, 1967). When rodents are socially isolated for prolonged periods, they exhibit hyperactivity (Garzon and del Rio, 1987) and aggression towards intruders (Garathus et al, 1967), such behaviour being reversed by antidepressant treatment (Garzon and del Rio, 1981). Thus social isolation causes symptoms that resemble those caused by destruction of serotonergic pathways in the forebrain, which may reflect the aggressiveness and impulsive behaviour reported to occur in a subgroup of depressed patients who have a low cerebrospinal fluid concentration of 5-hydroxyindole acetic acid. Such changes in serotonergic function that follow prolonged social isolation are long-lasting, and differ from the rapid returns of the serotonergic system to normal following exposure to acute stress (Anisman and Zacharko, 1982).

While social isolation as such has not been implicated in the aetiology of depression in animals, social isolation may model the failure of social function that can result from adverse events occurring in childhood (such as family discord, loss of a parent) and which may predispose to depression (Rutter and Madge, 1976). Low cerebrospinal fluid 5-hydroxyindole acetic acid concentrations are associated with low scores on socialization scales (Taskman-Benz et al, 1986). The concept that isolation-induced serotonin depletion may serve as an animal model for some aspects of depression is supported by the studies of social cooperation in rats (Schuster et al, 1982). In these studies, it was found that cooperative behaviour could be disrupted by destruction of forebrain serotonergic pathways but could be restored by the administration of the serotonin agonist fluperazine. It seems possible that one of the main functions of serotonin is to enhance the sensitivity of the animal to social cues. Willner (1989) has postulated that the activity of forebrain serotonin is controlled by social reinforcement. Thus serotonin turnover decreases if the social environment of the child or young animal fails to provide adequate reinforcement. This results in lack of self-control and the development of impulsive adults that exhibit antisocial behaviour; frequently such behaviour is associated with depression in the adult. Effective treatment with antidepressants corrects these behavioural deficits by correcting the serotonergic dysfunction and thereby also enhancing the sensitivity of the patient to social cues. Thus the developmental models of depression, and the social isolation models, could be valuable for understanding the developmental aspects of depression and the role of serotonin in social isolation.

Learned helplessness models

Seligman (1975) developed a model of learned helplessness which mimics some of the main features of depression, particularly of the kind that are precipitated by unfavourable environmental events. Dogs exposed to an unavoidable electrical shock were subsequently found to be unable to learn to avoid an aversive stimulus and remained motionless and 'helpless' in such a situation. Studies by Glazer and Weiss (1976) using the rat also showed that this species could exhibit 'behavioural despair'. These investigators analysed the changes elicited by unavoidable shock and showed that the relatively short-term stress (as shown by freezing behaviour increasing sympathoadrenal activity, etc.) carries over into the learning phase, which may account for the initial immobility. These investigators then showed that the persistent inability of the animal to respond is confined to the learned immobility that has been acquired during the unavoidable shock situation. Thus the 'learned helplessness' behaviour does not generalize to other types of behaviour that had been learned in the absence of the shock. Such findings have led to a serious reappraisal of the relevance of this model to depression.

Even though the relevance of the 'learned helplessness' model of depression may be questioned, short-term unresponsiveness to stress may provide a useful model for the detection of antidepressant drugs. The method developed by Porsolt et al (1978) involves placing rodents individually into a water-filled glass cylinder at 25°C from which they cannot escape. After a few minutes of vigorous swimming and attempted escape, the animals remain quiet, only making movements sufficient to keep their heads above water. Exposure to the same environment 24 h later shows that the animals have 'learned' not to try to escape from the container and therefore they remain immobile. Porsolt et al (1978) used this model as a test for antidepressant activity. They showed that both 'standard' tricyclic antidepressants such as amitriptyline and imipramine, and atypical antidepressants such as mianserin and iprindole, increase the time for which the animals struggle to escape from the container on being placed in it on the second occasion. Clearly, drugs that cause marked sedation or reduce the muscle tone will produce 'false positives' in such a test situation, but Porsolt et al (1978) did show that low doses of anxiolytics and neuroleptics were ineffective in this test. Despite the widespread use of the Porsolt 'learned immobility' test as a screening method for antidepressants, a critical evaluation of the test by O'Neill and Valentino (1982) suggests that it suffers from the same fundamental problems as the original Seligman (1975) model. Thus, it was shown that rodents exhibit 'behavioural despair' independently of their ability to escape from the cylinder of water and that the phenomenon did not generalize to a shock escape task. O'Neill and Valentino (1982) therefore conclude that the immobility may reflect either an adaptive response to the particular situation, physical fatigue, or a combination of these factors. Such criticism, together with the observation of Wallace and Hedley that such psychotropic drugs as caffeine, antihistamines and pentobarbital also reverse the 'behavioural despair' behaviour, suggests that such a model is an inadequate representation of depression and is of limited value in the detection of antidepressant drugs. Thierry et al (1984) have suggested that both the infant response to maternal separation in monkeys and the 'behavioural despair' in rodents show a searching–waiting strategy which, though not equivalent to depression, may be a model of adaptive behaviour of which depression is a pathological state.

Prolonged restraint stress as a rodent model of depression

Kennett et al (1985) have developed a rodent model of depression in which restraint stress causes a failure of adaptive protective responses to aversive stimulation. In this model, adult rats are restrained by taping their feet to a wire grid for 2 h. The animals are then released and allowed to recover for approximately 24 h. On being placed in the 'open field' apparatus the following day, the rats were hyperactive, but chronic (14 days) pretreatment with desipramine or sertaline reversed the stress-induced hypoactivity. These investigators also showed that $5-HT_{1A}$ full (e.g. 8-hydroxy-D-amino acridine and ipsapirone) act like antidepressants in this model. These behavioural changes are unlikely to be due to direct action of the drugs on serotonin receptors, as the antidepressant-like effects are evident long after the drugs have been eliminated. In addition to the hypoactivity, hypophagia and hypersecretion of corticosterone also occur (Kennett and Curzon, 1989). After exposure of the rats to restraint stress for consecutive days, tolerance occurs to the hypoactivity (and other symptoms). This tolerance was shown to be associated with increased functional activity of $5-HT_{1A}$ receptors. It was interesting to note in this model that stressed female rats showed a more marked maladaptive response to restraint stress than male rats. The plasma corticosterone concentration was also much higher than in male rats exposed to the same degree of restraint stress. The possible connection between brain serotonergic function (possibly involving $5-HT_{1A}$ receptors) and the hypersecretion of glucocorticoids was shown by the normalization of the maladaptive behaviour by the $5-HT_1$ agonist 5-methoxy-dimethyltryptamine which occurred following the administration of the glucocorticoid synthesis inhibitor metyrapone (Kennett and Curzon, 1989).

This model of depression differs from most other rodent models in that female rats show more marked behavioural deficits than male rats and thereby simulates the clinical situation whereby women appear to be more prone to depression than men. In addition, this model suggests that effective antidepressants desensitize presynaptic $5-HT_{1A}$ receptors, thereby leading to enhanced serotonergic transmission (Blier and de Montigny, 1985). The highest density of 5-HT$_{1A}$ receptors occurs in the hippocampus, an area of the brain that is rich in glucocorticoid receptors. The glucocorticoid receptors are crucially involved in the adaptation to stress; there is clinical evidence to suggest that these receptors are hyposensitive to glucocorticoid stimulation in depression, and this leads to hypersecretion of cortisol (Dinan, 1994). Thus the behavioural, endocrine and serotonergic function changes in the brain of rats subject to chronic restraint stress simulate many of the changes seen in depression. However, the prolonged (2-h) restraint stress that is used to induce this maladaptive behaviour is open to serious ethical objections.

Reserpine-induced depression

The serendipitous discovery that imipramine reversed the symptoms of ptosis and hypothermia induced in rodents by reserpine pretreatment led to the development of the reserpine reversal test as a model for the detection of antidepressants. As a result of the almost universal use of this test by the pharmaceutical industry, a plethora of tricyclic antidepressants have been discovered over the past two decades, all of which have qualitatively similar pharmacological and therapeutic profiles to that of imipramine. Such drugs are assumed to reverse reserpine-induced symptoms by elevating the intersynaptic concentrations of biogenic amines, largely as a result of the drugs impeding the reuptake of biogenic amines for the synaptic cleft. Monoamine oxidase inhibitors (MAOIs) also reverse the acute effects of reserpine, primarily by blocking the intraneuronal catabolism of the biogenic amines. The very success of the reserpine antagonism test in the development of a variety of both tricyclic antidepressants, such as desipramine, clomipramine, dothiepin and doxepin, and some of the newer antidepressants which lack the tricyclic structure (e.g. nomifensine, viloxazine, zimeldine and citalopram) has tended to restrict the development of other animal models of depression. Furthermore, as both the conventional reserpine antagonism test and the 'learned helplessness' test of Porsolt et al (1978) could select tricyclic antidepressants after their acute administration, the development of animal models which enabled antidepressants to be selected only following their chronic administration was also hampered. Thus atypical antidepressants such as iprindole, mianserin, salbutamol and flupenthixol, which did not affect the amine reuptake mechanism and were therefore inactive in reserpine antagonism tests, were only discovered to be antidepressants following their clinical assessment, often for other psychiatric and non-psychiatric conditions. Such findings stress the need to develop new animal models that do not rely on a specific structure or acute biochemical profile involving an inhibition of amine reuptake.

Muricidal rat model of depression

Lesions of the olfactory bulbs increase the incidence of mouse-killing behaviours in strains of rat that would not normally exhibit this behaviour (Vergnes and Karli, 1963). Increased irritability has also been shown to occur when specific serotonin neurotoxins, such as 5,7-dihydroxytrypta-mine, are injected bilaterally into the olfactory bulbs (Cairncross et al, 1979), a situation that may explain the enhanced muricidal behaviour in rats which have been surgically bulbectomized. Several investigators have shown that a deficit in brain serotonin function is associated with muricidal behaviour. Thus, administration of the tryptophan hydroxylase inhibitor parachlorophenylalanine (Sheard, 1969) and the administration of serotonin neurotoxins (Vergnes and Kempf, 1982) have been shown to induce muricidal behaviour. Conversely, drugs facilitating central sero-tonergic neurotransmission attenuate muricidal behaviour. Antidepres-sant drugs, which are specific serotonin uptake inhibitors following their acute administration, e.g. fluoxetine (Gibbons and Glusman, 1978), the serotonin agonists quipazine and 5-hydroxytrophan (Bocknik and Kulka-rni, 1974) and the releasing agent fenfluramine (Gibbons and Glusman, 1978), all antagonize spontaneous or neurotoxin-induced muricidal behaviour. As such tricyclic antidepressants as imipramine, desipramine and amitriptyline also attenuate muricidal behaviour (Eisenstein et al, 1982), the effects of drugs on such behaviour have been used as a rapid screening test for potential antidepressants. However, it is now well established that many centrally acting drugs which do not have an anti-depressant activity in humans also show positive 'antidepressant' activity in this test. Besides fenfluramine, amphetamine and antihistamines have also been shown to be active in the muricidal rat model (see Eisenstein et al, 1982). Thus, from these experimental studies it may be concluded that the muricidal rat model may be useful for defining the effects of a cen-trally acting drug on serotonin metabolism but cannot be used as a reli-able model for the detection of antidepressants.

The apomorphine antagonism model for the detection of antidepressants

Interest in the possible involvement of the dopaminergic system in the mode of action of antidepressants has arisen from the observation that many antidepressants inhibit the reuptake of tritiated dopamine into synaptosomes from the rat brain (Randrup and Braestrup, 1977). Although antidepressants have traditionally been assumed to exert their therapeutic action by modulating noradrenergic and serotonergic trans-mission in the brain, there is now evidence that chronically administered antidepressants increase the density of D_2 and D_3 receptors in the nucleus accumbens of the rat (Willner, 1989). In the chronic mild shock test of Willner (1991), the anhedonia that occurs is postulated to be an expression of decreased dopaminergic function. Most classes of antidepressants appear to reverse the chronic mild stress-induced anhedonia. In earlier studies, Serra et al (1979) showed that chronic mianserin or amitriptyline treatment prevents the hypomotility of rats that are subsequently injected with a low (0.05 mg/kg) acute dose of apomorphine. These findings have been extended by Chiodo and Antelman (1980), who showed that the ability of apomorphine to selectively depress the spontaneous electrical activity of dopaminergic neurons in the zona compacta of the substantia nigra was attenuated following the chronic administration of tricyclic antidepressants or iprindole. It can be concluded from such studies that prolonged antidepressant treatment results in subsensitivity of dopamine autoreceptors.

An investigation of the effects of chronic treatment (14 days) of rats with citalopram, nomifensine, salbutamol, α-flupenthixol and sulpiride in antagonizing the hypomotility induced by the acute administration of apomorphine has been summarized elsewhere (Hasan and Leonard, 1983). In this study, it was shown that those drugs with proven antidepressant activity attenuate the hypomotility of apomorphine, whereas those lacking such activity (e.g. reserpine) do not.

Like the bulbectomy model, the apomorphine antagonism model only appears to select antidepressants following their chronic administration, and irrespective of their structure or presumed acute effects on one or more neurotransmitter systems.

Chronic mild stress model of depression

This model was developed by Willner (1990) in an attempt to use relatively realistic but stressful conditions that may act as trigger factors for depression in humans. In this model, rats or mice are exposed in a sequential manner to a variety of mild stressors (such as continuous illumination, wet bedding, background noise, changes of cage mates, cage tilted) which change every few hours for several weeks. This procedure has been found to decrease the sensitivity to reward as indicated by a reduction in the consumption of a weak sucrose selection (Willner, 1987). Normal sucrose consumption is restored when the rodent is treated chronically with an antidepressant. Most classes of antidepressants which have been tested in the chronic mild stress model have been found to be effective, as has electroconvulsive shock, lithium and the 5-HT$_{1A}$ partial agonist buspirone. Stimulants, neuroleptics, anxiolytics and opiates are ineffective in reversing the anhedonia (reduced sucrose consumption). Willner (1995) has reasoned that the chronic mild stress model has reasonable construct, face and predictive validity.

Changes in behaviour following olfactory bulbectomy

The North American psychologist Watson was probably the first investigator to comment on the behavioural effects of bilateral bulbectomy in rats. Most experimenters have reported an increased irritability and aggressiveness in rats following bulbectomy. More recent evidence suggest that hyperemotionality and aggressiveness do not appear in rats handled frequently before and during the postoperative period and are not primarily effects of the lesions per se (Richman et al, 1972; Thorne et al, 1973; Leonard and Tuite, 1981).

An increased incidence of muricidal (mouse-killing) behaviour has also been reported to occur following bilateral bulbectomy (Albert et al, 1981). While such behaviour is relatively uncommon in most strains of intact rats, the frequency of such behaviour is reported to increase dramatically following bulbectomy. However, the pattern of the mouse-killing behaviour is quite different to that seen in spontaneously muricidal strains. Thus, the latency to attack the mouse following bulbectomy is much longer and the killing is less efficient (e.g. more bites are inflicted by the bulbectomized rat compared to the spontaneously muricidal rat). This behaviour of the bulbectomized rat has been termed 'irritable aggression' and has been discussed in more detail elsewhere (Leonard and Tuite, 1981). Moreover, when spontaneously muricidal rats are bulbectomized, muricidal behaviour is considerably attenuated.

An increased incidence of cannibalism in female rats following bulbectomy, intermale aggression, territorial aggression and an alteration in sexual behaviour (Tyler and Gorski, 1980; Lumia et al, 1987) all suggest that such behavioural abnormalities are caused by the absence of more than just the essential olfactory cues following the lesions (see Leonard and Tuite (1981) for details).

In rodents, bulbectomy is followed by an increase in locomotor activity in a novel environment (Richman et al, 1972; Sieck, 1972; Jancsar and Leonard, 1983). These changes in locomotor activity and in other types of behaviour are not likely to be due to anosmia, because the reversible inhibition of the functioning of the olfactory nerve in the nasal cavity by zinc sulphate solution does not result in such behavioural changes. The hyperactivity shown by bulbectomized animals in the 'open field' must be considered as a failure of adaptation and risk assessment (Blanchard and Blanchard, 1983), and this 'deficit' can be attenuated by the chronic administration of antidepressants (Table 6.1). It should be noted that drugs lacking antidepressant activity do not attenuate this behaviour and neither will antidepressants following their acute administration (Leonard, 1984).

Differences have been found between the active and passive avoidance performance of the bulbectomized rat. Thus, bulbectomized rats have been shown to be deficient in the acquisition of a passive

Table 6.1   Some behavioural tests in which bulbectomized rats have been shown to differ from sham-operated controls.

Type of behaviour	Type of change by bulbectomy[b]	Reference
Muricidal behaviour	+	Cain (1974)
Cannibalism	+	Fleming and Rosenblatt (1974)
Sexual behaviour	−	Larsson (1971)
Exploratory behaviour	+	Sieck (1972)
Passive avoidance learning	−	Thorne et al (1973, 1976)
Active avoidance learning	+	Thorne et al (1973)
Extinction of conditioned taste aversion	−	Jancsar and Leonard (1984)
Eating pattern[a]	+	La Rue and Le Magneu (1972)
Rapid eye movement sleep	−	Sakurada et al (1976)

[a] Eating pattern disrupted following bulbectomy: quantity of food consumed reduced, but frequency of eating is increased.

[b] Increased (+) and decreased (−) relative to sham-operated controls.

avoidance task, but superior to controls in the acquisition of a two-way active avoidance task (shuttle box) (Sieck and Gordon, 1972; Thomas, 1973; Sieck et al, 1974). However, other investigators have shown that one-way active avoidance learning is deficient after bulbectomy (Cairncross and King, 1971; Marks et al, 1971; King and Cairncross, 1974). Deficits in runway behaviour for a food reward (Egan et al, 1979; Jancsar and Leonard, 1984) and in conditioned taste aversion also occur in the bulbectomized rat. The main differences between the bulbectomized rat and its sham-operated control are summarized in Table 6.2.

Changes in social (e.g. increased aggression, both territorial and, in general, irritability), sexual (e.g. maternal and mating behaviour) and non-social behaviours such as exploratory activity of a novel environment have been shown to occur following bulbectomy (see Leonard and Tuite (1981) for details). O'Connor and Leonard (1988) have shown that, when placed on a holeboard apparatus, the ambulation score, head dipping (a measure of the exploratory activity indicated by the animal investigating a hole) and grooming were significantly reduced in bulbectomized rats when compared with their sham-operated controls.

Furthermore, in a novel test for neophobia, bulbectomy caused a total elimination of the neophobia response when compared with sham-operated controls. In this test, which was developed by Broekkamp et al (1986), glass marbles are introduced into the home cage of the bulbectomized or sham-operated animal. The marbles provide the aversive stimulus and the time taken for the animal to displace and/or scatter the marbles from their initial position in the cage was used as a measure of the neophobic response.

Table 6.2   Open field responses following chronic psychotropic drug treatments in the bulbectomized rat.

Antidepressant	Activity	Novel or putative antidepressant	Activity
Desipramine	+	Zalospirone	+
Lofepramine	+	Ipsapirone	+
Desmethyl lofepramine	+	8-OH-DPAT	+
Desmethyl desipramine	+	BIMT 17	+
Imipramine	+	ORG 12962	+
Amitriptyline	+	FG 5893	+
Milnacipran	+	Methysergide	+
Nomifensin	+	Methiothepin	+
4-Hydroxynomifensin	+	Glycine	+
Mianserin racemate	+	MK-801	+
+ Enantiomer	+	CII 988	+
− Enantiomer	−	Devazepide	−
Desmethylmianserin	−	Atipamezole	−
8-Hydroxymianserin	−	Yohimbine	+
Mirtazepine racemate	+	Clonidine	−
+ Enantiomer	+	Salbutamol	+
− Enantiomer	−	GBR 12909	−
Trazodone	−	Sulpiride	+
Paroxetine	+	E-Flupenthixol	+
Fluoxetine	−	Chlorpromazine	−
Sertraline	+	Adinazolam	+
Tianeptine	+	Alprazolam	+
Fluvoxamine	+	Diazepam	−
Moclobemide	+	Baclofen	+
Esuprone	−	Progabide	+
IM 24	+	Gamma vinyl GABA	+
Parglyline	−	Phenobarbitone	−
Levoprotiline	+	THIP	−
Lithium chloride	−	Reserpine	−
		Indomethacin	−
		Dexamethasone	−
		Bepridil	−
		Atropine	−
		NPY	+
		Interleukin 2	−

In all cases, rats were examined following chronic 14-day treatment with the test substance.
+, active; −, inactive.

Whereas the sham-operated animals either completely, or almost completely, buried most of the marbles, bulbectomized animals did not attempt to bury any of the marbles. From this experiment, it would appear that the neophobic response is markedly attenuated following bilateral bulbectomy.

In addition to the gross behavioural changes that occur following bulbectomy, physiological changes have also been reported. Such changes include decreased heart rate and blood pressure (Kawasaki et al, 1980a,b), decreases in the frequency of REM sleep (Sakurada et al, 1976; Sakurada and Kitara, 1977), altered thermoregulation (Forster et al, 1980) and polydipsia (Wren et al, 1977). The changes in thermoregulation and possibly in fluid intake may be indicative of altered hypothalamic function, which has also been implicated by Kawasaki et al (1980a,b); these investigators reported that the bulbectomized rat exhibited enhanced emotional responses to stimulation of the posterior hypothalamus. It is not without interest that this altered hypothalamic responsiveness developed gradually over a period of 10 days, which may be suggestive of the development of neurotransmitter receptor hypersensitivity, in this and/or other brain regions, as a consequence of the lesion.

O'Connor and Leonard (1986) have also reported changes in other physiological variables as a consequence of bilateral bulbectomy. Thus, hypernatraemia and hyperchlorhydria occur in both young (7-week-old) and adult (12-week-old) rats following bulbectomy. This effect is maintained for at least 4 weeks after surgery and is unaffected by chronic antidepressant treatment. Serum potassium and calcium levels are unaffected. Decreased sensitivity of the osmoreceptors to elevated sodium (Chiaraviglio, 1969), thalamic malfunctioning due to the brain lesion (Sweet et al, 1949), blood loss or hypotension may help to explain these changes in electrolyte balance.

Endocrine changes following olfactory bulbectomy

The earliest and most studied endocrine change in major depression is the hypersecretion of the glucocorticoid cortisol, which is not suppressed by the administration of dexamethasone (Carroll, 1982). More recent studies have suggested that there is hypersecretion of cortisol in depressed patients throughout the 24-h cycle (Linkowski et al, 1994). Glucocorticoid secretion has been investigated following olfactory bulbectomy, but has yielded conflicting results, with some reports of raised levels of both basal and stress-induced glucocorticoids (Cairncross et al, 1977), which are reversed by chronic antidepressant treatment (Cairncross et al, 1979), while others have found no such differences (Broekkamp et al, 1986). Normal secretion of corticosterone has been reported to occur in bulbectomized rats throughout the light phase, but extended hypersecretion has been observed during the dark phase of the light–dark cycle (Song et al, 1994). This nocturnal hypersecretion is apparent from 24 h following surgery. These results suggest an altered circadian secretion of corticosterone. This can be correlated with increased basal cyclic AMP concentration in the suprachiasmatic nuclei of the hypothalamus at a point of maximal accumulation 8 weeks following olfactory bulbectomy (Vagell et al, 1991).

Much less attention has been paid to the dexamethasone suppression test in bulbectomized rats, which has been examined only on one occasion 4 h following dexamethasone, at which time no differences were evident between bulbectomized rats and their sham-operated controls (O'Connor, 1985). Recently, a variation of the dexamethasone suppression test has been investigated under basal and stress-induced conditions in the bulbectomized rat. This simulates the clinical situation in that several hours elapse after dexamethasone administration and prior to blood sampling (Carroll, 1982). In both conditions, suppression of corticosterone secretion was evident 12 h after dexamethasone administration. However, under basal experimental conditions, the corticosterone drugs had returned 36 h after dexamethasone, whereas in the stress-induced experiment, there was still a significant blunting of this response at this time interval. As bulbectomized rats behaved in a similar manner to their sham-operated controls, it would suggest that the response in the bulbectomized rat to a moderately stressful stimulus is not impaired. More recently, we have examined dexamethasone suppression in bulbectomized rats 45 min following dexamethasone administration (Kelly, unpublished observations). Under these conditions, a significant suppression of corticosterone was found in the sham-operated animals which was not apparent in bulbectomized animals. This may indicate that the kinetics of the suppressive response to dexamethasone differ in the bulbectomized rat.

Immune changes following olfactory bulbectomy

Immunological changes occurring following olfactory bulbectomy have been the subject of a recent review (Song and Leonard, 1995) and will only be summarized here (Table 6.3).

The earliest reported change in the immune system associated with olfactory bulbectomy was a reduction in neutrophil phagocytic response (O'Neill et al, 1987; Song and Leonard, 1993), similar to that found in depression (O'Neill and Leonard, 1990). More recently, a reduction in neutrophil catalase and glutathione peroxidase and an increase in superoxidase dismutase have been found (Song et al, 1994). The altered glutathione peroxidase was attenuated by chronic desipramine treatment. A reduction in mitogen-stimulated lymphocyte proliferation occurred (Song and Leonard, 1994), which has also been reported with depressed patients (Kronfol and House, 1989). In contrast, increased monocyte proliferative (Song and Leonard, 1995) and mononuclear phagocytic (Kelly, 1991) responses are observed in the bulbectomized rat; the latter effect is also found in depressed patients (McAdams and Leonard, 1993). An increase in positive acute-phase proteins and a reduction in negative acute-phase proteins also occurs in bulbectomized rats (Song and

Table 6.3   Immune changes following olfactory bulbectomy

Changes
Reduced neutrophil phagocytosis
Increased mononuclear cell phagocytosis
Reduced lymphocyte proliferation
Increased monocyte proliferation
Increased positive acute phase proteins
Reduced negative acute phase proteins
Increased neutrophils
Reduced lymphocytes
Increased leucocyte adhesiveness/ aggregation
Reduced thymus weight
Reduced spleen weight
Increased α_1-acid glycoprotein levels

Adapted from Song C and Leonard BE (1995).

Leonard, 1994); these are similar to the acute-phase protein alterations that are observed in depression (Maes, 1995). Of the acute-phase proteins, α_1-acid glycoprotein levels are increased in both the bulbectomized rat (Arnold and Meyerson, 1990) and depressed patients (Nemeroff et al, 1990). It is known that α_1-acid glycoprotein will suppress immune function and that levels can be increased by monocyte activation, as well as by glucocorticoids (Arnold and Meyerson, 1990). The α_1-acid glycoprotein concentration is not increased significantly until 5 weeks after surgery (Arnold and Meyerson, 1990).

The differential white blood cell profile is also altered following olfactory bulbectomy. An increase in neutrophils and reduction in lymphocytes is found (Song and Leonard, 1994). LAA is a marker of stress (Arber et al, 1991), and has been shown to be increased following olfactory bulbectomy (Song et al, 1993). A reduction in plaque-forming cells has been observed in bulbectomized mice (Komori et al, 1991). Reductions in the relative weights of the immune-related organs, thymus gland and spleen, have been observed (Song and Leonard, 1995). The ICV route of administration has also been used with interleukin-2, which does not attenuate the hyperactivity of bulbectomized rats (Song and Leonard, 1995).

Effect of psychotropic drugs on behavioural changes associated with olfactory bulbectomy

From the previous sections, it can be seen that there are a variety of behavioural responses that occur following olfactory bulbectomy and that these are quantifiable and can be replicated. Such changes are useful behavioural indicators of antidepressant activity. The choice of test varies greatly between laboratories, but the most commonly employed behavioural tests are the 'open field' and passive avoidance tests. Other more elaborate tests, such as the Morris maze and conditioned taste aversion, have been used less frequently, but also show that antidepressants attenuate bulbectomy-induced behaviour. A detailed list of the psychotropic agents that have been examined in the bulbectomized rat is given in Table 6.1.

Behavioural changes in the bulbectomized rat are attenuated with traditional tricyclic antidepressants such as amitriptyline and desipramine, and also atypical antidepressants (mianserin, nomifensine, trazodone), and the more recently introduced SSRIs (paroxetine, sertraline, fluvoxamine, but not fluoxetine) and reversible inhibitors of monamine oxidase (RIMAs) such as moclobemide and the experimental compound IM 24 (Bellver et al, 1990). In addition, the serotonin uptake-enhancing agent tianeptine is active (Kelly and Leonard, 1994), as are the mixed noradrenaline/serotonin uptake inhibitor milnacipran (Redmond et al, 1995) and the novel tetracyclic antidepressant mirtazepine (Van Riezen and Leonard, 1990). Antidepressant activity of the demethylated metabolites of lofepramine and desipramine have also been demonstrated (Kelly, 1991). Comparison of racemate and individual enantiomers has shown that the R (+) enantiomer, but not the R (−) enantiomer of mianserin, is active, while the desmethyl and 8-hydroxy metabolites were inactive (Van Riezen and Leonard, 1990). This lack of activity of mianserin metabolites has also been demonstrated in the DRL 72-S schedule (Hand et al, 1991). The triazolobenzodiazepines alpraxolam and adinazolam have shown activity in the bulbectomy model, but not the benzodiazepine diazepam or the barbiturate phenobarbitone.

The antidepressant properties of $5-HT_{1A}$ agonists are believed to be due to their actions on the postsynaptic $5-HT_{1A}$ receptors. Several $5-HT_{1A}$ agonists have demonstrated antidepressant activity, including FG 5893, zalospirone, 8-OH-DPAT (McNamara et al, 1995a) and ipsapirone (McNamara et al, 1996). The $5-HT_2$ antagonist/$5-HT_{1A}$ agonist BIMT 17 CL has also demonstrated antidepressant potential (McNamara, 1995), as has the non-selective $5-HT_1$ antagonist methiothepin (McNamara et al, 1995b). Antidepressant properties have also been shown via antagonism of α_2-receptors with yohimbine (Jancsar, 1981), but not with the α_2-antagonist antipamezole (Kelly, 1991). Nomfensine shows activity, whereas the more selective dopamine uptake inhibitor GBR 12909 does not attenuate the hyperactive response of bulbectomized rats (Kelly, 1991). The non-peptide CCK-B antagonist CI 988 is effective (Kelly and Leonard, 1992), but not the non-peptide CCK-A antagonist devazepide. Consistent with the theory of an involvement of the N-methyl-D-aspartate (NMDA) receptor in the mechanism of action of antidepressants (Paul et al, 1994), modulators of this receptor, such as glycine and MK-801, have demonstrated antidepressant activity in the bulbectomy model (Redmond, 1995). The antidepressant properties of MK-801 have also been demonstrated in the chronic mild stress model of depression (Papp and Moryl, 1994).

Neuropeptide Y (NPY) is a 36 amino acid peptide that is widely distributed in the central and peripheral nervous systems (Wettstein et al, 1995). The concentration of NPY is increased in the central nervous system in bulbectomized rats (Widerlov et al, 1988). Subacute ICV infusion of NPY has been shown to partially reverse the behavioural deficits associated with olfactory bulbectomy (Song and Leonard, 1995).

The number of compounds tested in the passive avoidance paradigm is considerably less than the number examined in the open field test. One reason for this is that certain drugs, particularly those acting on the serotonergic system, can attenuate the passive avoidance deficit associated with olfactory bulbectomy following acute treatment (Van Riezen and Leonard, 1990). Thus, as a predictor of chronic antidepressant effects, it is not as specific as the 'open field', where attenuation is only observed following chronic treatment.

Recently, the bulbectomy model has been combined with the forced swim test and the 8-OH-DPAT hypothermia test to make a three-animal model study design (Kelly and Leonard, 1994). In this study, the antidepressant sertraline was found to be effective in reducing the immoblity in the forced swim test following acute treatment, and in the open field and the 8-OH-DPAT test following chronic (>14-day) treatment.

Conclusion

The animal models of depression which have been considered in this chapter have contributed to the development of new antidepressants, suggested possible mechanisms of their action and helped to expand our knowledge of the psychobiology of depression. However, major problems underlying the validity of animal models of any psychiatric condition reside in the uncertainty concerning the nature of the disease process which they are designed to simulate. Only more research on the biological basis of mental illness will help to improve this situation. Nevertheless, animal models have the practical advantage of allowing hypotheses that have been developed on the basis of clinical observation to be tested in animals. If the hypothesis is not refuted in the animal model, then clinical studies could be devised to assess the validity of the hypothesis in patients. Thus, despite the widely recognized limitations of the animal models currently available, it is self-evident that they will continue to have a major impact on the development of novel antidepressants and indirectly help in the understanding of the aetiology of mental illness.

References

Albert DJ, Nanji N, Crew GL (1981) Structures posterior to the olfactory bulb which are responsible for the mouse killing and hyperactivity following lesions of the olfactory bulb, *Physiol Behav* **26:**395–9.

Anisman H, Zackarko RM (1982) Depression: the predisposing influence of stress, *Behav Brain Sci* **5:**89–137.

Arber N, Beliner S, Rorenberg Z et al (1991) The detection of aggregated leucocytes in the circulatory blood during stress, *Acta Haematol* **36:** 20–34.

Arnold FJ, Meyerson LR (1990) Olfactory bulbectomy alters alpha 1-acid glycoprotein levels in rat plasma, *Brain Res Bull* **25:**259–62.

Bellver C, Rubio P, Tarrio P, Leonard BE (1990) Effects of some new antidepressants on learned helplessness and olfactory bulbectomy models of depression, *Eur J Pharmacol* **183:** 2056–7.

Blanchard DC, Blanchard RJ (1983) Etho experimental approaches to the biology of emotions, *Annu Rev Psychol* **39:**43–68.

Blier P, de Montigny C (1983) Electrophysiological investigations on the effects of repeated zimelidine administration on serotonergic neurotransmission, *J Neurosci* **3:**1270–8.

Bocknik SE, Kulkarni AS (1974) Effect of a decarboxylase inhibitor (RO4-4602) on 5-HTP induced muricide blockade in rats, *Neuropharmacology* **13:**279–87.

Bowlby J (1968) Grief and mourning in infancy and early childhood, *Psy-*

choanal Study Child **15:**9–52.

Broekkamp CL, O'Connor WT, Tonnaer JADM, Ruk HW, Van Delft AML (1986) Corticosterone, cholineacetyl transferase and noradrenaline levels in olfactory bulbectomised rats in relation to changes in passive avoidance acquisition and open field activity, *Physiol Behav* **37:**429–34.

Cain DP (1974) Olfactory bulbectomy: neural structures involved in irritability and aggression in the male rat, *J Comp Physiol Psychol* **86:**213–20.

Cairncross ID, Wren AF, Cox B, Schnieden H (1977) Effects of olfactory bulbectomy and domicile on stress induced corticosterone release on the rat, *Physiol Behav* **19:**485–7.

Cairncross KD, King MG (1971) Facilitation of avoidance learning in anosmic rats in amitriptyline, *Proc Aust Physiol Pharmacol Soc* **2:**25.

Cairncross KD, Cox B, Foster C, Wren AT (1979) Olfactory projection systems, drugs and behaviour: a review, *Psychoneuroendocrinology* **4:**253–72.

Carroll BJ (1982) The dexamethasone suppression test for melancholia, *Br J Psychiatry* **140:**292–303.

Chiaraviglio E (1969) Effects of lesions of the septal area and olfactory bulb on sodium chloride intake, *Physiol Behav* **4:**693–7.

Chiodo LA, Antelman SM (1980) Repeated tricyclic induce a progressive dopamine autoreceptor subsensitivity independent of daily dose, *Nature* **287:**451–4.

Dinan TG (1994) Glucocorticoids and the genesis of depressive illness—a psychobiological model, *Br J Psychia-*

try **164:**365–71.

Egan J, Earley CJ, Leonard BE (1979) The effect of amitriptyline and mianserin on food motivated behaviour of rats trained in a runway: possible correlation with biogenic amine concentrations in the limbic system, *Psychopharmacology* **61:**143–7.

Eistenstein N, Iorid LC, Cody DE (1982) Role of serotonin in the blockade of muricidal behaviour by tricyclic antidepressants, *Pharmacol Biochem Behav* **17:**847–9.

Fleming AS, Rosenblatt JS (1974) Olfactory regulation of maternal behaviour in rat: II. Effects of peripherally induced anosmia and lesions of the lateral olfactory tract in pup induced killing, *J Comp Physiol Psychol* **86:**233–46.

Foster C, Parker J, Cox B (1980) Effects of olfactory bulbectomy and peripherally induced anosmia on thermoregulation in the rat: susceptibility to antidepressant type drugs, *J Pharm Pharmacol* **32:**630–4.

Garattini S, Giacolone E, Valzelli L (1967) Isolation, aggressiveness and brain 5-hydroxytryptamine turnover, *J Pharm Pharmacol* **19:**338–9.

Garzon J, del Rio J (1981) Hypersensitivity induced in rats by long term isolation: further studies on a new animal model for the detection of antidepressants, *Eur J Pharmacol* **74:** 287–94.

Gibbons JL, Glusman M (1978) Effects of quipazine, fluoxetine and fenfluramine on muricide in rats, *Fed Proc Fed Assoc Soc Exp Biol* **39:**257.

Glazer HI, Weiss JM (1976) Long-term interference effect. An alternative to 'learned' helplessness, *J Exp Psychol Anim Behav Process* **2:**202–13.

Hand TM, Marek GT, Seiden LS (1991) Comparison of the effects of mianserin and its enantiomers and metabolites on a behavioural screen for antidepressant activity, *Psychopharmacology* **105:**453–8.

Harlow HF (1958) The nature of love, *Am J Psychol* **13:**673–85.

Hasan F, Leonard BE (1983) Changes in behaviour and neurotransmitter metabolism in the rat following acute and chronic sulpiride administration. In: Ackenheil M, Matussek N, eds, *Special Aspects of Psychopharmacology* (Expansion Scientifique Francaise: Paris) 67–82.

Henn F, McKinney WT (1987) Animal models in psychiatry. In: Meltzer HY, ed., *Psychopharmacology: The Third Generation of Progress* (Raven Press: New York) 697–704.

Jancsar S, Leonard BE (1983) The olfactory bulbectomized rat as a model of depression. In: Usdin E, Goldstein M, Friedhoff AJ, Georgotas A, eds, *Frontiers in Neuropsychiatric Research* (Macmillan: New York) 3570–2.

Jancsar S, Leonard BE (1984) Changes in neurotransmitter metabolism following olfactory bulbectomy in the rat, *Prog Neuropsychopharmacol Biol Psychiatry* **8:**263–9.

Kaufman CT (1974) Mother–infant relations in monkeys and humans. In: White NF, ed., *Ethiology and Psychiatry* (University of Toronto Press: Toronto) 47068.

Kawasaki H, Watanabe S, Ueki S (1980a) Potentiation of pressor and behavioural responses brain stimulation following bilateral olfactory bulbectomy in freely moving rats, *Brain Res Bull* **5:**711–16.

Kawasaki H, Watanabe S, Ueki S (1980b) Changes in blood pressure and heart rate following bilateral olfactory bulbectomy in rats, *Physiol Behav* **24:**51–6.

Kelly JP (1991) The olfactory bulbectomized rat as a model of depression: biochemical, behavioural and pharmacological correlates. PhD Thesis, National University of Ireland.

Kelly JP, Leonard BE (1992) An investiation of the hyperactive response of olfactory bulbectomized rats, *J Psychopharmacol Suppl* A13.

Kelly JP, Leonard BE (1994) The effect of tinaeptine and sertraline in three animal models of depression, *Neuropharmacology* **33:**1011–16.

Kennett GA, Gurzon G (1989) Mechanism of action of 8-OHDPAT as a rat model for human depression. In: Bevan P, Cools AR, Archer J, eds, *Behavioural Pharmacology of 5HT* (Erlbaum: Hillsdale, NJ) 225–9.

Kennett GA, Dickonson SL, Curzon G (1986) Enhancement of some 5-HT dependent behavioural responses following repeated immobilization in rats, *Brain Res* **330:**253–63.

King MG, Cairncross KD (1974) Effects of olfactory tract secretion on brain noradrenaline, corticosterone and conditioning in the rat, *Physiol Behav* **10:**347–53.

Komori T, Fujiwara R, Nomura J, Yokoyama MM (1991) Effects of restraint stress on plaque forming cell response in normal and olfactory bulbectomized mice, *Biol Psychiatry* **29:**695–8.

Kronfol Z, House JD (1989) Lymphocyte mitogenesis, immunoglobulin and complement levels in depressed patients and normal controls, *Acta Psychiat Scand* **80:**142–7.

Larsson K (1971) Impaired mating performance in male rats induced peripherally or centrally, *Brain Behav Evolut* **4:**463–71.

La Rue CG, Le Magneu J (1972) The olfactory control of meal pattern in rats, *Physiol Behav* **9:**817–21.

Leonard BE (1984) Pharmacology of new antidepressants, *Prog Neuropsychopharmacol Biol Psychiatry* **8:**97–108.

Leonard BE, Tuite M (1981) Anatomical, physiological and behavioural aspects of olfactory bulbectomy in the rat, *Int Rev Neurobiol* **22:**251–86.

Linkowski P, Vancauter E, Kerhofs M, Mendlewicz J (1994) Circadian hormonal profiles and sleep in affective disorders, *Neuropsychopharmacology* **10:**S16–21.

Lumia AR, Lebrowski AF, McGinnis MY (1987) Olfactory bulb removal decreases androgen receptor binding in amygdala and hypothalamus and disrupts masculine sexual behaviour, *Brain Res* **404:**121–6.

Maes M (1995) Evidence for an immune response in major depression—a review and hypothesis, *Prog Neuropsychopharmacol Biol Psychiatry* **19:**11–38.

Marks HE, Remley NR, Seago JD, Hastings DW (1971) Effects of bilateral lesions of the olfactory bulbs of rats on measures of learning and motivation, *Physiol Behav* **7:**1–6.

McKinney WT (1977) Biobehavioural models of depression in monkeys. In: Hanin I, Usdin E, eds, *Animal Models in Psychiatry and Neurology* (Oxford: Pergamon Press).

McKinney WJ, Young LD, Suomi ST, Davis JM (1973). Chlorprimazine treatment in disturbed monkeys, *Arch Gen Psychiatry* **29:**490–4.

McNamara MG, Kelly JP, Leonard BE (1995a) Effect of 8-OHDPAT in the olfactory bulbectomized rat model of depression, *J Serotonin Res* **2:**91–9.

McNamara MG, Kelly JP, Leonard BE (1995b) Some behavioural effects of methiothepin in the olfactory bulbectomised rat model of depression, *Med Sci Res* **23:**583–5.

McNamara MG, Kelly JP, Leonard BE (1996) Some behavioural and neurochemical effects of ipsirone in two rodent models of depression, *J Psychopharmacol* **10:**126–33.

Nemeroff CB, Krishnan KRR, Knight DL, Benjamin D, Meyerson LR (1990) Elevated plasma concentrations of alpha 1-acid glycoprotein, a putative endogenous inhibitor of 3-H-imipramine binding site in depressed patients, *Arch Gen Psychiatry* **47:**3337–40.

O'Connor WJ (1985) The olfactory bulbectomized rat model of depression: a physiological behavioural and neurochemical investigation. PhD Thesis,

National University of Ireland.

O'Connor WT, Leonard BE (1986) Behavioural and neuropharmacological properties of the dibenxepines, desipramine and lofepramine: studies in the olfactory bulbectomised rat model of depression, *Prog Neuropsychopharmacol Biol Psychiatry* **12:**41.

O'Connor WT, Earley B, Leonard BE (1985) Antidepressant properties of the triazolobenzodiazepines alprazolam and adinazolam: studies on the olfactory bulbectomized rat model of depression, *Br J Clin Pharmacol* **19:** 45S–6S.

O'Neill B, O'Connor WT, Leonard BE (1987) Depressed neutrophil phagocytosis in the rat following olfactory bulbectomy reversed by chronic desipramine treatment, *Med Sci Res* **15:**267–8.

O'Neill KA, Valentino D (1982) Escapability and generalization: effect on behavioural despair, *Eur J Pharmacol* **78:**379–80.

Overstreet DH, Russell RW, Crocker AD, Gillin JC, Janoskky DS (1988) Genetic and pharmacological models of cholinergic supersensitivity and affective disorders, *Experientia* **44:**465–72.

Papp M, Moryl E (1994) Antidepressant activity of non-competitive and competitive NMDA receptor anatagonists in a chronic mild stress model of depression, *Eur J Pharmacol* **263:**1–7.

Paul IA, Nowak G, Layer RT, Skolnic P (1994) Adaptation of the N-methyl-D-aspartate receptor complex following chronic antidepressant treatments, *J Pharmacol Exp Ther* **2:** 95–102.

Peroutka SJ, Snyder SA (1980) Long-term antidepressant treatment decreases spiroperidol-labelled serotonin receptor binding, *Science* **210:** 88–90.

Porsolt RD, Anton G, Blavet N, Jalfre M (1978) Behavioural despair in rats: a new model sensitive to antidepressant treatments, *Eur J Pharmacol* **47:**379–85.

Randrup A, Braestrup C (1977) Uptake inhibition of biogenic amines by newer antidepressant drugs: relevance to the dopamine hypothesis of depression, *Psychopharmacology* **53:**309–14.

Redmond AM (1995) The contribution of the serotonergic and glutamergic systems in animal models of depression. PhD thesis, National University of Ireland.

Redmond AM, Kelly JP, Leonard BE (1995) Effects of olfactory bulbectomy and chronic amitriptyline treatment on phencyclidine (PCP) induced hyperactivity, *Med Sci Res* **23:**351–2.

Richman CL, Gulkin R, Knoblock K (1972) Effects of bulbectomisation, strain and gentling on emotionality and exploratory behaviour in rats, *Physiol Behav* **8:**447–52.

Rutter M, Madge N (1976) *Cycles of Disadvantage* (Heinemann: London).

Sakurada T, Kitara K (1977) Effects of p-CPA on sleep in olfactory bulb lesioned rats, *Jpn J Pharmacol* **27:** 389–95.

Sakurada T, Shima K, Tadano T, Sakurada S, Kisara K (1976) Sleep wakefulness rhythms in the olfactory bulb lesioned rat, *Jpn J Pharmacol* **26:** 605–10.

Schuster RH, Rachlin H, Rom M, Berger D (1982) An animal model of dynamic social interaction: influence of isolation, competition and shock-induced aggression, *Aggress Behav* **8:**116–21.

Seligman MEP (1975) *Helplessness* (Freeman: San Francisco).

Serra G, Avgiolas V, Fadda F, Gessa GL (1979) Hyposensitivity of dopamine autoreceptors induced by chronic administration of tricyclic antidepressants, *Pharmacol Res Commun* **12:**619–24.

Sheard M (1969) The effect of p-chlorophenylamine on behaviour of rats: relation to brain serotonin and 5-hydroxyindoleacetic acid, *Brain Res* **15:**524–8.

Sieck MH (1972) The role of the olfactory system in avoidance learning and activity, *Physiol Behav* **9:**705–10.

Sieck MH, Gordon BL (1972) Selective olfactory bulb lesions: reactivity changes and avoidance learning in rats, *Physiol Behav* **9:**545–52.

Sieck MH, Baumback HD, Gordon BL, Tuner JF (1974) Changes in spontaneous, odor modulated and shock induced behavioural patterns following direct olfactory lesions, *Physiol Behav* **13:**427–39.

Smith CB, Hollingsworth PJ, Garcia-Sevilla JA, Zis AP (1983) Platelet alpha 2 adrenoceptors are decreased in number after antidepressant therapy, *Prog Neuropsychopharmacol Biol Psychiatry* **7:**241–7.

Song C, Leonard BE (1993) Effect of thymopeptides on the behaviour and some immunological responses in the olfactory bulbectomized rat, *Med Sci Res* **20:**929–30.

Song C, Leonard BE (1994) Serotonin reuptake inhibitors reverse the impairments in behaviour, neurotransmitter and immune functions in the olfactory bulbectomized rat, *Hum Psychopharmacol* **9:**135–46.

Song C, Leonard BE (1995) The effect of olfactory bulbectomy in the rat, alone or in combination with antidepressants and endogenous factors, on immune function, *Hum Psychopharmacol* **10:**7–18.

Song C, Killeen AA, Leonard BE (1994) Catalase, superoxidase-dismutase and glutathione peroxidase activity in neutrophils of sham operated and olfactory bulbectomized rats following chronic treatment with desipramine and lithium chloride, *Neuropsychobiology* **30:**24–8.

Sulser F, Vetulani J, Mobley PL (1978) Mode of action of antidepressant drugs, *Biochem Pharmacol* **27:**257–61.

Sweet WH, Cotzias GC, Seed J, Yakhover J (1949) Gastrointestinal haemorrhage, hyperglycaema, azoteamia, hypercholesteraemia and hypenatremia following lesions of the frontal lobe in man, *Ann Res Nerv Mental Disord* 795–822.

Thierry B, Steru L, Chermat R, Simon P (1984) Searching–waiting strategy: a candidate for an evolutionary model of depression? *Behav Neurol Biol* **41:**180–9.

Thomas JB (1973) Some behavioural effects of olfactory bulb damage in the rat, *J Comp Physiol Psychol* **83:**140–8.

Thorne BN, Aaron M, Lathan EE (1973) Effects of olfactory bulb ablation upon emotionality and muricidal behaviour in four rat strains, *J Comp Physiol Psychol* **34:**339–44.

Traskman-Benz L, Asberg M, Schalling D (1986) Serotonergic function and suicide behaviour in personality disorders, *Ann NY Acad Sci* **487:**168–74.

Tyler JL, Gorski RA (1980) Bulbectomy and sensitivity to estrogen: anatomical and functional specificity, *Physiol Behav* **24:**593–600.

Vagell ME, McGinnis MY, Possidente BP, Narasimhan VN, Lumia AR (1991) Olfactory bulbectomy increases basal suprachiasmatic cyclic AMP levels in male rats, *Brain Res Bull* **27:**838–42.

Van Riezen H, Leonard BE (1990) Effects of psychotropic drugs on the behaviour and neurochemistry of olfactory bulbectomized rats, *Pharmacol Ther* **47:**21–34.

Vergnes M, Karli P (1963) D'enclenchement du comportement, d'agression interspecifique. Rat et souris par ablation bilaterale des bulbes olfactifs, *CR Seance Soc Biol* **157:**1061–3.

Vergnes M, Kempf E (1982) Effect of hypothalamic injection of 5,7-dihydroxytryptamine on eliciation of mouse killing in rats, *Behav Brain Res* **5:**387–97.

Wettstein JG, Earley B, Junien JL (1995) Central nervous system pharmacology of neuropeptide Y, *J Pharmacol Ther* **65:**397–414.

Widerlov E, Helig M, Ekman R, Wahlestedt C (1988) Possible relationship between neuropeptide Y (NPY) and major depression: evidence from human and animal studies, *Nord J Psychiatry* **42:**131–7.

Willner P (1987) Sensitization to the actions of antidepressant drugs. In: Emmett-Oglesby MW, Goudie AJ, eds, *Tolerance and Sensitization to Psychoactive Drugs* (Human Press: Clifton, NJ) 116–24.

Willner P (1989) Towards a theory of serotonergic dysfunction in depression. In: Bevan P, Cools A, Archer T, eds, *Behavioural Pharmacology of 5-HT* (Erlbaum: Hillsdale, NJ) 157–78.

Willner P (1990) Animal models of depression: an overview, *Pharmacol Ther* **45:**425–55.

Willner P (1991) Animal models as simulators of depression, *TIPS* **12:** 131–6.

Willner P (1995) Animal models of depression: validity and applications. In: Gessa GL, Fratta W, Paris L, Serra G, eds, *Depression and Mania: From Neurobiology to Treatment* (Raven Press: New York) 19–42.

7

Disorder of synaptic homoeostasis as a cause of depression and a target for treatment

David G Grahame-Smith

Edelman evinced impatience with progress made in understanding the neuroscientific problem of brain development and function (Edelman, 1993). This led to his theory of neuronal group selection. I borrow his sentiments to state that it does not seem likely that neuroscientific research can lead to a substantial view of abnormal brain function in mental illness unless global theories and models based upon them are created to bridge clinical observations and experimental results obtained in neurobiological science. Such theories must be testable, allowing for an experimental approach to their investigation.

This leads to my hypothesis, which owes much to the work of Kandel on the neurobiology of memory (see Bailey et al, 1994) and to some of the concepts in Edelman's theory of neuronal group selection.

Hypothesis

Mood is dependent upon the numerical, structural and functional homoeostasis of sets of as yet indeterminate synapses. This homoeostasis is vulnerable to neurobiological forces created by the external and inner worlds of the individual, in which both physical and psychological factors usually combine. The strength of the processes maintaining this homoeostasis in synaptic function determine the regularity and appropriateness of mood.

Depressive illness results from a dysfunction of the processes maintaining homoeostasis in the function of the responsible sets of neurons. Recovery, whether spontaneous or treatment aided, signals re-establishment of the homoeostatic mechanism. Drugs and other modalities of treatment act to normalize the processes responsible for this homoeostasis in synaptic function.

In this hypothesis, the vulnerability of the individual lies in the security of the foundation of their homoeostatic processes, which themselves will be subject to genetic and epigenetic influences. The emphasis is that the function of this group of indeterminate synapses is under the control of a higher-order system and that synaptic function may be globally disturbed within that group. The primary abnormality would, then, not be in the group of synapses itself but in the system responsible for maintaining the homoeostasis of their function. This shifts the focus of the neurobiology of depression conceptually and experimentally.

I now examine whether this hypothesis is feasible.

The homoeostasis of synaptic function in respect of mood

First it is necessary to define the meaning of homoeostasis of synaptic function. I will assume that there is a discrete or diffuse synaptic map or maps in the brain upon which mood depends (see below).

Every synapse is in a highly dynamic state. Its function is to transmit signals from one neuron to another, and the processes involved are complex and subject to many levels of molecular control. Incoming signals must have some surety of both the likelihood and level of response. An action potential must lead through a cascade of biophysical and biochemical processes to an appropriate and predictable response, be it excitatory or inhibitory. This is the meaning of homoeostasis in this context.

Is the functional homoeostasis of an individual synapse the sole responsibility of that synapse or are there influences external to that synapse ensuring that its operation is appropriate? The evidence favours a combination of both. First, there is the dependence of future synaptic function on present activity (i.e. activity dependence). Second, there are neurotrophic mechanisms aiding the formation of functional synaptic connections and the homoeostasis of their function once they are established, many of which are probably as yet unknown. The neurobiological background for the hypothesis of disorder of synaptic homoeostasis and its relevance to mood is covered by many of the ideas propounded by Edelman. His theory of neuronal group selection has three phases (Figure 7.1):

1. *Primary repertoire.* This is a developmental phase during which primary neuronal wiring is laid down. This will be under genetic control and influenced by epigenetic factors operative in utero.
2. *Secondary repertoire.* As the neonate experiences the harsh world of extrauterine existence, its experiences will lay down neurobiological traces, and immediately the concept of memory has implications. The most objective impressive changes in this context are the adaptive (learning) responses occurring in the cortical visual system as the

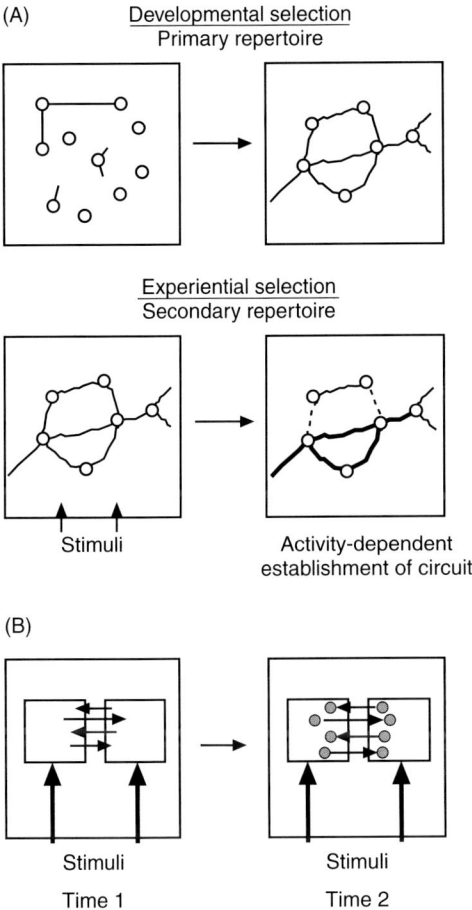

(A) Developmental selection
Primary repertoire

Experiential selection
Secondary repertoire

Stimuli   Activity-dependent
                          establishment of circuit

(B)

Stimuli   Stimuli

Time 1   Time 2

OVERLAPPING, INFILTRATING, MULTIUSER,
INTEGRATED, INDEPENDENT, MULTIACCESSIBLE

Figure 7.1

(A) Initially, Edelman conceives isolated neurons making rather random interconnections (top left). As development proceeds, many connections are made (the primary repertoire) (top right), some of which may be transient, because if they are not used they undo, and if they are used then, by the principle of activity dependence, they become established (the secondary repertoire) (bottom right). (B) Again, using the concept of activity dependence, groups of neurons make functional contacts, those contacts persisting if they prove to have functional worth (top boxes). This would lead to the development of groups of neurons (lower diagram), which, while functionally independent, overlap in respect of other groups, can be used in unison with a variety of other groups, and are accessible by many other groups. It is conceivable that, with such an organization, a specific group might be used in several different functions, depending on the team of neuronal groups in which it is playing. Adapted from Edelman (1993).

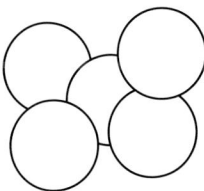

infant animal starts to categorize its visual experiences (see Rosenzweig, 1996). This results in new visual cortical maps. Edelman proposes that new synaptic connections are formed initially by random connection but are established by being used, i.e. activity dependence, a concept put forward by Hebb (1949).

3. *Re-entrant mapping.* The next level of complexity is produced by a process of re-entrant mapping. Groups of neurons with their synaptic connections are envisaged which connect through random synaptic contacts with other groups of neurons. This sets up a communication between groups and if activity of this group contact proves advantageous to the organism, it survives through activity dependence; hence the Darwinian analogy. It is possible to see that, contact having been made between two groups of neurons, such interconnection can grow by back and forth parallel communication to form a comprehensive neuronal group association. Edelman terms this process neuronal group selection, and it is potentially an extremely powerful tool for increasing the sophistication of brain function. Any one group of neurons may communicate with several other groups of neurons, singly or in concert, and thereby subserve several different functions acting in different partnerships.

Running through the whole of Edelman's theory is the neurobiological backbone of fluxile synaptogenesis and the epigenetic factors controlling it. A part of his hypothesis crucial to the discussion here is his assertion that there are no programmes, no sets of instructions, no overarching pedagogue explicitly controlling synaptic changes in neuronal systems. This allows for the development of brain function according to experience and the inner world, but at the same time implies a neurobiology which allows it all to happen in an ordered way. Should that neurobiology be disturbed, then serious defects in the adaptive capabilities of the brain result. The biological systems overseeing this organizational flux should be able to sense 'value' in the neuronal programmes set up by this process. By 'value' is meant the fitness of the changes appropriate for the adaptation needed. They must also enable it to occur by providing the wherewithall necessary for it to happen. Herein lies a paramount role for neuromodulating systems.

The task now is to apply the general ideas behind this theory to the understanding of depressive illness using the discipline of neurobiological science. To do this it is necessary to discuss some of the basic principles of synaptic and neuronal plasticity, before applying them to the phenomena of mood and its disorders.

Some fundamentals of synaptic structure and formation

The synapse is a very complicated structure and the process of its formation is still not well understood. Most interest in this has been on the part of those interested in the embryonic development of the nervous system, and many have used systems more simple to study than the central nervous system (e.g. the neuromuscular junction).

In our state of knowledge as it is, it is necessary to examine every source of information to help discover the mechanisms of synapse formation, continued survival and dissolution or death, to see what clues we can discover which might be relevant to synaptic homoeostasis and depression.

Haydon and Drapeau (1995) reviewed the early events in synaptogenesis. They identified three phases from contact to connection (Figure 7.2).

1. *Ready.* They propose that the essential release (presynaptic) and detection (postsynaptic) machinery is in place before contact.
2. *Set.* This rudimentary machinery has to be strengthened and further packaged later after contact. For instance, at the neuromuscular junction contact triggers a focusing of the acetylcholine receptors at the synaptic site. Basarsky et al (1994) examined synaptogenesis in primary cultures of neonatal hippocampal neurons. They found that as cultures progressed and synapses were formed, the distribution of synaptic markers such as rab 3a, synapsin 1 and synaptotagmin alters and these markers become restricted to varicose boutons in mature synaptic cultures. Studies of a special synapse in the leech (Haydon and Drapeau, 1995) have revealed a post-translational mechanism whereby receptors with different functions at the same postsynaptic site all sensitive to the neurotransmitter 5-HT can be

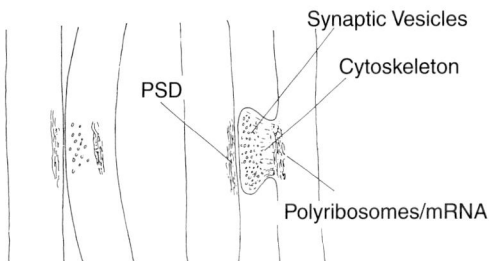

Synaptic Vesicles

Cytoskeleton

PSD

Polyribosomes/mRNA

Figure 7.2

Synaptogenesis. Here is depicted the formation of a synapse between two neural elements. It could be dendrodendritic, axoaxonic, or dendroaxonic. On the left are seen the two elements approaching contact. Already the fundamentals of the pre- and postsynaptic machinery are present. As the synapse forms, the postsynaptic density becomes more evident. Presynaptically, from rudimentary elements, there is increased production/clustering of synaptic vesicles. Cytoskeletal elements become more obvious, indicating ultrastructural organization, and polyribosomes cluster at the base of the presynaptic element. This illustrates the ready/steady/go concept discussed in the text.

selected during maturation of a synapse, thereby marking the functional phenotype of that synapse.

3. *Go.* In this phase, specificity is developed further by activity-dependent selection among previously formed synapses. In several systems there is evidence of the promiscuous formation of synapses during development which are then subject to selection by activity dependence. In other systems, target recognition and retrograde signalling determine the final assembly of the functional synaptic machinery.

Abraham and Bear (1996) recognize and give evidence for a state in which plasticity (i.e. change) does not actually occur but in which the threshold for induction of plasticity is lowered, making synaptic plasticity much easier to bring about under appropriate conditions (metaplasticity). The proposal is based upon the effect that prior synaptic activation has on the ease or difficulty of inducing long-term potentiation (LTP). Priming of a system or the induction of resistance to plasticity in it is another layer of control which could have important physiological and pathological implications, e.g. in the consideration of prior experience, current stress and the influence of hormonal status.

Our knowledge of the fundamental processes of synaptogenesis is rudimentary. Figure 7.2 is offered as a simplistic working model. It assumes that some of the components of a functional synapse are already present near or at the point of potential contact of the respective neuronal partners. Steward and his colleagues have been particularly active in promoting the exciting idea that the protein constituents of postsynaptic membranes are locally synthesized from mRNA which has been transported to the postsynaptic site (Steward et al, 1988). Polyribosomes are found beneath synaptic junctions in greatest density at the time of the initial formation of synaptic contact and probably play a role in the local synthesis of new proteins necessary for the establishment of the functional synapse. Südhof (1995) has comprehensively reviewed the cycle of the synaptic vesicle, an important synaptic component which has to be manufactured or imported for a new synapse to become functional. The number of protein components of synaptic vesicles which have to be synthesized for new synapses to function is astonishing. There are, at a minimum, 18 proteins integral to the vesicle, and over 10 associated with it. There are numerous synaptic plasma membrane proteins and a number of proteins reversibly associating with the plasma membrane. These are mentioned because synapsin, synaptophysin, synaptotagmins, and CAM kinases have all been suggested as putative markers for synaptogenesis and neuronal plasticity.

In Table 7.1 are shown some proteins thought to play a structural or functional role in synapse formation.

Table 7.1   Some proteins thought to play a part in synapse formation.

Proteins controlling gene expression
   Transcription factors, e.g. CREB
   Protein products of intermediate early genes, e.g. c-*fos*, c-*jun* (AP1)

Structural and functional proteins
   NCAMS and other adhesion molecules
   Synaptophysin and other synaptic vesicle proteins
   GAP43
   MAP-2
   Ion channel proteins
   Neurotrophic factors and their receptors

Synaptic and neuronal plasticity

Up- and downregulation of receptors, synthetic and metabolic enzymes, transporters and aspects of intracellular messenger cascades, as concomitants of neuroadaptation, is well accepted. The idea that synaptogenesis, neuronal growth and remodelling are still active in the adult brain is one that many are still not comfortable with. There is now abundant evidence that training or experience produces changes in the neurochemistry and anatomy of the adult cerebral cortex (see Rosenzweig, 1996) and that sensory and motor maps in adult mammals reorganize during recovery from CNS lesions. A number of examples is given to illustrate the relevant neurobiology of synaptic and neuronal plasticity.

Aplysia

The work of Kandel's group is particularly relevant (Bailey et al, 1994).

In the marine mollusc *Aplysia* there is a form of avoidance behaviour to noxious stimuli which involves a withdrawal reaction of the gill. *Aplysia* can learn by exposure to a noxious stimulus, usually electroshock, and shows its learning by a sensitization of its avoidance behaviour to a given stimulus. *Aplysia* has a simple nervous system, and one essential feature of it is a sensory neuron which synapses with a motor neuron controlling the withdrawal reflex of the gill. There are facilitatory neurons modulating synaptic traffic between the sensory neuron and the motor neuron, and 5-HT is an important neurotransmitter in these modulatory neurons. There are two different phases of memory formation in *Aplysia*: short-term and long-term. The short-term memory is dependent upon small but functionally important modifications of existing synaptic molecules, whereas long-term memory is dependent upon the production of new macromolecular components and synaptic remodelling. The opposite sequence of events occurs in the phenomenon of habituation, which implies that synaptic dissolution may occur.

In the production of long-term memory in *Aplysia*, 5-HT release from facilitatory neurons on to axoaxonal synapses of the sensory neurons acts to stimulate the production of cyclic AMP; this then stimulates a protein kinase A, which in turn phosphorylates transcription factors that act on promoters of the cAMP-inducible genes, expression of which results eventually in the production of a group of macromolecules known to be involved in synaptic remodelling. Later in this chapter, neural cell adhesion molecules (NCAMs) will be discussed, and it is worth noting that an NCAM specific to *Aplysia* (apCAM) is involved in the synaptic remodelling and sprouting observed during learning (Figure 7.3). Zhu et al (1995) have investigated how changes in the *Aplysia* cell adhesion molecule (apCAM) are related to the formation of new presynaptic varicosities by 5-HT. They found that 5-HT-induced formation of new sensory varicosities is directed by the presence of zones on the motor axon that are enriched in apCAM. 5-HT caused increased enrichment of apCAM levels at existing sensory varicosities contacting the motor neuron. Antibodies to apCAM blocked the long-term changes in synaptic efficacy and sensory neuron structure produced by 5-HT. 5-HT also causes a redistribution of

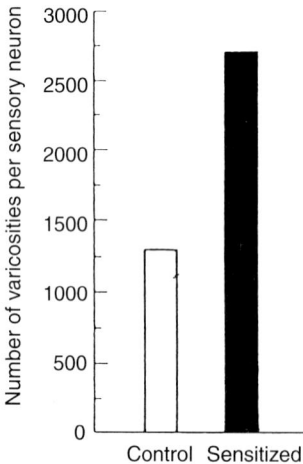

Figure 7.3

Changes occurring in the *Aplysia* nervous system during sensitization of the gill withdrawal reflex. Above are shown the number of varicosities per sensory neuron. They increase markedly during sensitization. Below is a diagram depicting the sprouting and increased synaptic contacts occurring between the sensory and motor neuron during sensitization. This illustrates the principle of axonal sprouting and synaptogenesis, partially under the control of 5-HT. Adapted from Kandel et al (1991).

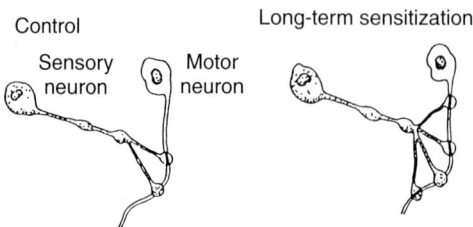

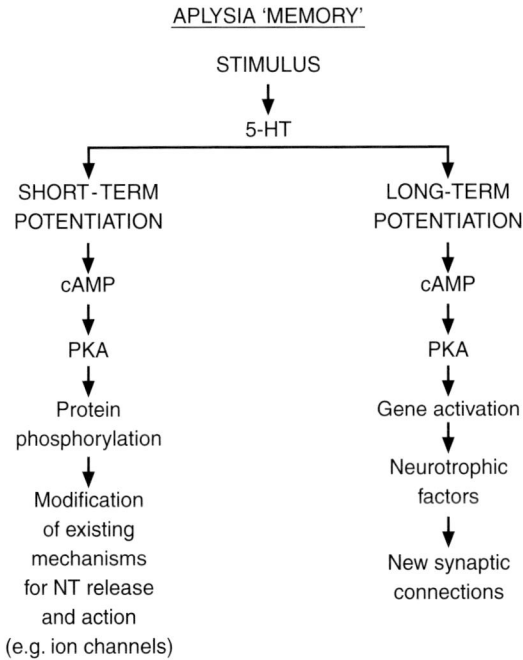

APLYSIA 'MEMORY'

STIMULUS

↓

5-HT

SHORT-TERM
POTENTIATION

↓

cAMP

↓

PKA

↓

Protein
phosphorylation

↓

Modification
of existing
mechanisms
for NT release
and action
(e.g. ion channels)

LONG-TERM
POTENTIATION

↓

cAMP

↓

PKA

↓

Gene activation

↓

Neurotrophic
factors

↓

New synaptic
connections

Figure 7.4

The cascades responsible for short-term and long-term memory in *Aplysia* are illustrated. The initial parts of the cascade are similar, a switch taking place after activation of protein kinase A (PKA). The short-term memory involves post-translational changes in existing molecules. The long-term memory requires gene activation, neurotrophic activity and structural alterations, i.e. neural plasticity and synaptic remodelling.

apCAM in a way expected to encourage sensory neuron growth and synapse formation. The broad features of the cascade involved are shown in Figure 7.4. This remodelling leads to alterations in the circuitry linking the sensory and motor neuron, such that during the process of sensitization there is a sprouting of the sensory axons and new synapse formation. Here in microcosm is a system illustrating the neurobiological phenomena involved in synaptic and neuronal plasticity. It is not unlikely that in broad conceptual terms, adaptive responses in the mammalian brain follow a similar course (Kandel and Hawkins, 1992).

Long-term potentiation

A repetitive train of stimuli delivered to one of the afferent pathways of the hippocampus produces a subsequent increase in the excitatory synaptic potential in the postsynaptic hippocampal neurons which, in vitro, lasts for hours, and in vivo in the rat for days or weeks. LTP requires coincident presynaptic and postsynaptic activity (Bliss and Lomo, 1973; Bliss and Collingridge, 1993).

LTP is an example of neuronal adaptation and plasticity which may be related to memory and learning. Its mechanism continues to receive much attention. There are at least two overlapping phases in the development of LTP, in principle not unlike the short- and long-term memory processes in *Aplysia*. First, the stimulation causes activation of postsynaptic NMDA receptors. This produces a rise in intracellular Ca^{2+} concentrations in the postsynaptic neuron. This results in activation of kinases and a range of post-translational biochemical changes which alter presynaptic and postsynaptic function in the short-term. Knock-out of the gene for the enzyme, protein kinase C, inhibits the establishment of LTP (Mayford et al, 1995). The initial transcriptional changes result in a biochemical cascade leading to changes in gene expression and subsequent protein synthesis which confer the much longer maintenance of LTP. The following is a brief account of some of the factors involved which are relevant to the later discussion.

Brain-derived neurotrophic factor (BDNF) mRNA expression is increased in dentate granule cells during LTP as a result of NMDA receptor stimulation (Dragunow et al, 1993) LTP elevates BDNF, NT-3, *trkB* and *trkC* gene expression, and expression of the intermediate early gene *zif*/268. These changes are dependent on NMDA receptor activation, show specific anatomical distribution and show variations in the time elapsed after induction of the LTP (Bramham et al, 1996). BDNF and NT-3 enhance synaptic strength at Schaffer collateral–CA1 synapses in the hippocampus through tyrosine kinase receptors (Kang and Schuman, 1995) and BDNF enhances LTP in hippocampal slices (Figurov et al, 1996). Protein synthesis is necessary for the maintenance of LTP (Otani and Abraham, 1989). NCAMs may play a part in the maintenance of LTP (Ronn et al, 1995). At some stage in the process of LTP it is likely that a diffusible messenger passes from postsynaptic to presynaptic neuron, being part of the mechanism for strengthening of the proximal synapse, e.g. nitric oxide (Schuman and Madison, 1994).

A strain of mice has been produced with a coding sequence deletion in the BDNF gene. Surprisingly, these mice survived but showed decreased LTP in the CA1 region of the hippocampus (Korte et al, 1995). There are now a number of studies showing structural changes in neuronal and synaptic architecture in the hippocampus accompanying LTP, suggesting that neuronal and synaptic remodelling form part of the biological process leading to the long-term changes in the physiological function of the hippocampus (Lipton and Kater, 1989; Geinisman et al, 1993; Edwards, 1995). Bliss et al (1983) showed that depletion of brain noradrenaline or 5-HT caused a decrease in the excitability of granule cells of the dentate gyrus and reduced the duration of LTP, and it is suggested that the monoamines may play a role in modulating the neuronal remodelling necessary for LTP.

Other situations in which neuronal and synaptic plasticity occur, apart from the developmental process, are seizures (Stewart et al, 1994; Yount et al, 1994; Lindefors et al, 1995) (including electroconvulsive shock), kindling (Geinisman et al, 1988), visual experience (Rosenzweig, 1996) and intracerebral lesions (Raisman and Field, 1990). In each of these examples there is evidence of either functional change (electrophysiological), immediate early and late gene expression for products likely to be involved in neural and synaptic plasticity, or structural changes proving plasticity. It is important to note that the neuronal plasticity observed in LTP, vision, kindling, seizures and lesioning occur in the adult brain, so that the phenomena we are considering are not confined to the young or developing brain. This is important in applying these concepts to depression.

Some molecules involved in neuronal and synaptic plasticity

Neural cell adhesion molecules (NCAMs)

If changes in neuronal connectivity are important for memory and for the hypothesis currently under examination, then the molecules involved in the adhesion of neuron to neuron would be expected to play a part. Their most obvious functional role is in establishing and stabilizing synaptic connections and configurations. However, if new synaptic connections are to be made and reconfiguration of synapses is to occur, then connectivity would have to be dismantled and re-established in a different format. Neural cell adhesion molecules (NCAMs) might be expected to play an important role in both the dissolution of old and formation of new synapses.

NCAMs are members of the general immunoglobulin-like family of cell adhesion molecules. They are particularly important during the embryonic development of the nervous system for the establishment of synaptic connections. For this role, NCAM undergoes post-translational modifications by polysialation of its extracellular domain. In the postnatal period this form of NCAM is widely dispersed throughout the brain. In the adult brain it is much less evident and is found in discrete areas undergoing continued synaptic rearrangement. There is also evidence that NCAMs may have other functionally active roles in promoting neural synaptic plasticity.

For instance, Keino-Masu et al (1996) suggest that an NCAM encoded by the DCC gene acts as a receptor for netrin-1, a chemoattractant or neuron guidance molecule for commissural neurons in spinal cord. There are at least two other major classes of molecules involved in neural cell adhesion which are also glycoproteins: these are the cadherins and the integrins, but little is known yet about their roles in the remodelling of neural connections in the adult brain.

Jorgensen (1995) has tried to devise an index of new neuronal sprouting and synaptic remodelling based upon NCAM function. He proposes that an elevated NCAM/D3 (SNAP-25) ratio may indicate synaptic remodelling. He has found no evidence for any change in this ratio in the post-mortem hippocampi of depressed patients. Ronn et al (1995) applied

NCAM antibodies to hippocampal slices and inhibited subsequent LTP induction in the CA1 region. They propose that NCAM is involved in the initial phase of LTP. There are several pieces of evidence that upregulation of polysialated-NCAM is associated with sprouting and synaptogenesis during the induction of LTP and other situations requiring strengthening of synaptic function in the hippocampus (Bahr, 1995).

Microtubular function and MAP-2

Microtubules are cylindrical polymers of α- and β-tubulin and a major component of the neuronal cytoskeleton. Associated with microtubules are a class of proteins known as microtubule-associated proteins (MAPs). It is believed that MAP-2 is involved in maintaining the structure of microtubulin. It does this by an interaction with the microtubular protein, which is functionally most effective when it is in the dephosphorylated state. Microtubular structure becomes unstable when MAP-2 is phosphorylated by MAP-2 protein kinase. Microtubular function is very important in maintaining neural structural integrity and in enabling remodelling, presumably by breaking down part of the neuronal cytoarchitecture and then building it afresh in a different form. Neurotransmission, which can modulate levels of intracellular cAMP and thereby affect the activity of MAP-2 kinases, can alter microtubular structure and promote remodelling.

MAP-2 is highly concentrated in dendrites and is almost absent from axons. This suggests that MAP-2 is important in determining the specific architecture of the neuron. MAP-2 mRNA is one of the mRNAs which is transported into dendrites of neurons undergoing differentiation in culture (see above; Steward et al, 1988). MAP-2 mRNA and protein has been used as an index of new dendritic growth, synaptogenesis and plasticity (Johnson and Jope, 1992).

Neurotrophic factors

The neurotrophic factors are extremely important for our understanding of the mechanisms of neuronal and synaptic plasticity. Lewin and Barde (1996), Segal and Greenberg (1996), Maness et al (1994), and Ibanez (1995) have reviewed many aspects of the neurotrophic factors. The first neurotrophic factor to be discovered was Nerve Growth Factor (NGF), and now the repertoire has expanded to include BDNF, Neurotrophin (NT-3), NT4/5 and Clinically Neurotrophic Factor (CNTF). These are synthesized and secreted by neurons and act upon a series of receptors specific for the individual neurotrophic factor. These receptors are tyrosine kinases (NGF-*trkA*, BDNF-*trkB*, NT-3-*trkC*, NT4/5-*trkA* and NT4/5-*trkB*). Stimulation of these receptors results in a series of intracellular signalling cascades which stimulate several post-transcriptional mechanisms, resulting in short-term synaptic strengthening (Levine et al, 1995).

Processes are also set in train which lead to gene expression resulting in long-term changes in neuronal morphology and connectivity.

Lo (1995) has reviewed the role of neurotrophic factors in synaptic plasticity. There is a link between electrical activity and neurotrophin mRNA levels in the hippocampus. There is also evidence that neurotrophins influence synaptic transmission and the intrinsic excitability of neurons both in the short- and long-term. One mechanism for this might involve activation of synapsins, which are proteins associated with synaptic vesicles and an important factor governing their release and regulating neurotransmitter-dependent neurotransmission. There is evidence in vivo and in vitro that a balance between glutamate (excitatory) and GABA (inhibitory) function determines the physiological levels of BDNF and NGF mRNAs in hippocampal neurons. If glutamate function predominates, then BDNF and NGF synthesis increase, and if GABA predominates, the reverse occurs. This provides a background for activity-dependent synaptic plasticity (Zafra et al, 1991). Bonhoeffer (1996) has reviewed the role of neurotrophins in the activity-dependent processes necessary for cortical connections and neuronal plasticity, not only in the developing brain but also in the adult brain (e.g. LTP).

The long-term effects of NGF on PC12 cells in culture are due to changes in gene expression, and it is interesting to note the array of changes produced, which involve voltage-gated sodium, calcium and potassium channels and neurotransmitter receptors such as nicotinic acetylcholine receptors.

This suggests that NGF stimulates a coherent programme of gene expression altering the phenotype of the neuron. Presumably the pre-existing neuronal phenotype will determine what genes are open to regulation, and this will differ with neuronal type.

This might suggest that if neurotrophic factors are involved in many of the situations (e.g. chronic antidepressant drug therapy) in which apparently isolated though apparently coherent up- and downregulation of receptors have been found, these changes may be the tip of an iceberg of a more widespread alteration of neuronal function and that more comprehensive changes in the neuronal functional phenotype may have been induced.

Functional aspects of BDNF

Several groups have studied the effect of BDNF on aspects of brain function or the effects of various brain stimuli on BDNF and other neurotrophic factors.

Neurotrophins can modulate stimulus-dependent activity in the adult cortex. Prakash et al (1996) quantified the effects of locally applied NGF and BDNF on the functional representation of a stimulated whisker in the barrel subdivision of the rat somatosensory cortex. BDNF caused a rapid and long-lasting decrease in the amplitude of the activity-dependent intrinsic signal, whereas NGF did the opposite. The chronic administration of electroconvulsive shock (ECS) or antidepressant drugs increases hippocampal BDNF mRNA and completely blocks the downregulation of BDNF mRNA in the hippocampus produced by restraint stress in rats (Nibuya et al, 1995). Intracortical BDNF infusions prevent p-chloro-amphetamine-induced loss of 5-HT neurons. It is believed that BDNF promotes the survival of 5-HT axons normally damaged by the toxin, and also causes the sprouting of mature uninjured 5-HT neurons (Mamounas et al, 1995). The expression of neurotrophins and their receptors can be altered by several brain insults, such as seizures, hypoglycaemia, ischaemia and trauma. Many of these insults probably act through glutamate release. It is suggested that increased neurotrophic activity might protect against neuronal damage and enable repair (Lindvall et al, 1994).

5-HT and its interrelationship with neurotrophism

Molecules used for communication in mature nervous systems also play important roles in development, maintenance and plasticity of individual neurons. Lipton and Kater (1989) reviewed the evidence that neurotransmitters, in addition to trans-synaptic signalling, can induce a spectrum of effects on neuronal cytoarchitecture, ranging from neurite sprouting to dendritic pruning and even cell death. Such profound alterations presumably constitute part of the normal ongoing modelling of the nervous system, disorders of which will contribute to pathology. Much of the work reviewed refers to developing nervous systems but the mechanisms and concepts are likely to apply in adult neuronal plasticity. In the context of developing the current hypothesis, they cite the case of the snail *Helisoma*. When embryonic *Helisoma* are depleted of 5-HT they grow into adults in which the neurons expected to be influenced by 5-HT (a group known as B15) show abnormal morphology and connectivity. Lipton and Kater conclude that in this instance 5-HT has modulating effects on cytoarchitecture. It is not clear whether such neurotransmitter action is exerted as a specific and direct modulating role on cytoarchitecture or whether alterations in synaptic function brought about by 5-HT depletion alter synaptic survival by reducing activity-dependent consolidation. Evidence is given for acetylcholine, dopamine, GABA, glutamate, noradrenaline, somatostatin and vasoactive intestinal peptide modulating neuronal plasticity in diverse systems.

There is evidence that $5\text{-HT}_{2A/2C}$ receptors play a modulatory role in learning and therefore perhaps in the neural plasticity underlying it. Agonists of these receptors enhance, and antagonists retard, the learning abilities of animals in certain tasks. LSD, methylene dioxymethamphetamine (MDMA) and quipazine were amongst the 5-HT 'agonists' that enhanced, while 8-hydroxy-2-(di-*n*-propylamino)-tetralin (8-OH-DPAT) either had no effect or retarded learning. 5-HT antagonists such as ritanserin retarded learning, while ketanserin and spiperone had no effect (Harvey, 1995).

Azmitia and his colleagues (Nishi et al, 1996) believe that the effect of 5-HT on neuronal plasticity may be mediated through 5-HT_{1A} receptors which are negatively coupled to adenylate cyclase and generally hyperpolarize membranes by opening K^+ channels. Synaptophysin and MAP-2 in the cortex and hippocampus of the adult rat are reduced by 5-HT depletion with PCA treatment and the loss of synaptophysin is reversed by in vivo treatment with ipsapirone, a 5-HT_{1A} agonist. In culture, a 5-HT_{1A} agonist enhances the maturation of neurons containing choline acetyltransferase (i.e. cholinergic neurons). Morphometric analysis was used to study the effect of ipsapirone on synaptophysin immunoreactivity in hippocampal neuronal cell cultures from 18–19-day-old rat fetuses. Ipsapirone caused an increase in synaptophysin in mainly the cell bodies of the neurons.

Although this evidence is a mixture of adult, fetal, cell culture and non-vertebrate data, it does provide a precedence for a neurotrophic role for 5-HT.

Jacobs and Azmitia (1992) reviewed the structure and function of the serotonin (5-HT) system. They made a number of interesting points. The extensive distribution of 5-HT neurons and terminals and their regular electrical activity is well suited to the establishment of activity-dependent synaptic contacts throughout the brain. They propose that 5-HT is involved in the verification and consolidation of interneuronal contacts, i.e. it exerts a categorizing neurotrophic effect. The non-synaptic disposition of many 5-HT terminals, as emphasized by Descarries and his colleagues over the years (Seguela et al, 1989), suggests a distant non-synaptic role for much of the 5-HT released, which would fit with a paracrine neurotrophic function. Whitaker-Azmitia et al (1996) and Emerit et al (1992) have also reviewed the mounting evidence that 5-HT function is of importance in brain development, playing a role in the organization of neuronal connectivity.

Branchek (1995) reviewed the 5-HT receptors ($5\text{-HT}_{4,6,7}$) which are linked to increased production of cAMP and which are therefore candidates for transducing 5-HT signals to gene expression. This does not exclude similar effects of 5-HT receptors linked to the phosphatidylinositol breakdown pathway (e.g. 5-HT_2), or indeed 5-HT_3 receptors linked to ion channels which could bring about lasting change through a Ca^{2+}-mediated cascade.

Siuciak et al (1996) found that intracerebral infusion of BDNF near the raphe nuclei increased 5-HT synthesis and/or turnover. These changes might be due to alterations in the firing of 5-HT neurons (Celada et al, 1996). These findings indicate some functional link between 5-HT and BDNF.

Biochemical cellular cascades controlling gene expression

If neurotransmission and neuromodulation cause long-lasting synaptic and neuronal plasticity, there must be intracellular signalling cascades to transmit signals from neuronal cell membranes to the genome, thereby influencing gene expression.

The scheme common to neurotransmitter and neuromodulater control of neuronal gene expression is shown in Figure 7.5, and it provides a background upon which one can build an understanding of the processes by which the brain adapts to experience, by which both short-term and long-term homoeostasis of neural programmes is controlled, and by which the long-term effects of psychotropic drugs and electro-convulsive therapy (ECT) can be explained. There are many details not yet understood but the essentials are in place. There are a number of 'ripple' mechanisms. For instance, antidepressants have been shown to cause the expression of BDNF mRNA. Assuming that this translates into protein, the BDNF will be secreted by neurons and will act on *trkB* receptors on its own and other neurons to activate a further specific cascade to cause gene expression in relation to its short-term and long-term neurotrophic effects.

Some of the details of these cascades and their relationship to neural plasticity in the context of mental illness are described by Duman et al (1994). They have proposed that the genetic abnormality leading to psychiatric illness may not be the production of abnormal gene products but instead an abnormality in genetic programmes regulating normal gene products, resulting in abnormal neural plasticity and adaptability. For instance, they propose that stress results in sustained increased firing of noradrenergic neurons in the locus coereleus, with increased release of noradrenaline. Activation of adenylate cyclase through β-adrenoreceptors linked to G proteins produces increased levels of cAMP. cAMP activates kinases, which modify by phosphorylation the structure and activity of certain protein factors modulating the expression of immediate early genes. These genes, such as c-*fos* and c-*jun*, produce proteins which act to orchestrate further regulated gene expression, such as the upregulation of the enzyme tyrosine hydroxylase, which is the rate-limiting step in the synthesis of noradrenaline. There are similar changes in respect of 5-HT and its controlling enzyme, tryptophan hydroxylase. The neuron is, then, into the mode of long-term adaptive plastic change. Before that occurs, the cAMP-activated kinases may also cause short-term adaptive changes by altering existing proteins such as enzymes and ion channels to produce acutely altered responses to stimuli. Both the short- and long-term responses attempt to adapt the nervous system to maintain homoeostasis as best they can to the demands of changed circumstances. There is an extraordinary similarity between *Aplysia* and the rat brain in respect of the steps in the cAMP signalling cascade to gene

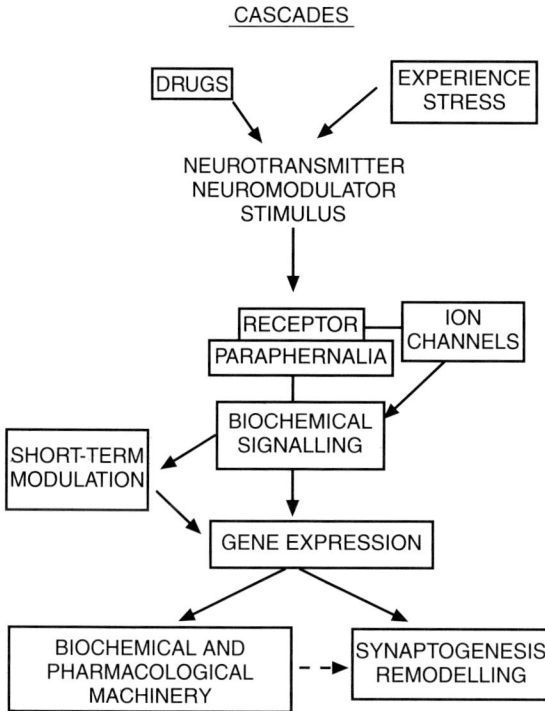

CASCADES

```
        ┌───────┐              ┌──────────────┐
        │ DRUGS │              │  EXPERIENCE  │
        └───────┘              │    STRESS    │
             ╲              ╱  └──────────────┘
              ╲            ╱
        NEUROTRANSMITTER
        NEUROMODULATOR
           STIMULUS
               │
               ▼
        ┌──────────┐   ┌──────────┐
        │ RECEPTOR │───│   ION    │
        │PARAPHERNALIA│ │ CHANNELS │
        └──────────┘   └──────────┘
               │
               ▼
        ┌────────────┐
        │ BIOCHEMICAL│
        │  SIGNALLING│
        └────────────┘
   ┌────────────┐
   │ SHORT-TERM │
   │ MODULATION │
   └────────────┘
               │
               ▼
        ┌────────────────┐
        │ GENE EXPRESSION│
        └────────────────┘
         ╱              ╲
┌──────────────────┐  ┌──────────────┐
│ BIOCHEMICAL AND  │  │SYNAPTOGENESIS│
│ PHARMACOLOGICAL  │--▶│ REMODELLING │
│   MACHINERY      │  │              │
└──────────────────┘  └──────────────┘
```

Figure 7.5

The general features of the cascades underlying synaptogenesis and neuronal remodelling resulting from the actions of drugs and also experience and stress. In broad principle, it also applies to the processes of memory. The similarities with Figure 7.4 can be noted.

expression and subsequent neural and synaptic plasticity (see Figures 7.4 and 7.5) (Duman et al, 1994).

Drugs of addiction produce long-term neuronal adaptive responses in the central nervous system which are responsible for the addictive state with its manifestations of craving and associated drug-seeking behaviour, withdrawal syndromes and tolerance. Biochemical cascades leading to similar changes in gene expression are involved (Nestler et al, 1993; Hyman and Nestler, 1996).

The mood–memory analogy

How might the neurobiology underlying memory (which has been emphasized in the preceding discussion) be related to the neurobiology of mood? Figure 7.6 is a convenient diagram on which to base a discussion of the matter. I do not imply that the two mental functions depend upon the same brain functions but I do wish to draw an analogy between the two in respect of the principles of the neurobiological mechanisms involved.

Memory has an afferent arm, i.e. experience. Although memory installation can be conscious or explicit (exam learning), in everyday experience much of it is implicit, and occurs without active attention (today's weather). Memory recall is the efferent arm and, again, although it is sometimes actively conscious, much of it is not.

Mood is similar. In everyday affairs mood is undoubtedly affected through the afferent arm of experience and, depending on the depth of experience, happiness or sadness ensuing from it may last a shorter or longer time (like memory). Again, in everyday affairs people with normal mood do not go around thinking, 'Am I happy, am I sad?' Mood is normally largely a subconscious phenomenon. Bend your mind to it though, or undergo psychometric testing of mood, and, like memory, it is there and can be quantified. Just as memory pervades all that we think, so does mood (normal and abnormal). Loss of memory in Alzheimer's disease is catastrophic, and so is severe endogenous depression.

This analysis is made to try and encompass mood and memory within the framework of a similar neurobiology, i.e. one of changing synaptic

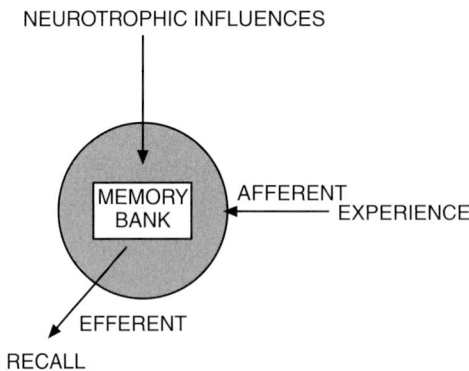

NEUROTROPHIC INFLUENCES

MEMORY BANK AFFERENT EXPERIENCE

EFFERENT

RECALL

Figure 7.6

A speculative attempt to straightjacket mood and memory into the same format to illustrate some of the superficial similarities and to allow the application of the same neurobiological principles to both (see text for further explanation).

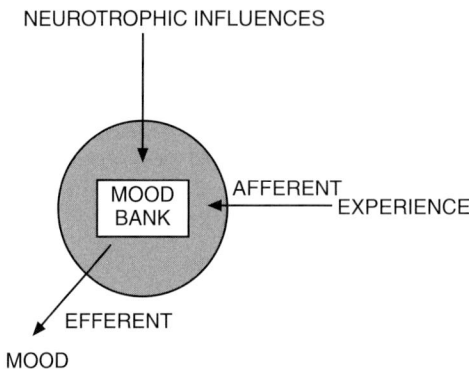

NEUROTROPHIC INFLUENCES

MOOD BANK AFFERENT EXPERIENCE

EFFERENT

MOOD

and neuronal function with homoeostatic mechanisms coping with necessary stimuli for change and adaptation. Using this analogy, I suggest that, as for memory, normal mood is maintained in the face of experience (stress) by neurobiological adaptive responses occurring in the relevant neuronal groups. The biology of the system has to be in balance to allow this adaptation to occur. If it is not, then mood will stray outside normal confines.

If indeed this analysis has some credence, then we can draw analogies between the neurobiology of memory and that of mood. There are three principles to emphasize at the outset:

1. There would always be an acute ongoing importance for synaptic function in mood (i.e. short-term processes) and then a long-term controlling process, on the background of which the short-term process occurs.
2. Both short-term and long-term modulation would depend upon neurotransmitter or neuromodulator action, and this would be signalled intracellularly by biochemical transducing cascades, the long-term effects involving gene expression and subsequent synaptic and neuronal plasticity.
3. While neurotransmitter or neuromodulator activity will have important activity-dependent effects in maintaining and encouraging synaptic homoeostasis, there would be a necessary role for neurotrophic influences to provide long-term homoeostasis of synaptic connections and function and associated neuronal plasticity.

Depression

Can we find any features of the clinical illness of depression or of its treatment which might fit this neurobiological model?

Table 7.2 shows features of the illness of depression which indicate a complex process, generally rather slow moving, programmed into the biology of the individual, often dependent upon a genetic background, and often triggered, at least in its early years, by stress, indicating a stress–biology link. There is a chronology to it, with mainly adult age of onset, an episodic natural history with the time between episodes often decreasing as the patient gets older, sometimes a seasonality (seasonal affective disorder), a diurnality of mood, and chronobiological circadian phase shifts in biological rhythms, including disturbed sleep patterns (Goodwin and Jamison, 1990; Gelder et al, 1996).

The genetic predisposition would be explained as follows. One would propose that an inherited genetic defect produces a defective biology in that individual which leads to a disorder of neuronal adaptation when the individual is faced with stress. Clinically, this results in a vulnerability to

Table 7.2   Clinical features of depression suggesting a complex programmed abnormality in gene expression.

Genetics
Natural history
Age of onset
Stress: life-events
Episodicity
Seasonality
Diurnality
Cycling
Biological rhythms
Sleep

depression associated with adverse life-events. Because of this predisposition, depression is frequently recurrent. The associated abnormalities in glucocorticoid control mechanisms are difficult to place in this context. The clear adverse effects of corticosteroids on the stability of neuronal connections and synaptic function makes their excess potentially a bad thing for the neurobiology of depression. Female sex hormones are important in synaptic and neuronal plasticity, and changes in their levels could contribute to the maternity blues, post-puerperal depression, premenstrual tension and the induction of depression by the contraceptive pill.

Antidepressant treatments

Most drugs, including the antidepressants, are developed on the basis of an acute pharmacology. All the antidepressants, the tricyclics, serotonin selective reuptake inhibitors (SSRIs), monoamine oxidase (MAO) inhibitors and the newer drugs such as nefazadone and trazodone have been developed on the basis of their acute actions on noradrenaline and/or 5-HT function. Antidepressant treatments take 2–4 weeks to produce a clear therapeutic effect. If they are discontinued quickly after recovery, relapse is more likely than if they are continued for several months.

ECT twice weekly requires three or four treatments before a therapeutic response is seen. Improvement then tends to occur quickly with subsequent treatments. Antidepressant drugs must be continued for a period of months after a course of ECT to decrease the likelihood of relapse, suggesting a synergy between ECT and antidepressants (Gelder et al, 1996).

These phenomena suggest something more than an acute simple and transient point-to-point pharmacological effect of the treatments. Why does it take so long for the therapeutic effect to appear, when, as can be safely predicted from what is known of the pharmacokinetics and pharmacodynamics of many of these drugs, monoamine function in the brain is affected within hours or less of the first dose? The delay in onset of the therapeutic

Table 7.3   Effects of repeated long-term administration of antidepressant drugs, MAO inhibitors, ECS and lithium upon 5-HT-mediated behavioural functions in the rat and mouse (Grahame-Smith, 1992).

	8-OH-DPAT rat 5-HT Behavioural (5-HT$_{1A}$ receptor)	8-OH-DPAT Hypothermia in the rat (5-HT$_{1A}$ receptor)	8-OH-DPAT Hypothermia in the mouse (5-HT$_{1A}$ receptor)	Mouse head-twitch (5-HT$_2$ receptor)
Anti-depressant drugs	All aspects decreased	Attenuated	Attenuated	Decreased
MAO inhibitors	All aspects decreased	Attenuated	Attenuated	Decreased
ECS	Stereotypes decreased Locomotor activity increased?	Attenuated	Attenuated	Increased
Lithium	All aspects increased	No change	Attenuated	Decreased

effect and the need for continuation of these treatments for a time suggests other than a simple continuation of an acute pharmacology. Because of this, my colleagues and I over several years have been studying the chronic adaptive pharmacology of antidepressant drugs, ECT (using repeated ECS in rats as an analogy) and also lithium, as it too may owe its therapeutic effects to an adaptive and chronic pharmacology.

A summary of our accumulated findings on the effects of antidepressant drugs, ECS and lithium on 5-HT function in rats and mice is given in Table 7.3.

Because of the methodological problems, it has been very difficult to mirror these animal experiments in humans and study the chronic adaptive pharmacology of tricyclic antidepressants in patients with depression. However, a number of clinical studies have been done in which 5-HT agonist strategies have been used to stimulate neuroendocrine function in normal people and patients with depression taking antidepressant drugs, and these do suggest neuroadaptive changes (Siever et al, 1983; Meltzer 1984, Meltzer et al, 1984; Glue et al, 1986; Price et al, 1988, 1989, 1990; Cowen et al, 1989; Sargent et al, 1997a,b).

Taking the animal studies and clinical studies together, two clear conclusions can be drawn:

1. Antidepressant drugs and ECS when administered to rats and mice cause delayed effects to various aspects of 5-HT function. Human

studies point to delayed effects of the treatments on monoamine function, particularly 5-HT.

2. Changes occur in the number of many neurotransmitter receptor binding sites and also signalling cascades during chronic antidepressant drug treatment, ECS and lithium treatment but so far these changes do not form a coherent explanation for the functional behavioural changes observed. It is the search for a coherent explanation which has prompted the formulation of the current hypothesis.

The application of molecular neurobiology

Recently we have employed the technique of differential display (Livesey and Hunt, 1996) to investigate the effects of SSRIs on gene expression in the brain of the rat.

Differential display of mRNA is a method which allows the systematic comparison of mRNAs expressed in tissues. If, for instance, one wishes to find out whether an antidepressant drug causes an adaptive response in the rat brain, then one compares the pattern of brain mRNA from treated rats with that from untreated rats. This is done by extracting the total mRNA from the tissue of interest (brain). This mRNA then undergoes reverse transcription to produce single-stranded cDNA. This cDNA is then amplified by polymerase chain reaction (PCR) incorporating ^{33}P-a-dATP. The amplified cDNA is then separated on a standard DNA sequencing gel and the products visualized by autoradiography (Livesey and Hunt, 1996). If a band of interest is found on the gel, then the cDNA is eluted, amplified by PCR and radioactively labelled. It can then be used as a probe in in situ hybridization or to probe northern blots to confirm differential expression, and cloned to discover its sequence and identity.

We have applied this technique to examine the differential expression of mRNAs in the brain during long-term treatment of rats with two SSRIs, fluoxetine and paroxetine. So far we have identified one band which appears to be upregulated by both drugs, though this conclusion has yet to be definitively verified. This band of mRNA codes for a NCAM which has homology with the so-called DCC gene (Pierceall et al, 1994; Keino-Masu et al, 1996). Several other differentially expressed bands common to both drugs have been identified and are being analysed.

This has suggested to us that SSRIs, through an action on 5-HT function, are causing the expression of a NCAM which is involved in synaptic plasticity, and we speculate that this is part of an orchestrated and coherent multiple gene expression response which results in synaptic/neuronal remodelling and re-establishment of synaptic homoeostasis.

Chronic, but not acute, treatment with fluoxetine or desmethylimipramine results in an increased expression of c-*fos* in the frontal cortex and hippocampus in response to the 5-HT$_{2A}$ agonist, 1-(2,5-dimethoxy-4-iodophenyl) 2-amino propene hydrochloride (DOI) (Tilakaratne et al, 1995). However, repeated ECS in the rat, while producing an increase in head-twitches in response to DOI, did not cause an increase in c-*fos* expression (Moorman et al, 1996). This is in contrast to the effects of chronic lithium administration, which greatly increases c-*fos* expression in response to DOI in the pyriform cortex (Leslie et al, 1993).

Chronic, but not acute, administration of antidepressant drugs increases the expression of the cAMP response element binding protein (CREB) mRNA in rat hippocampus. This is associated with evidence that CREB is functionally active. CREB could induce changes in gene expression, e.g. in BDNF mRNA expression, which might lead to neuronal and synaptic plasticity. Nibuya et al (1995) have shown that several antidepressant drugs administered chronically, but not acutely, increase BDNF and *trkB* mRNA in hippocampus and block the downregulation of BDNF mRNA in the hippocampus produced by restraint stress.

Repeated ECS given in a way that enhances 5-HT behavioural functions causes an upregulation of BDNF mRNA in hippocampus (Zëtterstrom et al, 1997). Pei et al (1997b) have shown that repeated ECS increases the expression of the MAP-2 mRNA in the dentate gyrus, and Moorman et al (1997) have shown that chronic SSRIs increase MAP-2 protein expression in various areas of cerebral cortex of the rat. MAP-2 protein is more or less restricted to dendrites. These findings suggest that, in certain areas of the brain, both SSRIs and repeated ECS promote dendritic sprouting and perhaps new synapse formation. Pei et al (1997a) have shown that repeated ECS causes selective changes in the expression of certain types of K$^+$ channel in hippocampus. For instance, chronic ECS causes an increase in the expression of the mRNA for the Kv4.2 channel, whereas the mRNA for this channel is decreased 6 h after one acute shock, a decrease not present 6 h after chronic shock. This is a clear example of adaptation in which early exposure to a treatment produces a different response to that in the adapted state. It is of interest that the Kv4.2 channel, like MAP-2, is mainly confined to dendrites, confirming that there may be dendritic growth.

We have also investigated the effects of acute and chronic ECS and the chronic effects of SSRIs on synaptophysin. Synaptophysin-like immunoreactivity measured by immunocytochemistry was increased in the ventromedial hypothalamus, amygdala and reuniens nucleus by chronic ECS (Moorman and Leslie, 1997). There were some small but significant increases in synaptophysin-LI measured by ELISA in response to SSRIs in certain brain areas.

Gradually, therefore, evidence is accumulating to suggest that antidepressant drugs and ECS (*vis-à-vis* ECT) are acting acutely via neurotransmitter function (i.e. antidepressant drugs via noradrenaline and/or 5-HT, and ECT probably via excitatory neurotransmitters such as glutamate) to set in train neurotrophic and synaptotrophic processes which result in the formation or strengthening of synapses and neuronal networks necessary for the maintenance of normal mood.

When one considers the incredibly intricate, widespread and heavy innervation of many areas of the brain with a web of fine 5-HT projection fibres and considers also the fact that many of these fibres do not form close synapses with target cells, implying that they release 5-HT in a 'cloud', it does seem that 5-HT is set up to act as a neuromodulatory system, one action of which might be to maintain synaptic homoeostasis by trophic effects. There is also evidence that many noradrenergic nerve terminals may not form strict synaptic contacts, again suggesting a neuromodulatory (paracrine) role for the noradrenergic system. This is intriguing considering the antidepressant effects of specific noradrenergic uptake-blocking drugs.

Conclusion

Translated into neurobiological terms (in contrast to its earlier neurophilosophical tone), the hypothesis proposed at the beginning of this paper is evolving as follows.

Mood, like memory, is dependent upon the numerical, structural and functional homoeostasis of sets of indeterminate synapses. This synaptic homoeostasis depends upon the normal physiological functioning of a neurotrophic system which involves the neuromodulatory/paracrine neurotrophic function of monoamines, particularly 5-HT but perhaps also noradrenaline, which may act, along with other factors, to release neurotrophic factors such as BDNF. 5-HT can have important short-term effects through biochemical cascades altering post-translational factors to maintain immediate synaptic function, but also has longer-term synaptotrophic and neurotrophic effects involving concerted and coherent changes in gene expression. The neurotrophic factors are also involved in enabling longer-term neurotrophic effects similarly through gene expression promoting synaptic cohesion and fine neuronal integrity.

This homoeostatic system is finely balanced and vulnerable to dysfunction. First, it must be able to react to external mental and physical stresses so as to maintain normality of function in those synapses involved in mood control. Adverse stress would be expected to require a balanced neuropsychobiological reaction to maintain psychological coping, as otherwise the organism might 'give up', which would be disadvantageous to survival (in Darwinian terms). Mood would be an essential factor in this coping reaction, as drive is a major component of mood and 'value of self' a component of the need to survive. These components of a neurotrophic system are under a higher-order control system involving many autonomic factors, including systemic endocrine function (e.g. thryoid, adrenal cortex, sex hormones) and other humoral and neuronal factors modulating the activity of monoamine systems, such as the regularity of firing of the raphe 5-HT neurons. The total system is genetically programmed, possibly through a hierarchical coordination of its parts. It is proposed that there is a genetic component which confers a phenotype having the neurobiological properties of the brain of a patient with depressive illness, producing the many chronological features of that illness, and therefore narrowing the genetic factor to a genetic programme controlling the security of this homoeostatic system over the span of the patient's lifetime. The genetically determined vulnerabliity would involve an inability to mount the neurobiological defence to stress (a neuroadaptive response) which normally allows psychological coping. Total breakdown of the homoeostatic system may occur such that recognizable stress may not be necessary to produce the antithesis of neurotrophism, which results in apparently unprovoked depressive illness.

Antidepressant treatment will act to enable the brain prone to a dysfunction of synaptic homoeostasis to mount an adequate synaptotrophic and neurotrophic response, whether this be through the monoamine systems, as with the current antidepressant drugs, or through excitatory neurotransmitter systems, perhaps secondarily affecting monoamine and/or neurotrophic factor function, as seems likely with ECT. It is clear that, in many patients, episodes of depression resolve naturally, and endogenous reversal of dysfunction or neurobiological coping mechanisms eventually cut in to terminate the illness. This self-limiting property of many medical pathologies is a common physical phenomenon and there is no reason why it should not also apply to the neurobiology of depressive illness. However, as with medical illness, the self-limiting property does not always manifest itself and serious destructive pathology may then ensue, as it may in depression. What of lithium? I would suggest that, whatever its point-to-point molecular target, it acts to promote the continued background neurotrophic effects of 5-HT, thereby reducing vulnerability to synaptic homoeostatic dysfunction and acting as a prophylactic in affective disorder.

References

Abraham WC, Bear MF (1996) Metaplasticity: the plasticity of synaptic plasticity, *Trends Neurosci* **19:**126–30.

Bahr BA (1995) Long-term hippocampal slices: a model system for investigating synaptic mechanisms and pathologic processes, *J Neurosci Res* **42:**294–305.

Bailey CH, Alberini C, Ghirardi M, Kandel ER (1994) Molecular and structural changes underlying long-term memory storage in Aplysia. In: Stjarne L, Greengard P, Griller SE, Hokfelt TGM, Ottoson DR, eds, *Molecular and Cellular Mechanisms of Neurotransmitter Release* (Raven Press: New York) 529–44.

Basarsky TA, Parpura V, Haydon PG (1994) Hippocampal synaptogenesis in cell culture: developmental time course of synapse formation, calcium influx, and synaptic protein distribution, *J Neurosci* **14:**6402–11.

Bliss TV, Collingridge GL (1993) A synaptic model of memory: long-term potentiation in the hippocampus, *Nature* **361**:31–9.

Bliss TV, Lomo T (1973) Long-lasting potentiation of synaptic transmission in the dentate area of the anaesthetized rabbit following stimulation of the perforant path, *J Physiol Lond* **232**:331–56.

Bliss TV, Goddard GV, Riives M (1983) Reduction of long-term potentiation in the dentate gyrus of the rat following selective depletion of monoamines, *J Physiol Lond* **334**: 475–91.

Bonhoeffer T (1996) Neurotrophins and activity-dependent development of the neocortex, *Curr Opin Neurobiol* **6**:119–26.

Bramham CR, Southard T, Sarvey JM, Herkenham M, Brady LS (1996) Unilateral LTP triggers bilateral increases in hippocampal neurotrophin and trk receptor mRNA expression in behaving rats: evidence for interhemispheric communication, *J Comp Neurol* **368**:371–82.

Branchek TA (1995) $5-HT_4$, $5-HT_6$, $5-HT_7$; molecular pharmacology of adenylate cyclase stimulating receptors, *Semin Neurosci* **7**:375–82.

Celada P, Siuciak JA, Tran TM, Altar CA, Tepper JM (1996) Local infusion of brain-derived neurotrophic factor modifies the firing pattern of dorsal raphe serotonergic neurons, *Brain Res* **712**:293–8.

Cowen PJ, McCance SL, Cohen PR, Julier DL (1989) Lithium increases 5-HT-mediated neuroendocrine responses in tricyclic resistant depression, *Psychopharmacol (Berl)* **99**: 230–2.

Dragunow M, Beilharz E, Mason B, Lawlor P, Abraham W, Gluckman P (1993) Brain-derived neurotrophic factor expression after long-term potentiation, *Neurosci Lett* **160**:232–6.

Duman RS, Heninger GR, Nestler EJ (1994) Molecular psychiatry. Adaptations of receptor-coupled signal transduction pathways underlying stress- and drug-induced neural plasticity, *J Nerv Ment Dis* **182**:692–700.

Edelman GM (1993) Neural Darwinism: selection and reentrant signaling in higher brain function, *Neuron* **10**:115–25.

Edwards FA (1995) Anatomy and electrophysiology of fast central synapses lead to a structural model for long-term potentiation, *Physiol Rev* **75**:759–87.

Emerit MB, Riad M, Hamon M (1992) Trophic effects of neurotransmitters during brain maturation, *Biol Neonate* **62**:193–201.

Figurov A, Pozzo-Miller LD, Olafsson P, Wang T, Lu B (1996) Regulation of synaptic responses to high-frequency stimulation and LTP by neurotrophins in the hippocampus, *Nature* **381**: 706–9.

Geinisman Y, Morrell F, de Toledo Morrell L (1988) Remodeling of synaptic architecture during hippocampal 'kindling', *Proc Natl Acad Sci USA* **85**:3260–4.

Geinisman Y, de Toledo Morrell L, Morrell F, Heller RE, Rossi M, Parshall RF (1993) Structural synaptic correlate of long-term potentiation: formation of axospinous synapses with multiple, completely partitioned transmission zones, *Hippocampus* **3**:435–45.

Gelder M, Gath D, Mayou R, Cowen P (1996) *Oxford Textbook of Psychiatry*, 3rd edn (Oxford University Press: Oxford and New York).

Glue PW, Cowen PJ, Nutt DJ, Kolakowska T, Grahame Smith DG (1986) The effect of lithium on 5-HT-mediated neuroendocrine responses and platelet 5-HT receptors, *Psychopharmacology (Berl)* **90**: 398–402.

Goodwin FK, Jamison KR (1990) *Manic-depressive Illness* (Oxford University Press: New York).

Grahame-Smith DG (1992) Serotonin in affective disorders, *Int Clin Psychopharmacol* **6:**5–13.

Harvey JA (1995) Serotonergic regulation of associative learning, *Behav Brain Res* **73:**47–50.

Haydon PG, Drapeau P (1995) From contact to connection: early events during synaptogenesis, *Trends Neurosci* **18:**196–201.

Hebb DO (1949) *The Organisation of Behaviour: a Neuropsychological Study* (Wiley: New York).

Hyman SE, Nestler EJ (1996) Initiation and adaptation: a paradigm for understanding psychotropic drug action, *Am J Psychiatry* **153:**151–62.

Ibanez CF (1995) Neurotrophic factors: from structure–function studies to designing effective therapeutics, *Trends Biotechnol* **13:**217–27.

Jacobs BL, Azmitia EC (1992) Structure and function of the brain serotonin system, *Physiol Rev* **72:**165–229.

Johnson GV, Jope RS (1992) The role of microtubule-associated protein 2 (MAP-2) in neuronal growth, plasticity, and degeneration, *J Neurosci Res* **33:**505–12.

Jorgensen OS (1995) Neural cell adhesion molecule (NCAM) as a quantitative marker in synaptic remodeling, *Neurochem Res* **20:**533–47.

Kandel ER, Schwartz JH, Jessell TM (1991) *Principles of Neural Science,* 3rd edn (Elsevier: New York).

Kandel ER, Hawkins RD (1992) The biological basis of learning and individuality, *Sci Am* **267:**53–60.

Kang H, Schuman EM (1995) Long-lasting neurotrophin-induced enhancement of synaptic transmission in the adult hippocampus, *Science* **267:** 1658–62.

Keino-Masu K, Masu M, Hinck L et al (1996) Deleted in colorectal cancer (DCC) encodes a netrin receptor, *Cell* **87:**175–85.

Korte M, Carroll P, Wolf E, Brem G, Thoenen H, Bonhoeffer T (1995) Hippocampal long-term potentiation is impaired in mice lacking brain-derived neurotrophic factor, *Proc Natl Acad Sci USA* **92:**8856–60.

Leslie RA, Moorman JM, Grahame Smith DG (1993) Lithium enhances 5-HT2A receptor-mediated c-fos expression in rat cerebral cortex, *Neuroreport* **5:**241–4.

Levine ES, Dreyfus CF, Black IB, Plummer MR (1995) Brain-derived neurotrophic factor rapidly enhances synaptic transmission in hippocampal neurons via postsynaptic tyrosine kinase receptors, *Proc Natl Acad Sci USA* **92:**8074–7.

Lewin GR, Barde YA (1996) Physiology of the neurotrophins, *Annu Rev Neurosci* **19:**289–317.

Lindefors N, Brodin E, Metsis M (1995) Spatiotemporal selective effects on brain-derived neurotrophic factor and trkB messenger RNA in rat hippocampus by electroconvulsive shock, *Neuroscience* **65:**661–70.

Lindvall O, Kokaia Z, Bengzon J, Elmer E, Kokaia M (1994) Neurotrophins and brain insults, *Trends Neurosci* **17:**490–6.

Lipton SA, Kater SB (1989) Neurotransmitter regulation of neuronal outgrowth, plasticity and survival, *Trends Neurosci* **12:**265–70.

Livesey FJ, Hunt SP (1996) Identifying changes in gene expression in the nervous system: mRNA differential display, *Trends Neurosci* **19:**84–8.

Lo DC (1995) Neurotrophic factors and synaptic plasticity, *Neuron* **15:**979–81.

Mamounas LA, Blue ME, Siuciak JA, Altar CA (1995) Brain-derived neurotrophic factor promotes the survival and sprouting of serotonergic axons in rat brain, *J Neurosci* **15:**7929–39.

Maness LM, Kastin AJ, Weber JT, Banks WA, Beckman BS, Zadina JE (1994) The neurotrophins and their receptors: structure, function, and neuropathology, *Neurosci Biobehav Rev* **18:**143–59.

Mayford M, Abel T, Kandel ER (1995) Transgenic approaches to cognition, *Curr Opin Neurobiol* **5**:141–8.

Meltzer HY (1984) Serotonergic function in the affective disorders: the effect of antidepressants and lithium on the 5-hydroxytryptophan-induced increase in serum cortisol, *Ann NY Acad Sci* **430**:115–37.

Meltzer HY, Lowy M, Robertson A, Goodnick P, Perline R (1984) Effect of 5-hydroxytryptophan on serum cortisol levels in major affective disorders. III. Effect of antidepressants and lithium carbonate, *Arch Gen Psychiatry* **41**:391–7.

Moorman JM, Leslie RA (1997) The effect of serotonin selective reuptake inhibitors on synaptophysin immunoreactive-like protein in rat brain. In preparation.

Moorman JM, Grahame-Smith DG, Smith SE, Leslie RA (1996) Chronic electroconvulsive shock enhances 5-HT$_2$ receptor-mediated head shakes but not brain c-fos induction, *Neuropharmacology* **35**:303–13.

Moorman JM, Leslie RA, Pei Q (1997) The effect of chronic treatment of rats with serotonin selective uptake inhibitors on MAP2 immuno-reactive like protein in rat brain. In preparation.

Nestler EJ, Hope BT, Widnell KL (1993) Drug addiction: a model for the molecular basis of neural plasticity, *Neuron* **11**:995–1006.

Nibuya M, Morinobu S, Duman RS (1995) Regulation of BDNF and trkB mRNA in rat brain by chronic electroconvulsive seizure and antidepressant drug treatments, *J Neurosci* **15**: 7539–47.

Nishi M, Whitakerazmitia PM, Azmitia EC (1996) Enhanced synaptophysin immunoreactivity in rat hippocampal culture by 5-HT1A agonist, S100b, and corticosteroid receptor agonists, *Synapse* **23**:1–9.

Otani S, Abraham WC (1989) Inhibition of protein synthesis in the dentate gyrus, but not the entorhinal cortex, blocks maintenance of long-term potentiation in rats, *Neurosci Lett* **106**:175–80.

Pei Q, Burnett PWJ, Grahame-Smith DG, Zetterstrom TSC (1997a) Differential effects of acute and chronic electroconvulsive shock on the abundance of messenger RNAs for voltage-dependent potassium channel subunits in the rat brain, *Neuroscience* **78**:343–50.

Pei Q, Burnett PWJ, Zetterstrom TSC (1997b) Changes in mRNA abundance of microtubule-associated protein in rat brain following electroconvulsive shock (submitted).

Pierceall WE, Reale MA, Candia AF, Wright CV, Cho KR, Fearon ER (1994) Expression of a homologue of the deleted colorectal cancer (DCC) gene in the nervous system of developong Xenopus embryos, *Dev Biol* **166**:654–65.

Prakash N, Cohen-Cory S, Frostig RD (1996) Rapid and opposite effects of BDNF and NGF on the functional organization of the adult cortex *in vivo*, *Nature* **381**:702–6.

Price LH, Charney DS, Delgado PL, Heninger GR (1990) Lithium and serotonin function: implications for the serotonin hypothesis of depression. *Psychopharmacology* **100**:3–12.

Price LH, Charney DS, Delgado PL, Anderson GM, Heninger GR (1989) Effects of desipramine and fluvoxamine treatment on the prolactin response to tryptophan. Serotonergic function and the mechanism of antidepressant action. *Arch Gen Psychiatry* **46**:625–31.

Price LH, Charney DS, Heninger GR (1988) Effects of trazodone treatment on serotonergic function in depressed patients, *Psychiatr Res* **24**:165–75.

Raisman G, Field PM (1990) Synapse formation in the adult brain after lesions and after transplantation of embryonic tissue, *J Exp Biol* **153**: 277–87.

Ronn LCB, Bock E, Linnemann D,

Jahnsen H (1995) NCAM-antibodies modulate induction of long-term potentiation in rat hippocampal CA1, *Brain Res* **677:**145–51.

Rosenzweig MR (1996) Aspects of the search for neural mechanisms of memory, *Annu Rev Psychol* **47:**1–32.

Sargent P, Williamson DJ, Cowen PJ (1997a) Brain 5-HT neurotransmission during paroxetine treatment, *Br J Psychol* (in press).

Sargent P, Williamson DJ, Pearson G, Odontiadis J, Cowen PJ (1997b) Effect of paroxetine and nefazodone on 5-HT$_{1A}$ receptor sensitivity, *Psychopharmacology* (in press).

Schuman EM, Madison DV (1994) Nitric oxide and synaptic function, *Annu Rev Neurosci* **17:**153–83.

Segal RA, Greenberg ME (1996) Intracellular signaling pathways activated by neurotrophic factors, *Annu Rev Neurosci* **19:**463–89.

Seguela P, Watkins KC, Descarries L (1989) Ultrastructural relationships of serotonin axon terminals in the cerebral cortex of the adult rat, *J Comp Neurol* **289:**129–42.

Siever LJ, Uhde TW, Jimerson DC et al (1983) Clinical studies of monoamine receptors in the affective disorders and receptor changes with antidepressant treatment, *Prog Neuropsychopharmacol Biol Psychiatry* **7:**249–61.

Siuciak JA, Boylan C, Fritsche M, Altar CA, Lindsay RM (1996) BDNF increases monoaminergic activity in rat brain following intracerebroventricular or intraparenchymal administration, *Brain Res* **710:**11–20.

Steward O, Davis L, Dotti C, Phillips LL, Rao A, Banker G (1988) Protein synthesis and processing in cytoplasmic microdomains beneath postsynaptic sites on CNS neurons. A mechanism for establishing and maintaining a mosaic postsynaptic receptive surface, *Mol Neurobiol* **2:**227–61.

Stewart C, Jeffery K, Reid I (1994) LTP-like synaptic efficacy changes following electroconvulsive stimulation, *Neuroreport* **5:**1041–4.

Südhof TC (1995) The synaptic vesicle cycle: a cascade of protein–protein interactions, *Nature* **375:**645–53.

Tilakaratne N, Yang ZL, Friedman E (1995) Chronic fluoxetine or desmethylimipramine treatment alters 5-HT2 receptor mediated c-fos gene expression, *Eur J Pharmacol Mol Pharmacol* **290:**263–6.

Whitaker-Azmitia PM, Druse M, Walker P, Lauder JM (1996) Serotonin as a developmental signal, *Behav Brain Res* **73:**19–29.

Yount GL, Ponsalle P, White JD (1994) Pentylenetetrazole-induced seizures stimulate transcription of early and late response genes, *Mol Brain Res* **21:**219–24.

Zafra F, Castren E, Thoenen H, Lindholm D (1991) Interplay between glutamate and gamma-aminobutyric acid transmitter systems in the physiological regulation of brain-derived neurotrophic factor and nerve growth factor synthesis in hippocampal neurons, *Proc Natl Acad Sci USA* **88:**10 037–41.

Zëtterstrom TSC, Pei Q, Grahame-Smith DG (1997) The effect of acute and chronic electroconvulsive shock on the abundance of messenger RNA for brain derived neurotrophic factor in the rat brain. In preparation.

Zhu H, Wu F, Schacher S (1995) Changes in expression and distribution of Aplysia cell adhesion molecules can influence synapse formation and elimination in vitro, *J Neurosci* **15:**4173–83.

8

Norepinephrine and serotonin in antidepressant action: evidence from neurotransmitter depletion studies

Pedro L Delgado, Francisco A Moreno, Rebecca Potter and Alan J Gelenberg

Historical perspective

While our understanding of the clinical aspects of the phenomenology, prevalence, course and treatment of major depression has advanced considerably, the neurobiological basis of depression remains unknown. For many years, the neurobiological basis of depression has been conceptually linked to the mechanism of antidepressant action. Most models have been largely two-dimensional, postulating either an actual or a functional deficiency in various monoamine neuronal systems (Bunney and Davis, 1965; Schildkraut, 1965; Coppen, 1967; Charney et al, 1981). Even though strong support exists for the role of monoamine systems in the therapeutic mechanism of antidepressant action (Heninger and Charney, 1987), intensive investigation has failed to find convincing evidence of a primary dysfunction of a specific monoamine system in patients with major depression (Delgado, 1995).

Past theories of the mechanism of action of antidepressants have focused on *restoration* of monoamine neurotransmitter function. However, more recent thinking has begun to focus on the adaptive changes induced in brain areas and circuits modulated by monoaminergic systems or within monoamine neurons themselves (Blier and de Montigny, 1994; Hyman and Nestler, 1996). It is now clear that the *rate of synthesis* of a wide variety of neuronal components, including receptors, ion channels, monoamine synthetic enzymes and G proteins, and the very rate of growth of neurons themselves, is under the tonic control of receptor-mediated interactions (Hyman and Nestler, 1996). These observations raise the possibility that the long-term effects of increased synaptic levels of monoamines may include a cascade of time-dependent changes that are responsible for the therapeutic effects of antidepressant drugs.

In part, progress in understanding the relationship of monoamine systems to therapeutic antidepressant responses and the neurobiology of depression has been inhibited by the lack of direct methods for testing hypotheses in humans. The advent of neurotransmitter depletion paradigms has begun to provide new data relevant to these issues. This chapter will review data from neurotransmitter depletion studies relevant to the role of the noradrenergic and serotonergic systems in the mechanisms underlying the therapeutic effects of antidepressants and the neurobiological basis of depression.

5-HT and norepinephrine in antidepressant action and the neurobiology of depression

Antidepressant action

Electrophysiologic studies in laboratory animals have suggested that most antidepressant drugs and electroconvulsive therapy (ECT) enhance neurotransmission across 5-HT synapses after long-term, but not after short-term, administration (de Montigny and Blier, 1984; Blier et al, 1990). Antidepressants appear to cause an enhancement of 5-HT function through different mechanisms. Tricyclic antidepressant drugs and ECT appear to sensitize postsynaptic neurons to the effects of 5-HT, while monoamine oxidase inhibitors (MAOIs) enhance availability of 5-HT, and 5-HT reuptake inhibitors desensitize presynaptic inhibitory 5-HT autoreceptors (Blier et al, 1990).

While some antidepressants alter levels of 5-HT_2 receptors, the most consistent finding in regard to the long-term effects of drugs that are known to have antidepressant properties is either a decrease in the sensitivity of presynaptic 5-HT_{1A} receptors or a sensitization of postsynaptic 5-HT_{1A} responses (Blier et al, 1990; Blier and de Montigny, 1994). Additional, 5-HT_{1A} receptors and 5-HT_{2A} receptors located on the same cells have been shown to antagonize each others' actions (Berendsen and Broekkamp, 1990). Hence, drugs such as nefazodone, which are 5-HT_{2A} receptor antagonists, have been hypothesized to mediate their antidepressant effects through an indirect increase in 5-HT_{1A} receptor function by blocking 5-HT_{2A} receptors. Blier and de Montigny (1994) have suggested that all drugs that have antidepressant effects in humans mediate their action through a final common pathway involving either directly or indirectly enhancing 5-HT_{1A} receptor-mediated neurotransmission in the hippocampus and/or frontal cortex.

There are also data suggesting an important role for noradrenergic mechanisms in antidepressant action. Many studies have identified decreased β-adrenoreceptor binding as well as increases in α_1- and decreases in α_2-adrenoreceptor binding after chronic antidepressant treatment (Sulser et al, 1977; Delgado et al, 1991a). Some authors have theorized that some noradrenergic antidepressants cause their therapeutic effects by enhancing excitatory and blocking inhibitory effects of norepinephrine (NE) on 5-HT neurons (Haddjeri et al, 1995; de Boer, 1996). Noradrenergic neurons maintain a dual modulation of 5-HT neurons. They tonically activate 5-HT neurotransmission through the effect of NE on excitatory α_1-adrenoreceptors located on 5-HT cell bodies (Mongeau et al, 1993). Noradrenergic neurons also tonically inhibit 5-HT release through inhibitory α_2-heteroreceptors located on 5-HT terminals. By enhancing postsynaptic α_1-adrenoreceptor activity, and/or blocking α_2-heteroreceptors, drugs can increase the firing rate of 5-HT neurons and the synaptic release of 5-HT (de Boer, 1996).

Thus, the preclinical and clinical data converge to suggest that enhancement of 5-HT neurotransmission may be a central component in the mechanism of antidepressant action. While noradrenergic mechanisms appear to be involved, the exact role of NE is less clear. What has not been addressed is why enhancement of 5-HT neurotransmission may be antidepressant, since treatments that acutely increase 5-HT availability do not lead to an immediate antidepressant effect (Heninger and Charney, 1987).

Neurobiology of depression

The deficiency hypotheses of the neurobiology of depression have been only partially supported. Deficiencies of NE or 5-HT or their metabolites in cerebrospinal fluid (CSF), blood or urine have not been consistently demonstrated in depressed patients, despite intensive efforts to do so (Charney et al, 1981; Heninger and Charney, 1987; Maes and Meltzer, 1995). A subgroup of depressed patients with a history of impulsivity or suicide do appear to have decreased CSF levels of the primary metabolite of 5-HT, 5-hydroxyindole acetic acid (5-HIAA); however, decreased CSF 5-HIAA is found in other diagnoses as well (Åsberg et al, 1987; Roy et al, 1990). Further evidence against the deficiency hypotheses is the lack of immediate efficacy of antidepressant treatments, given the rapid effect of various antidepressants in increasing synaptic NE and 5-HT concentrations.

Other data suggest that presynaptic 5-HT dysfunction may be present in some depressed patients. These data include the findings of lower plasma tryptophan (TRP) levels, reduced CSF 5-HIAA, decreased platelet 5-HT uptake, a blunted prolactin response to TRP and fenfluramine, as well as the preliminary report of a blunted hypothermic response to the 5-HT$_{1A}$ partial agonist ipsapirone (see Maes and Meltzer (1995) for comprehensive review).

Studies of NE function in affective disorder patients have suggested that postsynaptic abnormalities may be present in some depressed patients. Measures of postsynaptic noradrenergic activity suggest that there is a functional blunting of the responsiveness of hypothalamic

α_1- and α_2-adrenergic receptors and lymphocyte β-adrenergic receptors (Schatzberg and Schildkraut, 1995). Overall, it appears that differences in postsynaptic α_1- and α_2-adrenergic receptor function may exist in some depressed patients.

Unfortunately, it is impossible to know from the current literature whether the 'abnormalities' identified are in any way related to the etiology or symptoms of depression, or secondary characteristics related to some other primary abnormalities. Many of the differences identified could be secondary to non-specific differences between patients and controls such as differences in cortisol levels, weight loss, nutritional status, or prior exposure to psychotropic drugs. The most striking characteristic of the available literature is the failure to find consistent findings. Most investigators have taken this to mean that depression may involve several different etiologic subgroups (Schatzberg and Schildkraut, 1995).

Neurotransmitter depletion studies

Neurotransmitter depletion studies in humans provide an experimental paradigm for challenging our hypotheses regarding the role of monoamine systems in mental illness and the underlying pharmacologic mechanisms of therapeutic drug action. By transiently reducing the level of a particular neurotransmitter, we can begin to understand its importance to these processes in a living person.

5-HT depletion

The first clinical studies to use neurotransmitter depletion to investigate the role of monoamines in antidepressant action utilized p-chlorophenylalanine (PCPA). PCPA inhibits the rate-limiting step in 5-HT synthesis, inhibiting the enzyme tryptophan hydroxylase. In non-psychiatric patients with 5-HT-producing carcinoid tumors, PCPA acutely leads to a variety of behavioral changes, ranging from lethargy, irritability, anxiety and depression to psychosis, although many subjects demonstrate little behavioral change (Carpenter, 1970).

Two clinical studies published in the 1970s reported that PCPA appeared to rapidly reverse the antidepressant effects of both imipramine (Shopsin et al, 1975) and tranylcypromine (Shopsin et al, 1976) in patients with major depression. These studies demonstrated that antidepressant-remitted depressed patients experienced a depressive relapse within 24 h of the initiation of PCPA treatment, with a return to their remitted state again within 24 h of discontinuation of PCPA treatment (Shopsin et al, 1975, 1976). The Shopsin et al studies were highly criticized because of the lack of a placebo control and the small number of patients tested. No direct attempts at replication have been reported.

Most current research on 5-HT depletion has utilized depletion of tryptophan (TRP). The synthesis of 5-HT is entirely dependent on the availability of its precursor amino acid, TRP (Rose et al, 1954; Young et al, 1969, 1971, 1985, 1989; Fernstrom, 1977; Curzon, 1979, 1981; Delgado et al, 1989; Moja et al, 1989). Since TRP is an essential amino acid, mammals are dependent on dietary sources for it (Rose et al, 1954; Harper et al, 1970). Data now exist which suggest that dietary TRP depletion may specifically reduce brain 5-HT function (Moir and Eccleston, 1968; Fernstrom and Hirsch, 1975; Fernstrom, 1977; Curzon, 1979, 1981; Moja et al, 1989). Both increases (Moir and Eccleston, 1968; Fernstrom and Hirsch, 1975) and decreases (Curzon, 1979, 1981; Young et al, 1985, 1989; Delgado et al, 1989; Moja et al, 1989) in dietary TRP intake lead to corresponding changes in brain TRP, 5-HT and 5-HIAA levels in laboratory animals. Ingestion of TRP-free amino acid mixtures in vervet monkeys decreases plasma TRP and CSF TRP and 5-HIAA, with no change in CSF tyrosine, homovanillic acid (HVA) or 3-methoxy-4-hydroxyphenylethylene glycol (MHPG) (Young et al, 1989). Moreover, ingestion of TRP-free amino acid mixtures in laboratory animals leads to extremely rapid changes in both plasma TRP and brain 5-HT, with maximal reductions of brain 5-HT occurring within 2 h of ingestion of the TRP-free mixture (Moja et al, 1989; Young et al, 1989; Heslop et al, personal communication). A TRP-free amino acid drink causes a decrease in the release of brain 5-HT as measured by microdialysis (Heslop et al, personal communication; Artigas et al, 1993).

Dietary TRP depletion alters behavioral indices of 5-HT function in laboratory animals. It increases pain sensitivity (Lytle et al, 1975; Messing et al, 1976), acoustic startle (Walters et al, 1979) and muricidal behavior (Gibbons et al, 1979; Vergnes and Kempf, 1981), reducing rapid eye movement (REM) sleep (Moja et al, 1979) and enhancing the prolactin (PRL) response to 5-hydroxytryptophan (5-HTP) infusion (Clemens et al, 1980). The effects of TRP depletion on pain sensitivity, acoustic startle, muricidal behavior and REM sleep are reversed by TRP repletion, probably through alterations in central 5-HT function (Lytle et al, 1975; Messing et al, 1976; Gibbons et al, 1979; Walters et al, 1979; Vergnes and Kempf, 1981).

TRP-free or low-TRP diets administered to healthy humans cause reductions of plasma TRP levels (Rose et al, 1954; Young et al, 1969, 1971; Delgado et al, 1989; Moja et al, 1989). Maintenance for up to 1 month on such diets has been reported without serious medical or psychological consequences (Rose et al, 1954). Diets which reduce the plasma ratio of TRP to large neutral amino acids (LNAA) increase the competition of LNAA with TRP for passage across the blood–brain barrier, resulting in decreased levels of CSF 5-HIAA (Perez-Cruet et al, 1974). A 200 mg/day, low-TRP diet for 8 days enhanced the prolactin response to intravenous L-TRP in healthy humans, suggesting the development of postsynaptic 5-HT receptor supersensitivity (Delgado et al, 1989).

Reduction in plasma TRP of up to 80% can also be accomplished in 3–5 h by administering an oral TRP-free amino acid solution, which induces hepatic protein synthesis and thereby depletes available plasma TRP (Harper et al, 1970; Young et al, 1985, 1989; Moja et al, 1989). Such an amino acid mixture reduces night-time melatonin secretion in healthy subjects (Zimmerman et al, 1992) and the rate of serotonin synthesis in the brains of healthy subjects as measured by positron emission tomography (PET) (Nishizawa et al, 1997).

A variety of modifications of the TRP depletion paradigm have been used in clinical studies. These include administration of a TRP-free, 102.5-g 15-amino acid drink compared with a 2.3-g TRP-supplemented, 104.8-g 16-amino acid drink (Young et al, 1985); a 24-h low-TRP/low-protein diet followed by a TRP-free, 102.5-g 15-amino acid drink compared with a TRP-supplemented diet and drink (Delgado et al, 1990); and a TRP-free, 102.5-g 15-amino acid drink compared with a TRP-free, 25-g 15-amino acid drink (Krahn et al, 1996). Each of these paradigms has been shown to cause significant biological effects in humans. Table 8.1 describes the effects of some of these combinations on plasma free TRP and total TRP. Due to the simplicity of design, ability to maintain excellent double-blind conditions, and similarity of effect seen in clinical studies, most investigators, including our group, are now using the original amino acid mixture described by Young without the low-TRP diet (Young et al, 1985).

Weltzin et al (1994) suggest that while the 2.3-g TRP-supplemented drink leads to an increase in plasma total and free TRP levels, it causes a decrease in the TRP/LNAA ratio. Because TRP competes with LNAAs for

Table 8.1   Alternative TRP depletion paradigms.

Test Condition	Variation	Tryptophan	Baseline (µg/ml)	Five hours (µg/ml)	% Change
Depletion	Diet + Drink (N = 11)	Total	9.9 ± 2.3	1.5 ± 0.8	−85
		Free	1.9 ± 0.4	0.4 ± 0.2	−79
	Drink Alone (N = 15)	Total	9.9 ± 3.3	2.0 ± 2.0	−80
		Free	2.1 ± 0.4	0.8 ± 0.3	−62
Control	Diet + TRP Supplemented drink (N = 11)	Total	10.1 ± 2.0	23.1 ± 8.9	+230
		Free	2.0 ± 0.6	5.6 ± 2.6	+300
	Quarter-strength drink (N = 15)	Total	9.5 ± 1.0	5.4 ± 1.7	−44
		Free	2.0 ± 0.5	1.4 ± 0.5	−30

a common carrier across the blood–brain barrier, this might have some effect on decreasing brain TRP and 5-HT. However, behavioral effects have not been noted with the 2.3-g TRP-supplemented control test (Young et al, 1985; Smith et al, 1987; Delgado et al, 1990, 1991b, 1994; Benkelfat et al, 1994).

TRP depletion in antidepressant-remitted depressed patients

The first published study using the TRP depletion method in depressed patients (Delgado et al, 1990) showed that 67% of 21 depressed patients having achieved a therapeutic response to antidepressant medications within 2 weeks prior to testing experienced an acute but transient relapse of depressive symptoms during TRP depletion. Depressive relapse was defined as a 50% increase in the Hamilton Depression Scale (Ham-D) score with total score ≥ 17. None of the 21 patients in that study experienced a depressive relapse during control testing. While the Ham-D score 5 h after the TRP-depleting amino acid drink was significantly correlated with the minimum plasma free TRP level after the amino acid drink, other factors were also related to relapse during TRP depletion. Patients successfully treated with the relatively selective NE reuptake inhibitor desipramine were much less likely to relapse (only 20% relapse rate) than patients successfully treated with a selective 5-HT reuptake inhibitor or MAOI (90% relapse rate). Having failed to respond to more than one previous antidepressant trial also significantly increased the probability of relapse during TRP depletion. In other words, patients who were more treatment resistant, who were diagnosed with melancholia, and who had responded to either a 5-HT reuptake inhibitor or an MAOI, were more likely to relapse than patients who were relatively more treatment responsive, were non-melancholic, and had responded to desipramine.

In order to discern whether the differences in rates of depressive relapse in response to TRP depletion were specific to the antidepressant type to which the patient had responded, we conducted a second study (Delgado et al, 1997). This study entered only non-melancholic depressed patients who were either antidepressant treatment naive or who had previously had therapeutic antidepressant responses. These patients were randomly assigned to an open trial of either desipramine or fluoxetine. Patients who, after a minimum of 4 weeks of treatment, demonstrated a $\geq 50\%$ decrease from baseline in Ham-D score with a total score of ≤ 15 were tested with TRP depletion and control testing in a double-blind fashion. Forty-three patients (33 outpatient, 10 inpatient; mean age 40 years) with major depressive episodes (DSM-III-R) were tested. Thirty-two patients were treatment naive and 11 had a history of a previously successful antidepressant trial. Fifteen of 20 patients assigned to desipramine treatment and 15 of 18 assigned to fluoxetine treatment had therapeutic responses within an 8-week treatment trial. Twenty-five of

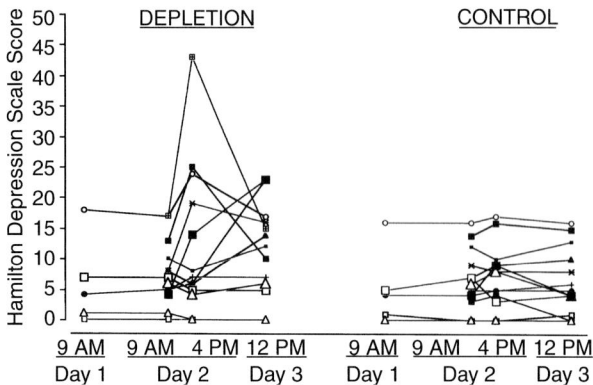

Figure 8.1

Change in Ham-D with TRP depletion in fluoxetine responders. (The symbols represent individual patients.)

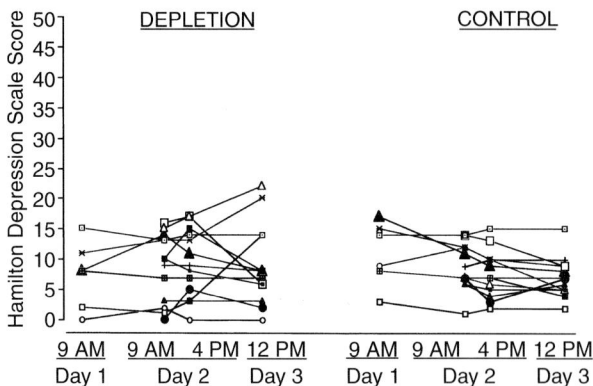

Figure 8.2

Change in Ham-D with TRP depletion in desipramine responders. (The symbols represent individual patients.)

the treatment-responding patients (13 desipramine; 13 fluoxetine) went on to TRP depletion testing after having maintained a therapeutic response for at least 2 weeks.

While 6 of 13 fluoxetine responders experienced a depressive relapse, only 1 of 13 desipramine responders did (Delgado et al, 1997). Figures 8.1 and 8.2 depict the Ham-D scores for fluoxetine and desipramine responders as they underwent TRP depletion and control testing. These data strongly suggest that desipramine may be less acutely dependent on 5-HT availability for its therapeutic effects. When all subjects taking desipramine in all studies (Delgado et al, 1990, 1993, 1997) are considered, the rate of relapse during TRP depletion is 20%. Given that it is a highly potent and selective NE reuptake inhibitor, the therapeutic effects of desipramine in depression may be more related to its effects on the noradrenergic system.

Recent work suggests that TRP depletion may not induce depression in depressed patients who have been in remission on antidepressants for a long time. In a retrospective review of data from several studies using the TRP depletion paradigm, Berman et al (1996) reported that one of the factors negatively correlated with rates of depressive relapse in specific serotonin reuptake inhibitor (SSRI)-treated depressed patients during TRP depletion is length of time on medication. Depressed patients who had been treated with SSRIs for longer were much less likely to relapse during TRP depletion compared to those who had been in remission for shorter times. Other investigators have reported similar findings. Benkelfat reported no effects of TRP depletion in bipolar patients maintained for over 1 year on lithium, while a recent report (Cappiello et al, 1996) showed a reversal of the antimanic effects of lithium in bipolar manic patients who had reached euthymia for 2 weeks or less prior to testing. Gillin (1995) reported significant changes in sleep EEG parameters, but no effects on mood in SSRI-treated depressed patients who had been maintained on medication for 2–13 months. In contrast, Lam et al (1995) showed that patients with seasonal affective disorder who had just achieved clinical remission from depression with phototherapy showed rates of relapse $\geqslant 80\%$. These studies suggest that the high rates of depressive relapse seen with TRP depletion in some prior studies may have been due to the fact that all of these patients were depleted within the first 2 weeks after they had achieved clinical remission.

TRP depletion in medication-free, symptomatic depressed patients

Our original hypothesis in this patient group was that they would feel more depressed during TRP depletion. We did not observe this (Delgado et al, 1994). TRP depletion was administered in a double-blind, placebo-controlled crossover fashion using the original low-TRP diet and amino acid drink procedure to 43 drug-free depressed patients (Delgado et al, 1990, 1994). Change in depressive symptoms on the Ham-D was assessed by categorization of the data in an attempt to define clinically meaningful changes in depression. The categories constructed were based on our clinical experience using the Ham-D. Change in depressive symptoms was categorized as much better ($\geqslant 10$-point decrease in total Ham-D score), better (5–9-point decrease), no change (0–4-point change), worse (5–9-point increase) or much worse ($\geqslant 10$-point increase in Ham-D).

Figure 8.3, which depicts a placebo-subtracted (depletion minus control) frequency histogram of the change in Ham-D score during TRP depletion testing, shows that there was minimal change in Ham-D score on the amino acid drink day (day 2).

Change in Ham-D score during the TRP depletion testing was not

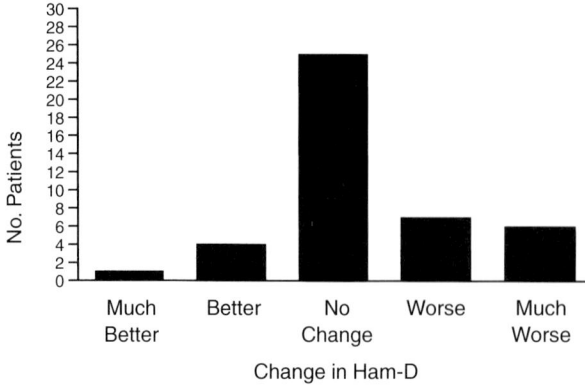

Figure 8.3

Ham-D score during TRP depletion in medication-free symptomatic depressed patients.

related to melancholic subtype, polarity, previous treatment history, age, gender or inpatient/outpatient status. There was no correlation between change in plasma total or free TRP and change in Ham-D score for these drug-free depressed patients during the entire 3-day test sequence on the day of the depletion or on the day after the depletion.

TRP depletion and vulnerability to depression

Benkelfat et al (1994) first investigated the effects of TRP depletion in subjects at risk for depression. These investigators found that TRP depletion caused minimal symptoms in healthy male subjects with no personal or family history of any mental disorder. In contrast, about 30% of subjects with a multigenerational family history of affective disorders had a 10-point or greater increase in the depression subscale of the profile of mood states during TRP depletion but not control testing (Benkelfat et al, 1994).

We have followed up this work with a study designed to assess the effects of TRP depletion on mood in subjects who were off medication and in clinical remission but had a past history of an episode of major depression (history-positive subjects) (Moreno et al, 1996, 1997). In order to qualify for the study, these history-positive subjects had to be drug-free for a minimum of 3 months prior to enrollment into the study. Subjects were excluded if they met DSM-IV criteria for any current Axis I disorder, including dysthymia and substance abuse or dependence. Further, they had to have a total score ≤10 on the Ham-D at screening. Subjects with a lifetime diagnosis of any Axis I disorder other than major depression, psychosis or suicidal behavior, or any current or lifetime diagnosis of any Axis II condition, were also excluded. Healthy subjects could not have a current or lifetime diagnosis of any mental disorder, and

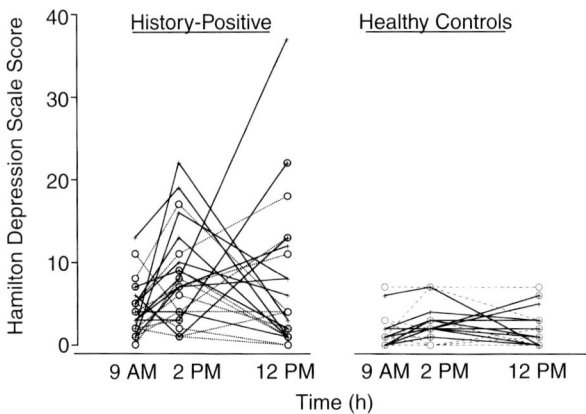

Figure 8.4

Ham-D score during TRP depletion in history-positive and healthy subjects. X depicts changes during a TRP-free, 102-g 15-amino acid drink, and circles depict changes during a TRP-free, 25-g 15-amino acid drink.

nor could they have a family history of any mental disorder or substance abuse. We hypothesized that these history-positive subjects would demonstrate transient, clinically meaningful depressive symptoms during TRP depletion while healthy subjects would not.

As can be seen in Figure 8.4, TRP depletion caused significant increases in depressive symptoms as reflected by the Ham-D score in the 12 history-positive subjects but not in the 12 controls. While the data presented clearly demonstrate a dramatic difference between the healthy and the history-positive subjects, the rate of full depressive relapse during TRP depletion for the history-positive subjects was considerably lower than what has been observed in our prior work with SSRI-treated depressives. Only 25% of the history-positive subjects met the criteria for depressive relapse (50% increase in Ham-D with total score ≥17). There was no effect of age, gender, age of onset of depression or prior number of depressive episodes on mood response to TRP depletion. There was an association of time in remission with depressive response, with the subjects having been well the least time being more likely to demonstrate a depressive response to TRP depletion.

Based on phone interviews using the Ham-D and DSM-IV criteria, eight of the 12 history-positive and one of the healthy subjects have gone on to develop symptoms consistent with a new episode of major depression in the year after TRP depletion. Interestingly, the healthy subject with some of the most prominent symptoms is the one who went on to develop an episode of major depression. In post hoc analysis, the most sensitive cut-off score on the Ham-D that distinguishes between history-positive and healthy subjects is ≥5-point increase in Ham-D with final score ≥8. While

Table 8.2   Depressive responses to TRP depletion and vulnerability to depression.

	Relapse on follow-up	No relapse on follow-up
Positive depletion response	7	3
Negative depletion response	2	12

these values seem low, the pilot data suggest that this criterion may be sufficiently sensitive to identify individuals at risk for future depression. Table 8.2 depicts the relationship between depressive response to TRP depletion (as defined above) and future depression. These values allow us to estimate the predictive value of the mood response to TRP depletion for future depressive episodes, including a sensitivity of 78%, specificity of 80%, positive predictive value of 70% and negative predictive value of 86%.

Catecholamine depletion

The synthesis of NE and DA can be reduced by administration of the drug α-methyl-*p*-tyrosine (AMPT). AMPT is an inhibitor of the first and rate-limiting step in catecholamine synthesis. AMPT reversibly inhibits the enzyme tyrosine hydroxylase. AMPT treatment in humans (600–4000 mg/day) decreases urinary excretion of catecholamine metabolites by up to 75% (Engelman et al, 1968). A 3 g/day dose of AMPT reliably reduces urinary MHPG by 70% and reduces CSF levels of the dopamine (DA) metabolite HVA by 61%, with no change in the 5-HT metabolite 5-HIAA (Bunney et al, 1971). Maximum reduction of catecholamine metabolites during AMPT treatment occurs within 2–3 days of initiation of treatment and returns to normal within 3–4 days after withdrawal of the drug (Engelman et al, 1968; Bunney et al, 1971).

AMPT has been administered in doses up to 4 g/day to various patients (for periods of time up to several months), including patients with essential hypertension, migraine headache, hyperthyroidism and pheochromocytoma (Engelman et al, 1968), Tourette's syndrome (Sweet et al, 1974) and tardive dyskinesia (Gerlach and Thorsen, 1976), heroin and amphetamine addicts (Pozuelo, 1976), psychotic depressives and manics (Brodie et al, 1970; Bunney et al, 1971), and depressed patients being treated with imipramine (Shopsin et al, 1975). AMPT has in general been well tolerated within the 2000–3000 mg/day dose range by patients in published studies. The limiting factor in determining the dose of AMPT utilized has been the occurrence of either sedation or the potential for the drug to crystallize in the urine. Because of these side effects, the average dose utilized in most studies has been approximately 3000 mg/day (Engelman et al, 1968; Bunney et al, 1971; Shopsin et al, 1975). The major side effects of AMPT are sedation, fatigue, crystalluria, extrapyramidal side effects, anxiety, depression and diarrhea. A potential side effect is the development of AMPT urine crystals (Engelman et al, 1968). Because of the potential for this, it is recommended that patients on AMPT be monitored with urinalysis daily, creatinine clearance, and a fluid maintenance of at least 2000 ml/day.

Even after administration to non-psychiatric patients over several months, AMPT does not seem to cause significant changes in mood in the majority of patients (Engelman et al, 1968). Most non-psychiatric patients and healthy subjects demonstrate little behavioral change other than sedation during AMPT treatment, with rebound insomnia frequently seen for 1–2 days after AMPT discontinuation (Engelman et al, 1968; Bunney et al, 1971; McCann et al, 1990). AMPT has been reported in open trials to decrease craving for opiates and amphetamines (Pozuelo, 1976), decrease tic movements in Tourette's syndrome (Sweet et al, 1974), reduce oral tardive dyskinesia (Gerlach and Thorsen, 1976), and potentiate antipsychotic efficacy in schizophrenia (Carlsson et al, 1972).

AMPT may have more behavioral effects in individuals with affective disorders than in other persons. In an open treatment trial of AMPT in patients with essential hypertension, 6 of 20 hypertensive patients had a history of a previous depressive episode. Three of these six became agitated on AMPT, requiring drug discontinuation (Engelman et al, 1968). In a double-blind trial, AMPT reduced manic symptoms in five of seven bipolar patients in the manic phase but two had an increase in manic symptoms (Brodie et al, 1970; Bunney et al, 1971). In the same study, three of four psychotic depressed patients became more depressed after AMPT treatment (Brodie et al, 1970; Bunney et al, 1971).

Catecholamine depletion in antidepressant-remitted depressed patients

One early study assessed the behavioral effects of AMPT in antidepressant-treated depressed patients. In three depressed patients having had a therapeutic response to imipramine, AMPT had no significant effect on the antidepressant response (Shopsin et al, 1975). In one of these patients, AMPT was started prior to initiation of antidepressant treatment, and that patient went on to have a therapeutic response to imipramine (Shopsin et al, 1975). Although these data are provocative, the small number of patients, the lack of placebo control and the fact that imipramine is a potent 5-HT reuptake inhibitor as well as a potent NE reuptake inhibitor mean that no broad conclusions can be drawn from this study.

Based on the contrast in the effects of TRP depletion between desipramine- and SSRI-treated depressed patients, we initiated a study investigating the effects of AMPT in antidepressant-treated depressed patients (Delgado et al, 1996; Miller et al, 1996a). Depressed patients (DSM-III-R criteria) were recruited and tested with AMPT and control tests while drug-free, and then again after successful antidepressant treatment. After drug-free testing, patients were randomly assigned to either desipramine or fluoxetine, and antidepressant treatment was performed with open routine clinical dosing over a maximum of 10 weeks. Treatment responders were scheduled for repeat testing within 2 weeks of meeting the response criteria.

Each test included a four-day sequence with a baseline day and two depletion days involving administration of AMPT 1 g t.i.d. (AMPT test) or diphenhydramine 50 mg t.i.d. (control test). The fourth day was a follow-up day. Diphenhydramine was used as an 'active placebo' because of the sedation associated with AMPT. Behavioral ratings of mood and plasma for MHPG and HVA levels were obtained throughout the 4-day test sequence.

Fifty-seven patients were randomized to treatment and 39 met response criteria. Eighteen of 27 desipramine-treated patients responded (67%) and 21 of 30 fluoxetine-treated patients responded (70% response). Sixteen desipramine responders and 21 fluoxetine responders completed repeat catecholamine depletion testing (Figures 8.5 and 8.6). Plasma levels of MHPG decreased by 50% and HVA decreased by 80% during AMPT administration. For statistical analysis, depressive relapse is defined as in our prior studies as a $\geq 50\%$ increase in Ham-D score with a final score ≥ 17. Eighty-one per cent (13/16) of desipramine responders met the criteria for depressive relapse during AMPT testing, and only 1 of 16 did during diphenhydramine testing ($p < 0.0001$, Fisher's exact test). In contrast, 20% of fluoxetine responders met relapse criteria during AMPT testing (4/21) and 3 of 21 did during diphenhydramine testing (non-significant). The difference in rate of relapse during AMPT testing between desipramine responders and fluoxetine responders is also highly significant ($p < 0.001$, Fisher's exact test).

Behavioral effects of baseline testing were not correlated with subsequent antidepressant response, or behavioral effects during depletion. There was no correlation between change in MHPG or HVA and behavioral response to AMPT, there were no significant differences between desipramine responders and fluoxetine responders in plasma MHPG and HVA levels at any time point, and there was no correlation between behavioral response to AMPT in either group or a change in either MHPG or HVA.

Catecholamine depletion in medication-free depressed patients
We predicted that if noradrenergic function was involved in the pathophysiology of depression, then there should be some exacerbation of depressive symptoms during AMPT-induced catecholamine depletion in

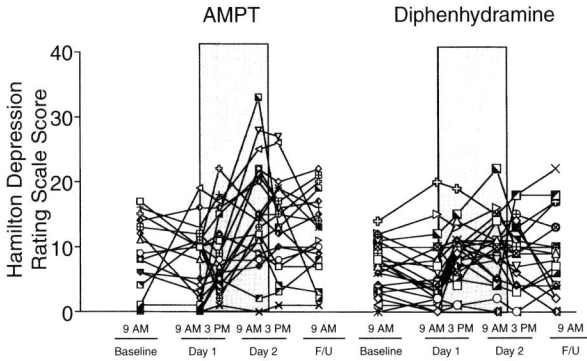

Figure 8.5

Ham-D score during catecholamine depletion in fluoxetine responders. (The symbols represent individual patients.)

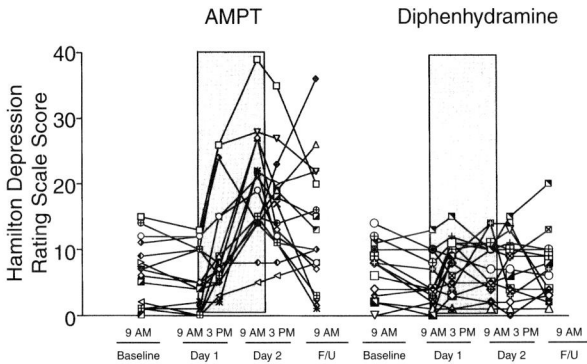

Figure 8.6

Ham-D score during catecholamine depletion in desipramine responders. (The symbols represent individual patients.)

drug-free symptomatic depressed patients. Instead of the predicted exacerbation, we saw minimal change in mood during or after AMPT or diphenhydramine administration in these subjects (Miller et al, 1996b). Analysis of the Ham-D scores for 50 of these patients as they underwent depletion and sham testing shows that there were no significant differences between AMPT and diphenhydramine testing and there was no exacerbation (Figure 8.7).

Conclusions

The results of neurotransmitter depletion studies suggest that TRP depletion and catecholamine depletion more strongly affect patients having

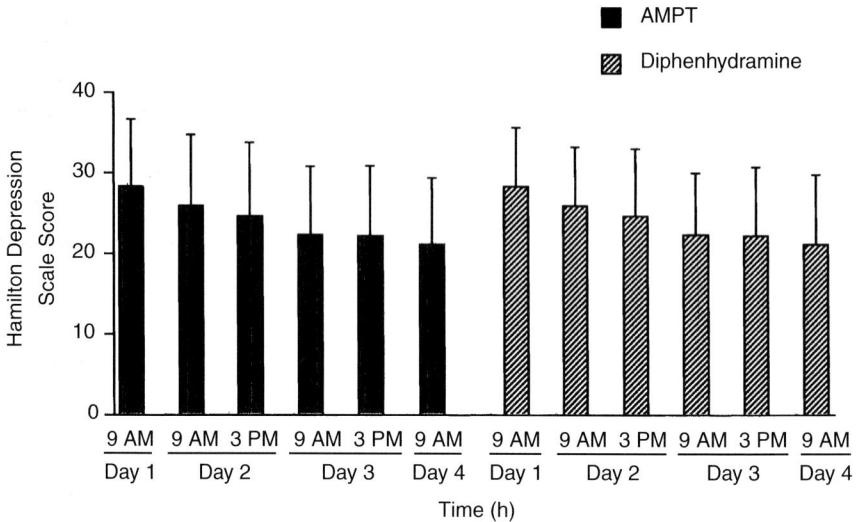

Figure 8.7

Ham-D score during catecholamine depletion in medication-free, symptomatic depressed patients.

recently responded to and being maintained on SSRIs and desipramine, respectively, although it is clear that some patients will have depressive responses with either TRP depletion or AMPT, regardless of the drug they are taking. These findings are consistent with the possibility that the neurotransmitter systems through which desipramine and SSRIs work are different, suggesting that at least two parallel mechanisms of antidepressant action may exist. The fact that some patients might be affected by either 5-HT or NE depletion is not completely surprising, given that the 5-HT and noradrenergic systems are intimately involved with each other (Pryor and Sulser, 1991).

The failure to see significant effects with depletion in medication-free symptomatic patients and healthy subjects implies that neither 5-HT nor noradrenergic dysfunction may be the simple cause of depression, although the possibility of a 'floor effect' cannot be ruled out. The finding that history-positive subjects have depressive symptoms more often than healthy subjects, but are less likely to have a full depressive relapse during TRP depletion than acutely remitted SSRI-treated patients, suggests that while these subjects are more dependent on 5-HT availability to maintain mood than healthy subjects, they are less dependent on the availability of 5-HT than are SSRI-treated patients.

The data suggesting that patients who have been in remission on antidepressants for a longer time prior to TRP depletion do not relapse as frequently or at all is consistent with our findings in the history-positive subjects. This suggests that 5-HT levels may be most important during the early phases of the antidepressant response. Rapid 5-HT depletion may only lead to a depressive relapse in individuals who have not yet consolidated the antidepressant response.

If antidepressant drugs are in fact initiating a time-dependent process by enhancing synaptic levels of monoamines, then understanding the details of that process may lead to a treatment which can provide an immediate antidepressant response. One of the most interesting observations in this regard is the fact that the release of several neurotrophic factors, including NT_3 (Smith et al, 1995), brain derived neurotrophic factor (BDNF) (Duman et al, 1997) and $S\text{-}100\beta$ (Whitaker-Azmitia, 1993) can be altered by increased levels of 5-HT or NE. A very recent report suggests that BDNF has antidepressant-like effects in rats (Siuciak et al, 1997). These observations, and the results of our depletion studies, have led us to suggest (Delgado, 1995) that antidepressant effects may involve adaptive changes induced by monoamines in the neurons which they modulate. Such a model could explain why antidepressant drugs are effective in such a wide variety of other mental conditions (e.g. panic disorder and obsessive-compulsive disorder) and in depressive syndromes that occur in individuals with parkinsonism or Alzheimer's disease (review: Delgado, 1995). This suggests that the focus of future study should shift to understanding the adaptive changes induced by antidepressants.

References

Artigas F, Bel N, Ferrer A and Cortes R (1993) Increased cortical extracellular 5-HT after repeated, but not acute, treatment with low doses of antidepressants. Reduction after tryptophan depletions. 23rd Annual Meeting of the Society for Neuroscience, Washington DC, Abstract 126.6, November 7–12.

Åsberg M, Schalling D, Traskman-Bendz L, Wagner A (1987) Psychobiology of suicide, impulsivity, and related phenomena. In: Meltzer HY, ed., *Psychopharmacology: The Third Generation of Progress* (Raven Press: New York) 655–68.

Benkelfat C, Seletti E, Mark A, Dean P, Palmour RM, Young SN (1994) Mood-lowering effects of tryptophan depletion: enhanced susceptibility in young man at genetic risk for major affective disorders, *Arch Gen Psychiatry* **51:** 687–97, Abstract 811.10, November 7–12.

Berendsen HHG, Broekkamp CLE (1990) Behavioral evidence for functional interactions between 5-HT receptor subtypes in rats and mice, *Br J Pharmacol* **101:**667–73.

Berman RM, Delgado PL, Miller HL, Price LH, Heninger GR, Charney DS (1996) Correlates of depressive relapse in medicated depressed subjects undergoing acute tryptophan depletion. In: *26th Annual Meeting of the Society for Neuroscience*, November, Washington, DC, Abstract 811.10, November 2.

Blier P, de Montigny C (1994) Current advances in the treatment of depression, *Trends Pharmacol Sci* **15:**220–6.

Blier P, de Montigny C, Chaput Y (1990) A role for the serotonin system in the mechanism of action of antidepressant treatments: preclinical evidence, *J Clin Psychiatry* **51**(4S): 14–20.

Brodie KH, Murphy DL, Goodwin FK, Bunney WE (1970) Catecholamines and mania: the effect of alpha-methyl-para-tyrosine on manic behavior and catecholamine metabolism, *Clin Pharmacol Ther* **12**(2):218–24.

Bunney WE Jr, Davis JM (1965) Norepinephrine in depressive reactions: a review, *Arch Gen Psychiatry* **13:** 483–94.

Bunney WE, Keith H, Brodie H, Murphy DL, Goodwin FK (1971) Studies of alpha-methyl-para-tyrosine in depression and mania, *Am J Psychiatry* **127**(7):872–81.

Cappiello A, Sernyak M, Malison RT, McDougle CJ, Heninger GR, Price LH (1996) Effects of acute tryptophan depletion in lithium remitted manic patients. In: *34th Annual Meeting of the American College of Neuropsychopharmacology*, 11–15 December, San Juan, Puerto Rico.

Carlsson A, Persson T, Roos BE, Walinder J (1972) Potentiation of phenothiazines by methyltyrosine in treatment of chronic schizophrenia, *J Neur Trans* **33:**83–90.

Carpenter WT (1970) Serotonin now: clinical implications of inhibiting its synthesis with para-chlorophenylalanine, *Ann Intern Med* **73:**607–29.

Charney DS, Menkes DB, Heninger GR (1981) Receptor sensitivity and the mechanism of action of antidepressant treatment, *Arch Gen Psychiatry* **38:** 1160–80.

Clemens JA, Bennett DR, Fuller RW (1980) The effect of a tryptophan-free diet on prolactin and corticosterone release by serotonergic stimuli, *Horm Metab Res* **12:**35–8.

Coppen A (1967) The biochemistry of affective disorders, *Br J Psychiatry* **113:**1237–64.

Curzon G (1979) Relationships between plasma, CSF and brain tryptophan, *J Neural Transm* **S.15:**93–105.

Curzon G (1981) Influence of plasma tryptophan on brain 5HT synthesis and serotonergic activity. In: Haber B, Gabay S, eds, *Serotonin: Current Aspects of Neurochemistry and Function* (Plenum Press: New York, London) 207–19.

De Boer Th (1996) The pharmacological profile of mirtazapine, *J Clin Psychiatry* **57**(4):19–25.

de Montigny C, Blier P (1984) Effects of antidepressant treatment on 5-HT neurotransmission: electrophysiological and clinical studies, *Adv Biochem Psychopharmacol* **39:**223–40.

Delgado PL (1995) Neurobiological basis of depression, *Adv Biol Psychiatry* **1:**161–214.

Delgado PL, Charney DS, Price LH, Landis H, Heninger GR (1989) Neuroendocrine and behavioral effects of dietary tryptophan depletion in healthy subjects, *Life Sci* **45**(24):2323–32.

Delgado PL, Charney DS, Price LH, Aghajanian GK, Landis H, Heninger GR (1990) Serotonin function and the mechanism of antidepressant action: reversal of antidepressant induced remission by rapid depletion of plasma tryptophan, *Arch Gen Psychiatry* **47:**411–18.

Delgado PL, Price LH, Heninger GR, Charney DS (1991a) Neurochemistry of affective disorders: implications for the amine hypotheses. In: Paykel ES, ed., *Handbook of Affective Disorders*, 2nd edn (Churchill Livingstone: London) 219–53.

Delgado PL, Price LH, Miller HM et al (1991b) Rapid serotonin depletion as a provocative challenge test for patients with major depression: relevance to antidepressant action and the neurobiology of depression, *Psychopharmacol Bull* **27**(3):321–30.

Delgado PL, Miller HM, Salomon RM, Licinio J, Gelenberg AJ, Charney DS (1993) Monoamines and the mechanism of antidepressant action: effects of catecholamine depletion on mood in patients treated with antidepressants, *Psychopharmacol Bull* **29**(3): 389–96.

Delgado PL, Price LH, Aghajanian et al (1994) Serotonin and the neurobiology of depression: effects of tryptophan depletion in drug-free depressed patients, *Arch Gen Psychiatry* **51**:865–74.

Delgado PL, Moreno FA, Buonopane A, Gelenberg AJ, Potter R (1996) Catecholamine depletion in desipramine- and fluoxetine-responders. In: *149th Annual Meeting of the American Psychiatric Association*, New York, New Research Abstracts, NR 334.

Delgado PL, Miller HM, Salomon RM et al (1997) Tryptophan depletion challenge in depressed patients treated with desipramine or paroxetine: implications for the role of serotonin in the mechanism of antidepressant action (submitted).

Duman RS, Heninger GR, Nestler EJ (1997) A molecular and cellular theory of depression, *Arch Gen Psych* **54**:597–606.

Engelman K, Horwitz D, Jequier E, Sjoerdsma A (1968) Biochemical and pharmacologic effects of α-methyltyrosine in man, *J Clin Invest* **47**:577–94.

Fernstrom JD (1977) Effects of the diet on brain neurotransmitters, *Metabolism* **26**(2):207–23.

Fernstrom JD, Hirsch MJ (1975) Rapid repletion of brain serotonin in malnourished corn-fed rats following L-tryptophan injection, *Life Sci* **17**:455–64.

Gerlach J, Thorsen K (1976) The movement pattern of oral tardive dyskinesia in relation to anticholinergic and antidopaminergic treatment, *Int Pharmacopsychiatry* **11**:1–7.

Gibbons JL, Barr GA, Bridger WH, Leibowitz SF (1979) Manipulations of dietary tryptophan: effects on mouse killing and brain serotonin in the rat, *Brain Res* **169**:139–53.

Gillin JC (1995) Rapid tryptophan depletion affects sleep EEG but not mood in fully remitted depressed patients on serotonin reuptake inhibitors. In: *Second International Congress of the World Federation of Sleep Research Societies*, Nassau, Bahamas (submitted).

Haddjeri N, Blier P, de Montigny C (1995) Noradrenergic modulation of central serotonergic neurotransmission: acute and long-term actions of mirtazapine, *Int Clin Psychopharmacol* **10**(4):11–17.

Harper AE, Benevenga NJ, Wohlhueter RM (1970) Effects of ingestion of disproportionate amounts of amino acids, *Physiol Rev* **50**: 428–548.

Heninger GR, Charney DS (1987) Mechanism of action of antidepressant treatments: implications for the etiology and treatment of depressive disorders. In: Meltzer HY, ed., *Psychopharmacology: The Third Generation of Progress* (Raven Press: New York) 535–44.

Hyman SE, Nestler EJ (1996) Initiation and adaptation: a paradigm for understanding psychotropic drug action, *Am J Psychiatry* **153**:151–62.

Krahn LE, Lu PY, Klee G, Delgado PL, Lin S-C, Zimmerman RC (1996) Examining serotonin function: a modified technique for rapid tryptophan depletion, *Neuropsychopharmacology* **15**: 325–8.

Lam RW, Zis AP, Grewal A, Delgado PL, Charney DS, Krystal JH (1995) Effects of acute tryptophan depletion in seasonal affective disorder in remission with light therapy, *Arch Gen Psychiatry* **53**(1):41–4.

Lytle LD, Messing RB, Fisher L, Phebus L (1975) Effects of long-term corn consumption on brain serotonin and the response to electric shock, *Science* **190**:692–4.

Maes M, Meltzer HY (1995) The serotonin hypothesis of major depression. In: Bloom FE, Kupfer DJ, eds, *Psychopharmacology: The Fourth Generation of Progress* (Raven Press: New York) 933–44.

McCann U, Penetar D, Shaham Y et al (1993) Effects of catecholamine depletion on alertness and mood in rested and sleep deprived normal volunteers, *Neuropsychopharmacol* **8:**345–56.

Messing RB, Fisher LA, Phebus L, Lytle LD (1976) Interaction of diet and drugs in the regulation of brain 5-hydroxyindoles and the response to painful electric shock, *Life Sci* **18:** 707–14.

Miller HL, Delgado PL, Salomon RM et al (1996a) Clinical and biochemical effects of catecholamine depletion on antidepressant-induced remission of depression, *Arch Gen Psychiatry* **53:**117–28.

Miller HL, Delgado PL, Salomon RM, Heninger GR, Charney DS (1996b) Effects of alpha-methyl-para-tyrosine (AMPT) in drug-free depressed patients, *Neuropsychopharmacology* **14**(3):151–8.

Moir ATB, Eccleston D (1968) The effects of precursor loading in the cerebral metabolism of 5-hydroxyindoles, *J Neurochem* **15:**1093–108.

Moja EA, Mendelson WB, Stoff DM, Gillin JC, Wyatt RJ (1979) Reduction of REM sleep by a tryptophan-free amino acid diet, *Life Sci* **24:**1467–70.

Moja EA, Cipollo P, Castoldi D, Tofanetti O (1989) Dose–response decrease in plasma tryptophan and in brain tryptophan and serotonin after tryptophan-free amino acid mixtures in rats, *Life Sci* **44:**971–6.

Mongeau R, Blier P, de Montigny C (1993) In vivo electrophysiological evidence for tonic activation by endogenous noradrenaline on α-2 adrenoreceptors of 5-hydroxytryptamine terminals in rat hippocampus, *Naunyn Scmiedebergs Arch Pharmacol* **347:**266–72.

Moreno FA, Gelenberg AJ, Potter R, Heninger GR, Buonopane A, Delgado PL (1996) Tryptophan depletion: a potential predictor of depressive episodes. 26th Annual Meeting of the

Society for Neuroscience, Washington DC, Abstract 811.9 November 21.

Moreno FA, McKnight K, Gelenberg AJ, Potter R, Heninger GR, Delgado PL (1997) Tryptophan depletion and vulnerability to depression (in review).

Nishizawa S, Benkelfat C, Young SN et al (1997) Differences between males and females in rates of serotonin synthesis in human brain. *Proc Natl Acad Sci* **94:**5308–13.

Perez-Cruet J, Chase TN, Murphy DL (1974) Dietary regulation of brain tryptophan metabolism by plasma ratio of free tryptophan and neutral amino acids in humans, *Nature* **248:**693–5.

Pozuelo J (1976) Suppression of craving and withdrawal in humans addicted to narcotics or amphetamines by administration of alpha-methyl-para-tyrosine (AMPT) and 5-butylpicolinic acid (fusaric acid), *Cleve Clin Q* **43**(2):89–94.

Pryor JC, Sulser F (1991) Evolution of the monoamine hypothesis of depression. In: Horton R, Katona C, eds, *Biological Aspects of Affective Disorders* (Academic Press: New York) 77–95.

Rose WC, Haines WJ, Warner DT (1954) The amino acid requirements of man, *J Biol Chem* **206**(1):421–30.

Roy A, Virkkunen M, Linnoila M (1990) Serotonin in suicide, violence and alcoholism. In Coccaro EF, Murphy DL (eds) *Serotonin in Major Psychiatric Disorders* (American Psychiatric Press, Washington DC) 187–208.

Schatzberg AF, Schildkraut JJ (1995) Recent studies on norepinephrine systems in mood disorders. In: Bloom FE, Kupfer DJ, eds, *Psychopharmacology: The Fourth Generation of Progress* (Raven Press: New York) 911–20.

Schildkraut JJ (1965) The catecholamine hypothesis of affective disorders: a review of supporting evidence, *Am J Psychiatry* **122:** 509–22.

Shopsin B, Gershon S, Goldstein M, Friedman E, Wilk S (1975) Use of synthesis inhibitors in defining a role for biogenic amines during imipramine treatment in depressed patients, *Psychopharmacol Commun* **2:**239–49.

Shopsin B, Friedman E, Gershon S (1976) Parachlorophenylalanine reversal of tranylcypromine effects in depressed patients, *Arch Gen Psychiatry* **33:**811–91.

Siuciak JA, Lewis DR, Wiegand SJ, Lindsay RM (1997) Antidepressant-like effect of brain-derived neurotrophic factor, *Pharmacol Biochem Behav* **56:**131–7.

Smeraldi E, Diaferia G, Erzegovesi S, Lucca A (1996) Tryptophan depletion in obsessive compulsive patients, *Biol Psych* **40:**398–402.

Smith MA, Makino S, Altemus M et al (1995) Stress and antidepressants differentially regulate neurotrophin-3 mRNA expression in the locus coeruleus, *Proc Natl Acad Sci USA* **92:**8788–92.

Sulser F (1987) Serotonin-norepinephrine receptor interactions in the brain: implications for the pharmacology and pathophysiology of affective disorders, *J Clin Psych* **48:**12–18.

Sulser F, Vetulani J, Mobley PL (1978) Mode of action of antidepressant drugs, *Biochem Pharmacol* **27:** 257–71.

Sweet RD, Bruun R, Shapiro E, Shapiro AK (1974) Presynaptic catecholamine antagonists as treatment for Tourette's syndrome: effects of alpha methyl para tyrosine and tetrabenazine, *Arch Gen Psychiatry* **31:**857–61.

Vergnes M, Kempf E (1981) Tryptophan deprivation: effects on mouse-killing and reactivity in the rat, *Psychopharmacol Aggr Soc Behav* **14:**19–23.

Walters JK, Davis M, Sheard MH (1979) Tryptophan-free diet: effects on the acoustic startle reflex in rats, *Psychopharmacology* **62:**103–9.

Weltzin TE, Fernstrom JD, McConaha C, Kaye WH (1994) Acute tryptophan depletion in bulimia: effects on large neutral amino acids, *Biol Psychiatry* **35:**388–97.

Whitaker-Azmitia PM, Clarke C, Azmitia EC (1993) Localization of 5-HT1A receptors to astroglial cells in adult rats: implications for neuronal-glial interactions and psychoactive drug mechanism of action. *Synapse* **14:**201–5.

Young SN, Smith SE, Pihl R, Ervin FR (1985) Tryptophan depletion causes a rapid lowering of mood in normal males, *Psychopharmacology* **87:** 173–7.

Young SN, Ervin FR, Pihl RO, Finn P (1989) Biochemical aspects of tryptophan depletion in primates, *Psychopharmacology* **98**(4):508–11.

Young VR, Hussein MA, Murray E, Scrimshaw NS (1969) Tryptophan intake, spacing of meals, and diurnal fluctuations of plasma tryptophan in men, *Am J Clin Nutr* **22:**1563–7.

Young VR, Hussein MA, Murray E, Scrimshaw NS (1971) Plasma tryptophan response curve and its relation to tryptophan requirements in young adult men, *J Nutr* **101:**45–60.

Zimmerman RC, Svoboda J, McDougle CJ et al (1992) The effect of acute tryptophan depletion on human melatonin secretion. In: *36th Symposium of the Deutsche Gesellschaft fur Endokrinologie*

9
Serotonin, impulse control and alcoholism

Markku Linnoila, J Dee Higley and Matti Virkkunen

Genetics and subtyping of alcoholism

Alcoholism, like many mental disorders, is a heterogeneous condition. It is the most common mental disorder among men in the Western industrialized countries, with a lifetime prevalence in excess of 10% (Robins et al, 1984). Some of the best studies on subtyping alcoholism, which have great heuristic value, were conducted in two cities in Sweden; the first one in Stockholm (Cloninger et al, 1981), and the replication study in Gothenburg (Sigvardsson et al, 1996). The investigators described two types of alcoholism: type I affects both men and women. An environmental provocation in the form of a dysfunctional adoptive family is required for the expression of the genetic vulnerability background. If an individual with the vulnerability background is raised in a dysfunctional adoptive family, then he or she will have roughly a three-fold increased risk to become alcoholic when compared to the general population. This form of alcoholism affects all women alcoholics in Sweden, by and large, and 75% of men. The age of onset of type I alcoholism is relatively late, after 25 years of age. Type I alcoholism is not associated with overt serotonergic dysfunction. The other form of alcoholism, called type II, affects only men. In the Cloninger et al studies, 25% of the male alcoholics had this form of the disease. Type II alcoholism is inherited from fathers to sons, and the patients are not only alcoholic, but also have antisocial behavioral traits. Type II alcoholism is one of the most heritable mental disorders. If an individual has the biological background of an antisocial alcoholic father, his risk to become an antisocial alcoholic, even when reared apart from his parents, is almost nine-fold, compared to the general male population. However, it is very important to realize that if we ask how many of the sons who have antisocial alcoholic fathers and are adopted as babies become antisocial alcoholics, the answer is less than one in five. This figure has important implications for prevention strategies.

An issue which is important to note in evaluating the likelihood that the vulnerability risk will actually lead to the development of any kind of alcoholism is the fact that, during the time over which the Cloninger et al studies were conducted, adoptive families in Sweden were carefully screened to exclude psychopathology. Therefore, the numbers derived by Cloninger et al probably represent an underestimation of the risk under prevailing conditions in most Western countries. In essence, they already include the beneficial effects of a prevention strategy—the careful screening of adoptive couples. Data by Cadoret et al (1995) from Iowa (reviewed below) may support this notion.

Clinically, type II alcoholism starts early in life. It is associated with frequent spontaneous alcohol seeking, fighting and arrests when drinking, but psychological dependence is infrequent. These patients are said to consume alcohol primarily because of its euphoric effects. Guilt and fear about the consequences of alcohol dependence and abuse are infrequent among type II alcoholics. In contrast, the patients with type I alcoholism have anxious personality traits. They are said to consume alcohol for its anxiolytic effects. Therefore, they are believed to become more severely dependent than type II alcoholics. Subtyping of alcoholics in treatment-seeking patient samples according to the Cloninger classification is complex, because the disease can skip generations and assortative mating is common among alcoholics (Lamparski et al, 1991).

Role of central serotonin in alcoholism

Prior to the publication of the Cloninger et al typology, Ballenger et al (1979) studied central serotonin metabolism by quantitating 5-hydroxyindole acetic acid (5-HIAA; the major metabolite of serotonin) in the cerebrospinal fluid (CSF) of young male alcoholics at the Bethesda Naval Medical Center. These investigators demonstrated that after a supervised abstinence of a minimum duration of 4 weeks on a locked ward, the patients had reduced CSF 5-HIAA, as compared to controls. Because of the demographics of the patients, there is a great likelihood that the sample consisted primarily of type II alcoholics. We investigated directly the impact of the Cloninger et al classification on central serotonin metabolism among alcoholics on The National Institute on Alcohol Abuse and Alcoholism research ward at the NIH Clinical Center (Fils-Aime et al, 1996). We used the von Knorring et al (1985) criteria to classify the alcoholics. We compared early-onset to late-onset male alcoholics after carefully screening out anybody who fulfilled the criteria for antisocial personality disorder. Indeed, we found that the patients with early-onset alcoholism had a lower mean CSF 5-HIAA concentration than the patients with late-onset alcoholism. There was, however, marked overlap between the CSF 5-HIAA distributions of the two groups. If we were to include patients with antisocial personality disorder and alcoholism in the sample, we would increase the number of patients at the low end of the distribution among the early-onset alcoholics.

Thus, it appears that early-onset male alcoholics are characterized by reduced central serotonin turnover rate. Reduced central serotonin turnover rate has been associated with an increased risk of attempted and completed suicide among many diagnostic groups of psychiatric patients (Roy and Linnoila, 1986). Therefore, it is important for clinicians to remember that among patients on whom psychological autopsies have been performed, the second most common antemortem diagnosis prior to completed suicide is alcoholism. It is second only to unipolar depression. Clinicians may do an inadequate job when evaluating young antisocial male alcoholics for suicide potential. It may be higher than is generally thought, and it may be related to reduced central serotonin turnover rate.

Central serotonin and antisocial behaviors

The findings of Cloninger et al (1981) and Sigvardsson et al (1996) were based on Swedish adoptees who were born in the late 1940s and early 1950s. Recent studies by Cadoret et al (1995) on adopted sons of antisocial biological fathers in Iowa present outcomes which are somewhat different from the findings of Cloninger et al. There is an interesting cluster of outcomes among the sons of antisocial fathers in Iowa, which consists of an overrepresentation of them among patients with early-onset alcohol abuse, antisocial personality disorder and drug abuse. The question these findings poses is: does this cluster of diagnoses have a general genetic vulnerability background, or are there specific vulnerability genes for each one of these disorders? The results in Iowa are intriguing, because they differ from the Swedish results, in that they show a role for the quality of the early developmental environment in contributing to the risk for the development of early-onset alcoholism and substance abuse among the sons. This difference may be due to the adoptive families in Iowa being less thoroughly screened for dysfunctionality than they were in Sweden 50 years ago.

What the findings by Cadoret et al suggest is that the antisocial genetic background sensitizes the young boys to the adversity in the adoptive family. The adversity in the adoptive family disproportionately increases the risk of the development of early-onset inappropriate aggressiveness and conduct disorder among the adopted sons of the antisocial fathers, as compared to sons of non-antisocial fathers. To understand precisely the adverse gene–environment interactions which are conducive to the development of this cluster of disorders requires the identification of the specific genes involved in causing the vulnerability. Such an understanding, in turn, will facilitate the design of targeted prevention strategies to forestall the untoward outcomes.

Is central serotonin turnover rate a familial trait?

There are data obtained in family studies which suggest that central sero-tonin turnover rate may play a role in this process. Studies by Winokur (1979) in Iowa introduced the concepts of pure unipolar depression and depression spectrum disorder. The former refers to families which have only unipolar depression among the family members, whereas in the fam-ilies with the latter, men have an overrepresentation of antisocial traits and alcoholism, and the women have unipolar depressions. Investigating this concept, Rosenthal et al (1980) found that depressed patients with alcoholic relatives, as compared to depressed patients without alcoholic relatives, have reduced central serotonin turnover rate.

In a family study, Coccaro et al (1994) used prolactin response to fen-fluramine challenge as an index of central serotonergic activity in patients with personality disorders. They found that a history of impulsive aggres-siveness in blood relatives was associated with blunted responses in the probands. In a recent study on violent Finnish alcoholics in Helsinki (Virkkunen et al, 1996), we observed that paternal violence, combined with paternal alcoholism, primarily contributes to the reduced central serotonin turnover rate, whereas paternal alcoholism without paternal vio-lence does not lead to reduced central serotonin turnover rate. This is interesting, because there is an emerging literature which documents paternal violence as a predictor of the son's early, inappropriate aggres-siveness, which, in turn, is a good predictor of conduct disorder and sub-stance abuse (Virkkunen and Linnoila, 1997). It is intriguing that paternal violence plays a role even in a situation when the father and the son have never shared the home. Virkkunen et al (1996) had a large enough num-ber of such father–son pairs in the sample that we can say that there may be a genetically transmitted vulnerability in these pedigrees. One vari-able affecting such vulnerability may be a reduced central serotonin turnover rate.

Studies on rhesus monkeys

We have investigated this issue with J Dee Higley and Steven Suomi in rhesus monkeys (Higley et al, 1993). The study included more than 270 monkeys. One group was reared in a peer-rearing paradigm without their parents, one group was reared by their own mothers and one group was cross-fostered to lactating but unrelated female monkeys. We found that during the first 6 months of life, 87% of the central serotonin turnover rate was genetically determined in the monkeys. Only 3% was environmen-tally determined. However, when we followed these monkeys past puberty, which may roughly represent about 15 years of human life, we observed that at this time about 50% of the variance in the central serotonin turnover rate was inherited, and the other 50% was environmentally determined (Higley et al, 1996a).

This finding raised the question: what are the environmental variables which contribute to the central serotonin turnover rate in a late-adolescent individual? From the study by Cadoret et al (1995), we can deduce that, among humans, adversity in an adopted family can in biologically predisposed individuals lead to behavioral outcomes which in clinical studies are often associated with reduced central serotonin turnover rate. Therefore, Higley et al (1996a) investigated the effects of parental deprivation on the development of the central serotonin system in the non-human primates. In these studies, the monkeys were never isolated, but they were reared in peer groups with monkeys of similar age without the presence of adults. It was discovered that peer rearing (i.e. parental neglect during early development) is conducive to an exacerbation of the general reduction in central serotonin turnover rate, which proceeds from infancy to puberty. The bulk of the reduction in the turnover rate took place around puberty, when severe aggression appeared. Thus, there may be a delayed effect of early parental neglect on central serotonin turnover rate during adolescence.

There are untoward social consequences to the monkeys due to the reduced central serotonin turnover rate, whether genetically or environmentally determined. One of them is that when these animals are introduced to social groups, the ones with low CSF 5-HIAA concentrations are predominantly relegated to low social dominance rankings. The dominant rhesus monkeys are not particularly aggressive, but they are very adept in building alliances and having the other monkeys do the fighting for them. This is something that the low-5-HIAA monkeys have a great deal of difficulty accomplishing, because they tend to go very quickly from stimulus to action, without actually evaluating the meaning of the stimulus (Higley and Linnoila, 1997). In other words, the monkeys with reduced central serotonin turnover rates exhibit signs of impaired impulse control.

In nature, the consequences of reduced central serotonin turnover rates among the monkeys are quite dramatic. We have investigated the issue under naturalistic conditions in a colony of 5500 monkeys on an island off the South Carolina coast. We followed a group of male monkeys from birth past puberty. The rhesus monkeys prevent inbreeding by expelling males from their social groups of origin at the time of puberty. Thus, the males have to negotiate their way to a different social group. This is very stressful and almost one half to the males end up being killed during the process. The low 5-HIAA monkeys get killed disproportionately. Fifty-five per cent of the lowest quartile are dead 1 year after puberty, whereas 0% of the highest quartile are dead at that time. The immediate question which arises is: how does this genetic background survive in nature when there is this kind of pressure against it? This matter is currently under investigation.

Serotonin and impulse control—testosterone and aggressiveness

CSF 5-HIAA concentration, as we have reported in several studies and others have confirmed, is primarily behaviorally related to impulse control; it is not directly related to aggressiveness (Higley and Linnoila, 1997; Virkkunen and Linnoila, 1997). This observation raises the question, where does the aggressive drive come from? A source may be testosterone. Finnish, alcoholic, violent offenders, whether impulsive or non-impulsive, tend to have increased CSF free testosterone concentrations, as compared to age- and sex-matched healthy volunteers (Virkkunen et al, 1994). Among the monkeys, there is an interesting interaction between CSF testosterone and 5-HIAA concentrations. Indeed, the most aggressive monkeys have a low CSF 5-HIAA concentration in combination with a high CSF free testosterone concentration (Higley et al, 1996b). These biochemical findings may also shed some light on the apparently curious finding that many patients with antisocial personality disorder who survive until their forties 'burn out' (i.e. they change their behaviors for the better) (Robins, 1966). Biochemically, two processes take place. Central serotonin turnover rate goes up (Brown and Linnoila, 1990) and testosterone production goes down. The relative importance of these two processes to behavioral changes among middle-aged patients with antisocial personality disorder is a subject for further studies. We have patients currently in longitudinal follow-up studies designed to elucidate this issue. The goal is to find the mechanisms conducive to the proposed natural change. Such an understanding may make it possible to facilitate this natural process and reduce the adverse consequences associated with antisocial behaviors earlier in life.

Central serotonin and activity of neuronal circuitry

The next issue that arises is: which central neuronal circuits are differently activated in individuals with reduced central serotonin turnover rates as compared to individuals with average to high central serotonin turnover rates? The first tentative answer to this question was obtained in a study conducted by Stanley et al (1985) at the medical examiner's office in Detroit. The investigators performed lumbar punctures on fresh cadavers and dissected the brains. They quantitated 5-HIAA in the CSF and brain tissue. They found a strong positive correlation ($r = 0.78$) between the 5-HIAA concentrations in the lumbar CSF and in the frontal cortex.

In a study on patients with obsessive-compulsive disorder (OCD), Insel et al (1985) found that patients, as compared to age- and sex-matched healthy volunteers during the same season, had increased CSF 5-HIAA concentrations, a situation which may be the opposite of that in patients with antisocial behavioral traits. Interestingly, patients with OCD, in PET studies using fluorodeoxyglucose to quantitate regional neuronal activity, have been shown by Baxter et al (1992) to have increased neuronal activity in the circuits which include the orbitofrontal corices, heads of the caudate nucleus and dorsomedial thalamic nuclei. Furthermore, regardless of the therapeutic modality used to treat the patients, whether cognitive-behavioral or pharmacologic, the patients who responded showed a reduction in the neuronal activity in the same circuits.

Our recent PET data revealed that methylchloropiperazine (mCPP, a $5-HT_{2C}$ receptor partial agonist), when infused intravenously, activates these same circuits in healthy volunteers, who became anxious and dysphoric as a result of the infusion. They showed a more vigorous activation of these circuits than did alcoholics (Hommer et al, 1997). The alcoholics with an early age of onset, who showed very little activation of these neuronal circuits, often experienced a somewhat euphoric response to the mCPP infusion. They also exhibited blunted prolactin and adrenocorticotrophic hormone (ACTH) responses to the mCPP infusion, as compared to healthy volunteers (George et al, 1997). Intriguingly, the degree of activation of the orbitofrontal, head of the caudate and dorsomedial thalamus circuits correlated positively with the prolactin responses to mCPP. These results suggest that patients with early-onset alcoholism who have antisocial personality traits and reduced central serotonin turnover rate may exhibit reduced activation of these neuronal circuits and reduced neuroendocrine responsiveness to serotonergic agonists.

We were also interested in investigating the neuronal activities of these circuits in rhesus monkeys with known central serotonin turnover rates. The monkeys are a marvellous model for behavioral, biochemical, developmental and genetic studies, but they need to be anesthetized for brain imaging. In our first study (Doudet et al, 1995), we anesthetized them using the functional GABA-A receptor agonist isoflurane. We attempted to keep all the animals under anesthesia of equal depth. This was determined by pinching the big toe of the monkey and observing a similar increase in the heart rate of every monkey. We found a strong negative correlation between lifetime aggressiveness and CSF 5-HIAA in the monkeys. In addition, we found a very strong negative correlation between deoxyglucose uptake, particularly in the orbital frontal cortex, CSF 5-HIAA concentration and aggressiveness. This finding, in combination with the observations of Hommer et al (1997), suggested that serotonin may regulate GABAergic responsiveness via $5-HT_{2C}$ receptors in the neuronal circuits, which consist of the orbitofrontal cortex, head of the caudate nucleus and dorsomedial thalamus.

Central serotonin and alcohol sensitivity

These findings led us to investigate alcohol sensitivity in rhesus monkeys with known central serotonin turnover rates. Alcohol is a functional GABA-A receptor agonist (Suzdak et al, 1996). Moreover, reduced sensitivity to the intoxicating effects of alcohol is a strong predictor of later development of alcoholism among sons of alcoholics (Schuckit, 1994). At baseline, when Schuckit measured standing steadiness, sons of alcoholic fathers did not sway any more or less than sons of non-alcoholic fathers. After consuming an equivalent amount of alcohol, the sons of alcoholic fathers as a group became less intoxicated (i.e. they swayed less than the sons of non-alcoholic fathers). Among the sons of alcoholic fathers, alcohol sensitivity is a strong predictor of future development of alcoholism, because 56% of those who showed a reduced response became alcoholic, and only 14% of those who showed an average response became alcoholic 10 years later.

We investigated whether we could reproduce the findings of Schuckit among the rhesus monkeys, and whether initial alcohol sensitivity could be related to central serotonin function. In a still unpublished study, Higley et al infused alcohol intravenously to alcohol-naive rhesus monkeys. They discovered that the lower a monkey's CSF 5-HIAA concentration, the less intoxicated the monkey became when exposed for the first time to a standard dose of alcohol. Moreover, those monkeys, which became aggressive towards the investigator during the first alcohol exposure, became aggressive again under the influence of alcohol when given alcohol the second time. Thus, as with humans, not every monkey becomes aggressive under the influence of alcohol, but the subgroup which does is characterized by reduced central serotonin turnover rate. Furthermore, when the monkeys were provided free access to both an aspartame-sweetened solution without ethanol and an aspartame-sweetened solution with 8% ethanol content, the low-5-HIAA monkeys consumed much more ethanol than the high-5-HIAA monkeys. Therefore, central serotonin turnover rate, which regulates initial alcohol sensitivity among the monkeys, is a strong predictor of alcohol consumption among rhesus monkeys living in a social group provided with free access to a palatable alcohol solution. The parallels to the human condition are obvious.

Serotonin-related molecular genetics

Psychiatric molecular genetics comprise a particularly challenging field of inquiry. This is because mental disorders are very common in the general population, and the patients are much more likely than the general population to have more than one comorbid mental disorder. Furthermore, assortative mating is frequent among patients with mental disorders (i.e. patients with mental disorders are more likely to marry patients with mental disorders than are the general population). This set of circumstances poses several problems for the investigator. About 10 years ago, David Goldman and I devised a strategy to investigate population isolates with the assumption that the genetic vulnerability backgrounds would be more homogeneous among isolated populations than in the general US population. The isolated populations we chose were Finns and certain American Indian tribes. Among the Finns, we chose probands with reduced central serotonin turnover rate, as indicated by a low CSF 5-HIAA concentration. We oversampled sibling pairs, and we collected a random control sample of the population around Helsinki. Everybody received a structured interview by the same Finnish research psychiatrist, who was blind to the central serotonin turnover rate of the individual. The interviews were blind-rated by two research psychiatrists in Bethesda, and any discrepancies in opinion were settled in a conference with a senior research psychiatrist. In addition, everybody filled out two personality inventories, and a social worker used a structured interview to collect data on lifetime alcohol, illicit drug and tobacco consumption. We also had access to the individual hospital and criminal records.

Nielsen et al (1994) demonstrated an association between a tryptophan hydroxylase gene polymorphism, suicidality and CSF 5-HIAA concentration. More recently, we have replicated this finding in an independent sample, and, with the added statistical power derived from combining the two samples, have also found a linkage between suicidal behavior and the tryptophan hydroxylase polymorphism (Nielsen et al, unpublished).

In the 5-HT$_{2C}$ receptor gene, we discovered a polymorphism which leads to an amino acid substitution in the extracellular part of the protein molecule. Because the gene is located on the X chromosome, males are hemizygotes. Eighty-seven per cent of males have one allele, and 13% have the other allele. The rare allele offers protection against the development of alcoholism among the Finns (Lappalainen et al, 1995). Goldman's group has discovered several other serotonin gene polymorphisms, whose importance for vulnerability to various mental disorders is currently under investigation.

Impact of molecular genetics in the future

How will the availability of information concerning the serotonergic gene background of patients affect future psychiatric practice? The first point to remember is that the effects of the genes are not predetermined. They interact with developmental environments, and therefore the genetic profile of a patient alone will not suffice for clinical decision-making. The clinician will still need to obtain a good developmental history, to evaluate the severity of current stressors, and to assign the diagnosis according to validated and generally agreed upon criteria. However, the clinician will probably be better able to select specific drugs for individual patients.

The other point which it is important to remember is that the developmental data suggest that, at the level of society, we should pay a lot of attention to early developmental conditions. Furthermore, we should perhaps spend more societal resources to improve the developmental conditions, particularly for the individuals who have heavy genetic vulnerability backgrounds. Understanding the particular genes contributing to the vulnerability backgrounds will provide a tremendous opportunity for specific positive interventions.

References

Ballenger J, Goodwin F, Major L, Brown G (1979) Alcohol and central serotonin metabolism in man, *Arch Gen Psychiatry* **36:**224–7.

Baxter LR, Schwartz JM, Bergman KS et al (1992) Caudate glucose metabolic rate changes with both drug and behavior therapy for obsessive-compulsive disorder, *Arch Gen Psychiatry* **49:**681–9.

Brown CL, Linnoila M (1990) CSF serotonin metabolite (5-HIAA) studies in depression, impulsivity and violence, *J Clin Psychiatry* **51**(suppl 4): 31–41.

Cadoret RJ, Yates WR, Throughton E, Woodworth G, Stewart MA (1995) Genetic-environmental interaction in the genesis of aggressivity and conduct disorders, *Arch Gen Psychiatry* **52:**916–24.

Cloninger C, Bohman M, Sigvardsson S (1981) Inheritance of alcohol abuse: cross-fostering analysis of adopted men, *Arch Gen Psychiatry* **38:**861–8.

Coccaro EE, Silverman J, Klar HM, Horvath TB, Siever L (1994) Familial correlates of reduced central serotonergic system function in patients with personality disorder, *Arch Gen Psychiatry* **51:**318–46.

Doudet D, Hommer D, Higley JD et al (1995) Cerebral glucose metabolism, CSF 5HIAA and aggressive behavior in rhesus monkeys, *Am J Psychiatry* **152:**1782–7.

Fils-Aime M, Eckardt M, George D, Brown G, Mefford M, Linnoila M (1996) Early-onset alcoholics have lower CSF-5HIAA than late-onset alcoholics, *Arch Gen Psychiatry* **53:**211–16.

George DT, Benkelfat C, Rawlings R et al (1997) Behavioral and neuroendocrine responses to m-chlorophenylpiperazine in subtypes of alcoholics and in healthy comparison subjects, *Am J Psychiatry* **154:**81–7.

Higley JD, Linnoila M (1997) A nonhuman primate model of excessive alcohol intake: personality and neurobiological parallels of Type I and Type II-like alcoholism. In: Galanter M, ed., *Recent Developments in Alcoholism* (Plenum Press: New York) 192–219.

Higley JD, Thompson WT, Champoux M et al (1993) Paternal and maternal genetic and environmental contributions to CSF monoamine metabolite concentrations in rhesus monkeys (macaca mulatta), *Arch Gen Psychiatry* **50:**615–23.

Higley JD, Mehlman P, Taub D et al (1996a) Excessive mortality in young, free-ranging male nonhuman primates with low CSF-5HIAA concentrations, *Arch Gen Psychiatry* **53:**537–43.

Higley JD, Mehlman PT, Poland RE et al (1996b) CSF testosterone and 5HIAA correlate with types of aggressive behaviour, *Biol Psychiatry* **40:** 1067–82.

Hommer D, Andreason P, Rio D et al (1997) Effects of m-chlorophenylpiperazine on the regional brain glucose utilization: a positron emission tomographic comparison of alcoholics and control subjects, *J Neurosci* **18:** 2796–806.

Insel TR, Mueller EA, Alterman I, Linnoila M, Murphy DL (1985) Obsessive compulsive disorder and serotonin: is there a connection? *Biol Psychiatry* **20:**1174–88.

Lamparski DM, Roy A, Nutt DJ, Linnoila M (1991) The criteria of Cloninger et al and von Knorring et al for subgrouping alcoholics: a comparison in a clinical population, *Acta Psychiatr Scand* **84:**497–502.

Lappalainen J, Zhang L, Dean M et al (1995) Identification, expression and pharmacology of a cys23-ser23 substitution in the human 5HT2C receptor gene (HTR2C), *Genomics* **27:**274–9.

Nielsen DA, Goldman D, Virkkunen M, Tokola R, Rawlings R, Linnoila M (1994) Suicidality and 5-hydroxyindoleacetic acid concentration associated with tryptophan hydroxylase polymorphism, *Arch Gen Psychiatry* **51:**34–8.

Robins LN (1966) *Deviant Children Grown Up* (Williams & Wilkins: Baltimore).

Robins LN, Helzer JE, Weissman MM et al (1984) Lifetime prevalence of specific psychiatric disorders in three sites, *Arch Gen Psychiatry* **41:**949–58.

Rosenthal N, Davenport Y, Cowdry R, Webster M, Goodwin F (1980) Monoamine metabolites in cerebrospinal fluid of depressive subgroups, *Psychiatr Res* **2:**113–19.

Roy A, Linnoila M (1986) Alcoholism and suicide, *Suicide Life Threat Behav* **16:**162–91.

Schuckit MA (1994) Low level of response to alcohol as a predictor of future alcoholism, *Am J Psychiatry* **151:**184–9.

Sigvardsson S, Bohman M, Cloninger CR (1996) Duplication of the Stockholm adoption study of alcoholism: confirmatory cross-fostering analysis, *Arch Gen Psychiatry* **53:**681–7.

Stanley M, Traskman-Benz L, Dorovini-Zis K (1985) Correlations between aminergic metabolites simultaneously obtained from human CSF and brain, *Life Sci* **37:**1279–86.

Suzdak PD, Glowa JR, Crawley JM, Schwartz RD, Skolinick P, Paul SM (1986) A selective imidazobenzodiazepine antagonist of ethanol in the rat, *Science* **234:**1243–7.

Virkkunen M, Linnoila M (1997) Serotonin in early-onset alcoholism. In: Galanter M, ed., *Recent Developments in Alcoholism*, Vol. 13 (Plenum Press: New York) 173–89.

Virkkunen M, Rawlings R, Tokola R et al (1994) CSF biochemistries, glucose metabolism and diurnal activity rhythms in alcoholic, violent offenders, fire setters and healthy volunteers, *Arch Gen Psychiatry* **51:**20–8.

Virkkunen M, Eggert M, Rawlings R, Linnoila M (1996) A prospective follow-up study of alcoholic violent offenders and fire setters, *Arch Gen Psychiatry* **53:**523–9.

von Knorring AL, Bohman M, von Knorring L, Oreland L (1985) Platelet MAO activity as a biological marker in subgroups of alcoholism, *Psychiatr Scand* **72:**51–8.

Winokur G (1979) Unipolar depression: is it divisible into autonomous subtypes? *Arch Gen Psychiatry* **36:**47–52.

10
Pharmacological challenge tests and brain serotonin function in depression and during SSRI treatment

Philip J Cowen

Introduction

It has long been proposed that depressive disorders may be caused by a decrease in serotonin (5-HT) neurotransmission (Coppen, 1967). This hypothesis has been based in large measure on the ability of antidepressant drugs to increase brain 5-HT function. However, obtaining direct evidence that brain 5-HT function is lowered in depressed patients has proved very difficult. For example, postmortem studies of brain 5-HT metabolism are difficult to carry out and subject to many methodological uncertainties. Peripheral tissues such as plasma and blood cells can be used to investigate certain aspects of 5-HT metabolism and receptor sensitivity. However, the relevance of these peripheral models to 5-HT function in the central nervous system is uncertain (see Cowen, 1996).

For these reasons, there has been much interest in the application of pharmacological challenge tests to the study of brain 5-HT function in depression. These tests employ a selective drug to activate brain 5-HT pathways and then measure a functional endpoint. This is usually a change in the plasma concentration of a particular hormone (a neuroendocrine challenge test). However, it is also possible to measure other endpoints, such as body temperature, psychological state or change in regional cerebral blood flow (see Cowen, 1993; Grasby et al, 1992). Used with appropriate methodological rigour, pharmacological challenge tests can provide valuable information about dynamic aspects of 5-HT neurotransmission in the living brain. As the work discussed below illustrates, such tests have provided the most consistent body of evidence to date that major depression is indeed associated with impaired 5-HT neurotransmission.

Brain 5-HT function in major depression: 5-HT neuroendocrine tests

5-HT neuroendocrine challenge tests aim to provide a functional assessment of brain 5-HT neurotransmission. The hypothalamus receives a dense innervation from the raphe nuclei, and activation of brain 5-HT pathways produces reliable increases in plasma concentrations of various anterior pituitary hormones, notably prolactin (PRL), growth hormone (GH) and corticotrophin (ACTH). The increase in ACTH leads to elevated plasma levels of cortisol, which can also be used as a marker of 5-HT neuroendocrine response. The increase in plasma level of a particular hormone that follows a selective 5-HT challenge provides a measure of the functional activity of brain 5-HT pathways (see Power and Cowen, 1992; Cowen, 1993).

5-HT neuroendocrine probes

5-HT probes are usually classified into those that increase brain 5-HT function by facilitating presynaptic 5-HT function and those that act directly on 5-HT receptors. Direct receptor agonists of increasing specificity are now becoming available. This should enable the sensitivity of specific 5-HT receptor subtypes to be assessed.

In both animal and human studies, there is evidence that the release of certain anterior pituitary hormones is regulated by multiple postsynaptic 5-HT receptor subtypes. In the male rat, for example, ACTH release can be provoked by selective activation of 5-HT_{1A} and 5-HT_2 receptors (see van de Kar, 1991). From this it would be predicted that the effect of 5-HT precursors, such as 5-hydroxtryptophan (5-HTP), in increasing ACTH levels would be mediated via indirect activation of both subtypes of postsynaptic 5-HT receptor. This, however, does not seem to be the case. In the rat, for example, studies with selective 5-HT receptor antagonists have indicated that 5-HTP-induced ACTH release is mediated solely via indirect activation of 5-HT_2 receptors, despite the undoubted ability of 5-HT_{1A} receptors to stimulate ACTH release (Gartside and Cowen, 1990). The reason for this surprising selectivity in postsynaptic receptor responses to precursor loading is not known.

Endocrine responses to 5-HT precursors

Intravenous tryptophan (TRP) in doses of 5 g or greater reliably increases plasma concentrations of PRL and GH in humans. We have found that the PRL and GH responses to TRP are attenuated by pindolol, a β-adrenoceptor antagonist which also possesses 5-HT_{1A} receptor antagonist properties. However, the endocrine effects of TRP are not inhibited by pretreatment with selective 5-HT_2 or 5-HT_3 receptor antagonists (see

Cowen, 1993). At present, therefore, we have provisionally concluded that the PRL and GH responses to TRP are mediated via indirect activation of postsynaptic 5-HT$_{1A}$ receptors, although other 5-HT receptor subtypes will need to be examined when selective probes become available.

Five studies of drug-free depressed patients have reported blunted PRL and GH responses to intravenous TRP compared to healthy controls (see Power and Cowen, 1992). In one study, however, the difference in PRL responses in depressives could be accounted for by decreased TRP levels following infusion (Koyama and Meltzer, 1986), while in two others, diminished PRL responses could only be demonstrated when patients with recent acute weight loss were excluded (Cowen and Charig, 1987; Deakin et al, 1990). Such exclusions are reasonable because, in healthy volunteers who lose weight by dieting, there is an increase in the PRL response to TRP (Anderson et al, 1990). Accordingly, concomitant weight loss in depressed patients may obscure blunted PRL responses to TRP.

Upadhyaya et al (1991) studied a group of depressed patients with TRP before and following recovery from major depression. They found that following recovery and a drug-free period of at least 3 months, the PRL and GH responses of the patients had returned to normal. This suggests that the blunted endocrine responses to TRP in depressed patients constitute a state rather than a trait abnormality.

5-HTP is another 5-HT precursor. At doses that do not cause nausea, 5-HTP produces a rather modest increase in plasma cortisol. This response is attenuated by the 5-HT$_2$ receptor antagonist ritanserin, but not by pindolol, suggesting that 5-HTP-induced cortisol release is mediated via indirect activation of 5-HT$_2$ receptors (Lee et al, 1991; Meltzer and Maes, 1994). Findings in depressed patients are inconsistent, but increased cortisol responses to 5-HTP have been reported in two studies (see Power and Cowen, 1992). This might be consistent with upregulation of 5-HT$_2$ receptors consequent on decreased 5-HT release.

Endocrine responses to clomipramine

Clomipramine is a selective 5-HT reuptake inhibitor but is metabolized in vivo to desmethylclomipramine, a noradrenaline reuptake inhibitor. However, during the time period of an acute clomipramine neuroendocrine challenge, plasma desmethylclomipramine is not detectable (Anderson et al, 1992). Three studies in depressed patients have found that the PRL responses to clomipramine are blunted, compared to the responses of healthy controls (see Power and Cowen, 1992). The identity of the postsynaptic 5-HT receptor subtype(s) that may mediate the PRL response to clomipramine in humans is not known.

The findings with clomipramine support the TRP data in suggesting that major depression is associated with impaired 5-HT-mediated PRL release. Importantly, PRL responses to other pharmacological challenges, such as the dopamine D_2 receptor antagonist metoclopramide and the direct lactotroph stimulant thyrotropin-releasing hormone, are not reliably blunted in depressed patients (Anderson and Cowen, 1991; Anderson et al, 1992). This suggests that the impairment in 5-HT-mediated PRL release seen in depression is not attributable to a generalized decrease in PRL secretion.

Endocrine responses to fenfluramine

Fenfluramine is a 5-HT-releasing and uptake-inhibiting agent which has been used both as the racemate, *dl*-fenfluramine, and the more selective 5-HT releaser, *d*-fenfluramine (see McTavish and Heel, 1992). In both animals and humans, the PRL response to *d*-fenfluramine is abolished by the 5-HT$_2$ receptor antagonist ritanserin, but not by pindolol (Goodall et al, 1993; Park and Cowen, 1995). This suggests that fenfluramine-induced PRL release is mediated by indirect stimulation of postsynaptic 5-HT$_2$ receptors.

Blunted PRL responses to fenfluramine have been found in 6 of 12 studies of drug-free depressed patients (Park et al, 1996), so this abnormality does not seem to be as consistent as the finding of impaired PRL response to TRP. In general, blunting of responses to fenfluramine appears to be associated with two distinct kinds of patient population. The first tend to be inpatients, have severe depressive symptoms with melancholia and may demonstrate cortisol hypersecretion (Mitchell and Smythe, 1990; Lichtenberg et al, 1992). The second have aggressive and impulsive personality traits with a history of suicide attempts (Coccaro et al, 1989).

It is worthwhile noting that subjects in the latter group may manifest blunted PRL responses to fenfluramine in the absence of a current depressive disorder (Coccaro et al, 1989). Presumably, here the blunted PRL responses may represent a trait marker of 5-HT dysfunction and could, perhaps, correspond with the abnormalities in cerebrospinal fluid (CSF) 5-hydroxyindole acetic acid (5-HIAA) that have been reported in subjects who tend to behave in an aggressive and impulsive way (Roy et al, 1990). In the first group, however, where blunted PRL responses to fenfluramine are associated with severe depression and cortisol hypersecretion, the impaired endocrine response appears to be a state marker of depression which remits with clinical recovery (Shapira et al, 1993).

Both fenfluramine and 5-HTP appear to produce their endocrine effects through indirect activation of postsynaptic 5-HT$_2$ receptors. It is therefore paradoxical that cortisol responses to 5-HTP may be enhanced in depression, while the PRL response to fenfluramine appears to be attenuated. One possibility is that 5-HTP is a precursor which can presumably restore a deficit in 5-HT stores in nerve terminals. In contrast, fenfluramine is a 5-HT-releasing agent which presumably can release only the 5-HT that is actually present at the nerve terminal.

Endocrine responses to 5-HT$_{1A}$ receptor agonists

A number of selective 5-HT$_{1A}$ receptor ligands are now becoming available for clinical study. The endocrine responses of depressed patients to these agents is of considerable interest in view of the possible role of 5-HT$_{1A}$ receptors in mediating resilience to adversity (Deakin and Graeff, 1991).

Administration of 5-HT$_{1A}$ receptor agonists to humans produces a characteristic profile of endocrine and temperature effects. The most reliable changes are an increase in plasma GH and a decrease in body temperature (see Cowen, 1993). Given in sufficient doses, most 5-HT$_{1A}$ receptor agonists also increase plasma ACTH and cortisol. Studies with pindolol suggest that the ACTH, GH and hypothermic responses to 5-HT$_{1A}$ receptor agonists are mediated by activation of 5-HT$_{1A}$ receptors (Lesch, 1992; Cowen, 1993; Seletti et al, 1995). Some currently employed 5-HT$_{1A}$ receptor agonists, notably buspirone and flesinoxan, also increase plasma PRL levels. However, the role of 5-HT$_{1A}$ receptors in buspirone-induced PRL release is unclear, and blockade of dopamine D$_2$ receptors may be the more important mechanism (Meltzer et al, 1991).

Studies in animals suggest that endocrine responses to 5-HT$_{1A}$ receptor challenge are mediated by activation of postsynaptic 5-HT$_{1A}$ receptors (see Cowen, 1993). The hypothermic response appears to be a consequence of activation of cell body 5-HT$_{1A}$ autoreceptors, but in some species postsynaptic 5-HT$_{1A}$ receptors may be involved as well (Bill et al, 1991; Hillegaart, 1991).

Results of studies with 5-HT$_{1A}$ receptor agonists in drug-free depressed patients have yielded inconsistent findings. Two studies have found blunted hypothermic responses which could be consistent with lowered sensitivity of 5-HT$_{1A}$ autoreceptors (Lesch, 1992; Cowen et al, 1994). In addition, both of the studies that employed ipsapirone as a challenge found impaired cortisol responses (Lesch, 1992; Meltzer and Maes, 1995). While this is consistent with subsensitivity of postsynaptic 5-HT$_{1A}$ receptors, depressed patients may exhibit blunted cortisol responses to a variety of pharmacological and hormonal challenges, presumably because of underlying hypothalamic–pituitary–adrenal axis dysfunction (Amsterdam et al, 1987).

In contrast to the blunting of ipsapirone-induced cortisol release, the GH response to buspirone, another probable measure of postsynaptic 5-HT$_{1A}$ receptor sensitivity, was unchanged in depressed patients (Cowen et al, 1994). This is of interest because buspirone-induced GH release is a consequence of direct activation of postsynaptic 5-HT$_{1A}$ receptors, while the GH response to TRP, which is reliably blunted in depressed patients (see above), involves indirect activation of these receptors (via increased 5-HT release). Taken together, the data suggest that the impairment in TRP-induced GH release in depression is due to abnormal function of presynaptic 5-HT neurons and not to impaired sensitivity of postsynaptic 5-HT$_{1A}$ receptors.

Endocrine responses to other 5-HT receptor challenges

Few studies have been reported of other 5-HT receptor challenges in depressed patients. The endocrine and temperature responses to *m*-chlorophenylpiperazine (mCPP) and 6-chloro-2-(1-piperazinyl)-pyrazine (MK-212) probably involve activation of 5-HT$_2$ receptors (see Cowen, 1993). At present, there is no consistent evidence that depressed patients have altered endocrine responses to either of these drugs (see Power and Cowen, 1992; Anand et al, 1994).

Conclusions

At present there is a considerable body of evidence to suggest that the endocrine responses to presynaptic 5-HT challenges are impaired in major depression. This abnormality appears to be state dependent, suggesting that it is related to the presence of depressive illness. There is less evidence that postsynaptic 5-HT receptor sensitivity is lowered in depression (Table 10.1). However, further work in this area is needed.

The relationship of impaired brain 5-HT function to the pathophysiology of depression is not fully clear. However, recent studies of TRP depletion in recovered unmedicated patients suggest that in subjects vulnerable to depression, acute reductions in brain 5-HT neurotransmission can be sufficient to provoke an acute depressive syndrome (Smith et al, 1997).

Table 10.1   Neuroendocrine responses to 5-HT challenges in major depression versus healthy controls.

Drug	Mechanism	Response versus controls
TRP	5-HT precursor	↓ GH, ↓ PRL
5-HTP	5-HT precursor	? ↑ Cortisol
Fenfluramine	5-HT releaser	↓ PRL (in about 50% of studies)
Clomipramine	5-HT reuptake inhibitor	↓ PRL
Ipsapirone Buspirone	5-HT$_{1A}$ receptor agonist	↓ Cortisol, ↓ Hypothermia, =GH
mCPP	5-HT$_{2C}$ receptor agonist	=PRL, =Cortisol

SSRIs and brain 5-HT function

Another use of pharmacological challenge tests is to assess the effect of psychotropic drugs on brain neurotransmitter function. Here there are often animal experimental data to guide human investigations. Obviously, pharmacological challenge studies in animals can be particularly useful when extrapolating preclinical work to human investigations.

From the point of view of the indoleamine hypothesis of depression, specific serotonin reuptake inhibitors (SSRIs) are of particular interest because their acute pharmacological effects are essentially confined to blockade of 5-HT reuptake. The fact that such drugs are effective antidepressants supports the concept that depression is associated with diminished brain 5-HT function (see Cowen, 1990).

There are, however, several problems with this line of argument. First, the fact that a selective drug is effective in a particular condition does not necessarily mean that the drug acts by reversing an underlying neurochemical abnormality. The utility of anticholinergic drugs in Parkinson's disease offers an obvious example of this. Second, drugs with quite different acute pharmacological actions from those of SSRIs, e.g. selective noradrenaline reuptake inhibitors, are as effective as SSRIs in the treatment of major depression (Anderson, 1997). This seems to indicate that increasing brain 5-HT function can be *sufficient* to produce a clinical antidepressant effect but is not *necessary*. Third, the action of SSRIs to inhibit 5-HT reuptake occurs within hours of SSRI administration; however, the therapeutic effect of SSRIs can take several weeks to become manifest (Asberg et al, 1986).

The latter observation suggests that the acute effect of SSRIs in blocking 5-HT reuptake triggers a series of adaptive changes in 5-HT and other neurotransmitter pathways. It has been proposed that it is these adaptive changes that are responsible for the therapeutic effect of SSRIs (Blier and de Montigny, 1994). It is important to find out if this is the case, because it might lead to quicker-acting and more effective antidepressant treatments. This chapter will focus on neuroadaptive effects in 5-HT pathways. This does not mean that changes in other neurotransmitter pathways are unimportant. However, the ability of acute plasma TRP depletion (presumably by lowering brain 5-HT function) to cause acute depressive relapse in remitted depressed patients taking SSRIs suggests that facilitation of brain 5-HT function plays a critical role in the therapeutic effect of SSRIs (Delgado et al, 1990).

Neuroadaptive effects of SSRIs in pre-clinical studies

5-HT$_{1A}$ receptors
Adaptive changes in brain 5-HT$_{1A}$ receptors are of potential importance in the antidepressant effect of SSRIs (Blier and de Montigny, 1994). This is

because 5-HT$_{1A}$ receptors function both as autoreceptors on 5-HT cell bodies, where they inhibit 5-HT neuronal firing (Sprouse and Aghajanian, 1987), and as postsynaptic receptors in terminal fields, where they mediate the effects of 5-HT released from presynaptic terminals (Andrade and Nicoll, 1987).

In animal experimental studies, repeated administration of SSRIs produces adaptive changes in 5-HT$_{1A}$ receptors. For example, electrophysiological investigations indicate that repeated administration of SSRIs desensitizes 5-HT$_{1A}$ autoreceptors in the raphe nuclei, while leaving unaltered the responsivity of postsynaptic 5-HT$_{1A}$ receptors in the hippocampus (Chaput et al, 1988; Blier and de Montigny, 1994). The net effect of these adaptive changes is gradually to free 5-HT neurons from inhibitory feedback control and thereby produce a substantial increase in 5-HT neurotransmission at postsynaptic 5-HT$_{1A}$ receptors (Blier and de Montigny, 1994).

However, not all experimental models support the lack of effect of SSRIs on postsynaptic 5-HT$_{1A}$ receptors. For example, both behavioural and neuroendocrine studies suggest that repeated SSRI treatment may decrease the functional sensitivity of postsynaptic 5-HT$_{1A}$ receptors (Goodwin et al, 1987; Li et al, 1994).

5-HT$_{1B/1D}$ receptors

5-HT$_{1B/1D}$ receptors are located both on 5-HT nerve terminals, where they function as inhibitory autoreceptors, and at certain postsynaptic sites, particularly the basal ganglia (Chopin et al, 1994). Electrophysiological and neurochemical studies have indicated that repeated treatment with SSRIs may desensitize terminal autoreceptors on 5-HT neurons in various brain regions, including hippocampus and hypothalamus (Moret and Briley, 1990; Blier and Bouchard, 1994). This adaptive change would be expected to lessen feedback inhibition at 5-HT terminals, thereby facilitating 5-HT release. Whether SSRIs alter the sensitivity of postsynaptic 5-HT$_{1D}$ receptors is uncertain.

5-HT$_2$ receptors

There have been numerous ligand-binding and behavioural studies on the effect of SSRIs on 5-HT$_{2A}$ receptors. The data from ligand-binding studies are rather inconclusive but in some investigations repeated SSRI treatment appears to downregulate 5-HT$_{2A}$ receptor density (see Johnson, 1991). There is rather more consistent evidence that SSRIs decrease behavioural responses to 5-HT$_{2A}$ receptor agonists. This suggests that SSRI treatment decreases the responsivity of postsynaptic 5-HT$_{2A}$ receptors (see Johnson, 1991).

The effect of SSRIs on postsynaptic 5-HT$_{2C}$ receptors has been less studied. However, hypolocomotor responses to mCPP are decreased by repeated SSRI treatment (see Kennett et al, 1994). This suggests that SSRIs decrease the sensitivity of postsynaptic 5-HT$_{2C}$ receptors.

SSRIs and 5-HT neurotransmission

A key question is the effect of repeated SSRI treatment on overall neuro-transmission at 5-HT synapses. From the above account it can be seen that the net effect of SSRIs on 5-HT neurotransmission is likely to involve a balance between a series of neuroadaptive changes in both pre- and postsynaptic 5-HT receptors. The desensitization of 5-HT_{1A} and 5-HT_{1B} receptors would be expected to increase 5-HT neurotransmission, while the functional downregulation of postsynaptic 5-HT_{1A} and 5-HT_2 receptors would produce the opposite effect. The overall balance of these effects on 5-HT neurotransmission is unclear.

There have been few studies in animals of this question. However, the work of Blier and de Montigny (1994), in which stimulation of ascending 5-HT neurons is used to activate postsynaptic 5-HT receptors in the hip-pocampus, suggests that in this brain region the net effect of SSRIs is to increase brain 5-HT neurotransmission.

SSRIs and challenge studies in humans

5-HT receptors

There is good evidence from studies of patients and healthy subjects that repeated treatment with SSRIs decreases the cortisol and GH responses to 5-HT_{1A} receptor agonists such as ipsapirone, buspirone and gepirone (Lesch et al, 1991; Anderson et al, 1996) (Figure 10.1). These studies also indicate that SSRI treatment blunts the hypothermic response to 5-HT_{1A} receptor stimulation (Figure 10.2). Because this response appears, in part, to be mediated by presynaptic 5-HT_{1A} autoreceptors, this suggests that SSRI treatment in humans may desensitize 5-HT_{1A} autoreceptors. Thus these data indicate that SSRI treatment decreases the responsiveness of both pre- and postsynaptic 5-HT_{1A} receptors.

There is less work on the effect of SSRIs on other 5-HT receptor sub-types in humans. We found that the decrease in plasma PRL produced by the $5\text{-HT}_{1B/1D}$ receptor agonist sumatriptan was not altered by repeated SSRI treatment in healthy subjects (Wing et al, 1996). Because sumatriptan-induced decreases in plasma PRL may be mediated by 5-HT_{1B} terminal autoreceptors (Herdman et al, 1996), this suggests that SSRIs may not desensitize presynaptic 5-HT_{1B} receptors in humans.

There are no direct postsynaptic 5-HT_{2A} receptor agonists available for use in humans but, as noted above, mCPP can be used to probe 5-HT_{2C} receptors. One study examined the effect of repeated fluoxetine treat-ment on the PRL response to mCPP in patients with obsessive-compul-sive disorder (Hollander et al, 1991). However, in patients taking fluoxetine, levels of mCPP after oral administration were much higher than before treatment. PRL responses to mCPP were greater too, but interpretation of this effect was complicated by the pharmacokinetic inter-action between the fluoxetine and mCPP.

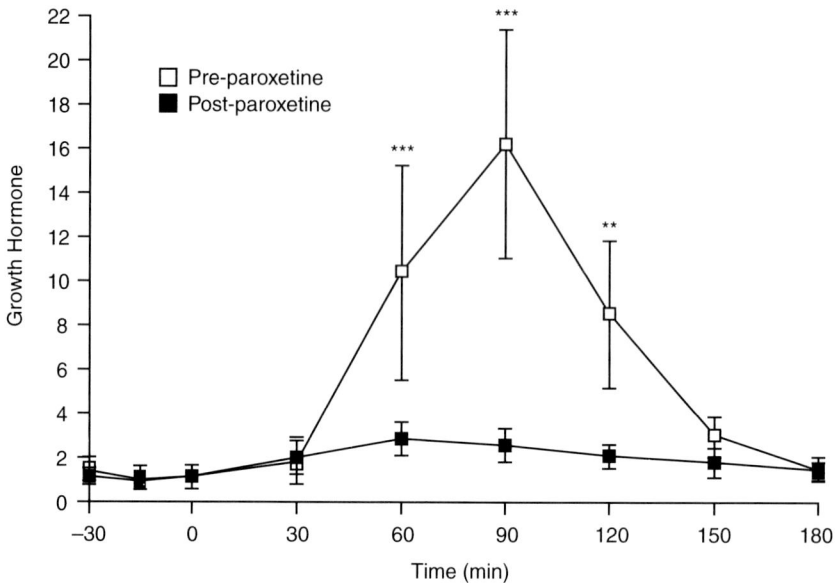

Figure 10.1

Mean plasma GH concentration following administration of gepirone (20 mg orally at time 0) in 12 healthy male subjects who were studied before (□) and at the end of 3 weeks of paroxetine treatment (30 mg daily) (■). GH levels following gepirone are significantly lower after paroxetine treatment.

We carried out a similar study in subjects taking paroxetine. Following repeated paroxetine administration, plasma mCPP levels after intravenous administration were no different to those seen before treatment. In contrast, PRL and hyperthermic responses to mCPP were significantly blunted (Figure 10.3). This suggests that in humans, as in animals, repeated SSRI treatment decreases the responsivity of postsynaptic 5-HT$_{2C}$ receptors.

SSRIs and 5-HT precursors

As noted above, the endocrine responses to 5-HT precursors depend both on the presynaptic release of 5-HT and on the sensitivity of postsynaptic 5-HT receptors. They may therefore provide an index of overall activity of 5-HT neurotransmission. In fact, studies in depressed patients with both TRP and the 5-HT precursor 5-HTP show that repeated SSRI treatment increases 5-HT-mediated endocrine responses to both these 5-HT precursors (Price et al, 1989) (Figure 10.4). This suggests that SSRIs increase overall neurotransmission at 5-HT$_{1A}$ and 5-HT$_{2}$ synapses despite a certain amount of downregulation of postsynaptic receptor responsiveness.

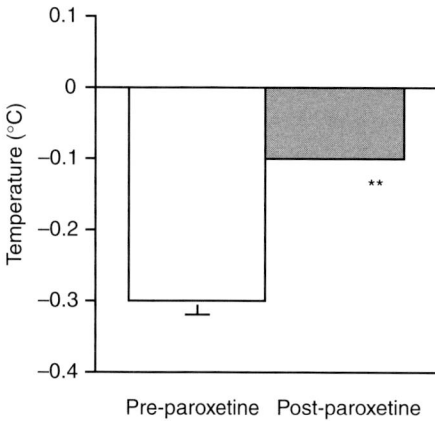

Figure 10.2

Mean oral temperature (measured as peak fall from baseline) following administration of gepirone (20 mg orally) in 12 healthy male subjects who were studied before (pre-paroxetine) and at the end of 3 weeks of paroxetine treatment (post-paroxetine). Hypothermic responses following gepirone are significantly lower after paroxetine treatment.

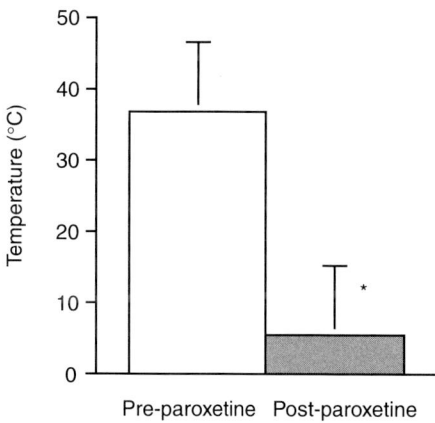

Figure 10.3

Hyperthermic response to mCPP (measured as area under the curve with placebo subtraction) in seven healthy subjects tested before (pre-paroxetine) and at the end of 3 weeks of paroxetine treatment (30 mg daily) (post-paroxetine). Hyperthermic responses post-paroxetine are significantly attenuated.

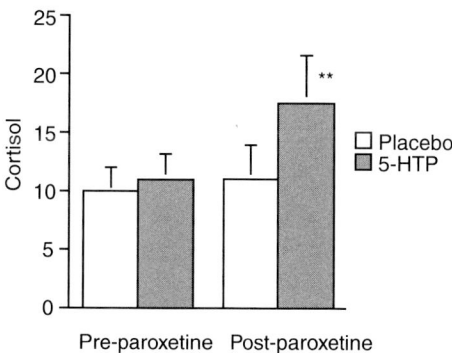

Figure 10.4

Cortisol response to 5-HTP (100 mg orally) and placebo (measured as area under the curve) in 10 depressed patients tested before (pre-paroxetine) and at the end of 8 weeks of paroxetine treatment. Cortisol responses to 5-HTP post-paroxetine are significantly enhanced.

Conclusions

Neuroendocrine studies in humans indicate that SSRIs do indeed produce adaptive changes in certain pre- and postsynaptic 5-HT receptors (Table 10.2). While the net effect of the various changes on 5-HT

Table 10.2   Effects of repeated SSRI treatment on neuroendocrine responses to 5-HT challenge.

Drug	Response
TRP	↑ PRL
5-HTP	↑ Cortisol
Buspirone	↓ GH, cortisol
Ipsapirone	↓ Hypothermia, cortisol
Gepirone	↓ Hypothermia, GH, cortisol
mCPP	↓ PRL, ↓ Hyperthermia
Sumatriptan	=PRL

neurotransmission is hard to predict, studies with 5-HT precursors suggest that, overall, SSRIs increase brain 5-HT function. This is consistent with the ability of techniques that lower brain 5-HT function, e.g. the process of TRP depletion, to produce a rapid reversal of the antidepressant effects of SSRIs in depressed patients (Delgado et al, 1990). Taken together, the evidence suggests that the ability of repeated SSRI treatment to enhance brain 5-HT neurotransmission is critical to their antidepressant effects.

● Acknowledgement

The author is an MRC Clinical Scientist.

References

Amsterdam JD, Maislin G, Winokur A et al (1987) Pituitary and adrenocortical responses to the ovine corticotropin releasing hormone in depressed patients and healthy volunteers, *Arch Gen Psychiatry* **44:**775–81.

Anand A, Charney DS, Delgado PL et al (1994) Neuroendocrine and behavioral responses to intravenous m-chlorophenylpiperazine (mCPP) in depressed patients and healthy comparison subjects, *Am J Psychiatry* **151:**1626–30.

Anderson IM (1997) Lessons to be learnt from meta-analyses of newer versus older antidepressants, *Adv Psychiatr Treat* **3:**57–62.

Anderson IM, Cowen PJ (1991) Prolactin response to the dopamine antagonist, metoclopramide, in depression, *Biol Psychiatry* **30:** 313–16.

Anderson IM, Parry-Billings M, Newsholme EA et al (1990) Dieting reduces plasma tryptophan and alters brain 5-HT function in women, *Psychol Med* **20:**785–91.

Anderson IM, Ware CJ, da Roza Davis JM et al (1992) Decreased 5-HT-mediated prolactin release in major depression, *Br J Psychiatry* **160:** 372–8.

Anderson IM, Deakin JFW, Miller ATJ (1996) The effects of chronic fluvoxamine on hormonal and psychological responses to buspirone in normal volunteers, *Psychopharmacology* **128:** 74–82.

Andrade R, Nicoll RA (1987) Pharmacologically distinct actions of serotonin on single pyramidal neurones of the rat hippocampus recorded in vitro, *J Physiol* **394:**99–124.

Asberg M, Erikkson B, Matensson B et al (1986) Therapeutic effects of serotonin uptake inhibitors in depression, *J Clin Psychiatry* **47:**23–35.

Bill DJ, Knight M, Forster EA et al (1991) Direct evidence for an important species difference in the mechanism of 8-OH-DPAT-induced hypothermia, *Br J Pharmacol* **103:**1857–64.

Blier P, Bouchard C (1994) Modulation of 5-HT release in the guinea-pig brain following long-term administration of antidepressant drugs, *Br J Pharmacol* **113:**485–95.

Blier P, de Montigny C (1994) Current advances and trends in the treatment of depression, *Trends Pharmacol Sci* **15:**220–6.

Chaput Y, Blier P, de Montigny C (1988) Acute and long-term effects of antidepressant 5-HT reuptake blocker on the efficacy of 5-HT neurotransmission: electrophysiological studies in the rat CNS, *Adv Biol Psychiatry* **17:**1–17.

Chopin P, Moret C, Briley M (1994) Neuropharmacology of 5-hydroxytryptamine, B/10 receptor byands, *Pharmacol Ther* **62:**385–405.

Coccaro EF, Siever LJ, Klar HM et al (1989) Serotonergic studies in patients with affective and personality disorders, *Arch Gen Psychiatry* **46:**587–99.

Coppen AJ (1967) The biochemistry of affective disorders, *Br J Psychiatry* **113:**1237–64.

Cowen PJ (1990) A role for 5-HT in the action of antidepressant drugs, *Pharmacol Ther* **46:**43–51.

Cowen PJ (1993) Serotonin receptor subtypes in depression: evidence from studies in neuroendocrine regulation, *Clin Neuropharmacol* **16**(suppl 3):S6–18.

Cowen PJ (1996) The serotonin hypothesis: necessary but not sufficient. In: Feighner JP, Boyer WF, eds, *Selective Serononin Re-uptake Inhibitors*, 2nd edn (John Wiley: Chichester) 63–86.

Cowen PJ, Charig EM (1987) Neuroendocrine responses to intravenous tryptophan in major depression, *Arch Gen Psychiatry* **44:**958–66.

Cowen PJ, Power AC, Ware CJ et al (1994) 5-HT$_{1A}$ receptor sensitivity in major depression: a neuroendocrine study with buspirone, *Br J Psychiatry* **164:**372–9.

Deakin JFW, Graeff FG (1991) 5-HT and mechanisms of defence, *J Psychopharmacol* **5:**305–15.

Deakin JFW, Pennell I, Upadhyaya AJ et al (1990) A neuroendocrine study of 5-HT function in depression: evidence for biological mechanisms of endogenous and psychosocial causation, *Psychopharmacology* **101:**85–92.

Delgado PL, Charney DS, Price LH et al (1990) Serotonin function and the mechanism of antidepressant action: reversal of antidepressant-induced remission by rapid depletion of plasma tryptophan, *Arch Gen Psychiatry* **47:**411–18.

Gartside SE, Cowen PJ (1990) Mediation of ACTH and prolactin responses to 5-HTP by 5-HT$_2$ receptors, *Eur J Pharmacol* **179:**103–9.

Goodall EM, Cowen PJ, Franklin M et al (1993) Ritanserin attenuates anorectic, endocrine and thermic responses to d-fenfluramine in human volunteers, *Psychopharmacology* **112:**461–6.

Goodwin GM, de Souza RJ, Green AR (1987) Attenuation by electroconvulsive shock and antidepressant drugs of the 5-HT$_{1A}$ receptor mediated hypothermia and serotonin syndrome produced by 8-OH-DPAT in the rat, *Psychopharmacology* **91:**500–5.

Grasby PM, Friston KJ, Bench C et al (1992) Effect of the 5-HT$_{1A}$ partial agonist buspirone on regional cerebral blood flow in man, *Psychopharmacology* **108:**380–6.

Herdman JRE, Delva NJ, Hockney RA et al (1994) Neuroendocrine effects of sumatriptan, *Psychopharmacology* **113:**561–4.

Hillegaart V (1991) Effects of local application of 5-HT and 8-OH-DPAT into the dorsal and medial raphe nuclei on core temperature in the rat, *Psychopharmacology* **103:**291–6.

Hollander E, de Caria C, Gully R et al (1991) Effects of chronic fluoxetine treatment on behavioural and neuroendocrine responses to meta-chlorophenylpiperazine in obsessive compulsive disorder, *Psychiatr Res* **36:**1–17.

Johnson AM (1991) The comparative pharmacological properties of selective serotonin re-uptake inhibitors in animals. In: Feighner JP, Boyer WF, eds, *Selective Serononin Re-uptake Inhibitors* (John Wiley: Chichester) 37–70.

Kennett GA, Lightowler S, de Biasi V et al (1994) Effect of chronic administration of selective 5-hydroxytryptamine and noradrenaline uptake inhibitors in a putative index of 5-HT$_{2C/2B}$ receptor function, *Neuropharmacology* **33:**1581–8.

Koyama T, Meltzer HY (1986) A biochemical and neuroendocrine study of the serotonergic system in depression. In: Hippius H, Klerman GL, Matussek N, eds, *New Results in Depression* (Springer: Berlin) 169–88.

Lee MA, Nash JF, Barnes M et al (1991) Inhibitory effect of ritanserin on the 5-hydroxytryptophan-mediated cortisol, ACTH and prolactin secretion in humans, *Psychopharmacology* **103:**258–64.

Lesch KP (1992) 5-HT$_{1A}$ receptor responsivity in anxiety disorders and depression, *Prog Neuropsychopharmacol Biol Psychiatry* **15:**723–33.

Lesch KP, Ho HA, Schulte HM et al (1991) Long-term fluoxetine treatment decreases 5-HT$_{1A}$ receptor responsivity in obsessive compulsive disorder, *Psychopharmacology* **105:**415–20.

Li Q, Brownfield MS, Levy AD et al (1994) Attenuation of hormone responses to the 5-HT$_{1A}$ agonist, ipsapirone, by long-term treatment with fluoxetine but not desipramine in male rats, *Biol Psychiatry* **36:**300–8.

Lichtenberg P, Shapira B, Gillon D et al (1992) Hormone responses to fenfluramine and placebo challenge in endogenous depression, *Psychiatr Res* **43:**137–46.

McTavish D, Heel RC (1992) Dexfenfuramine, *Drugs* **43:**713–33.

Meltzer HY, Maes M (1994) Effect of pindolol on the L-5-HTP-induced increase in plasma prolactin and cortisol concentrations in man, *Psychopharmacology* **114:**635–43.

Meltzer HY, Maes M (1995) Effect of ipsapirone on plasma cortisol and body temperature in major depression, *Biol Psychiatry* **38:**450–7.

Meltzer HY, Gudelsky GA, Lowy MT et al (1991) Neuroendocrine effects of buspirone: mediation by dopaminergic and serotonergic mechanisms. In: Tunnicliff G, Eison AS, Taylor OP, eds, *Buspirone: Mechanisms and Clinical Aspects* (Academic Press: San Diego) 177–92.

Mitchell P, Smythe G (1990) Hormonal responses to fenfluramine in depressed and control subjects, *J Affect Disord* **19:**43–51.

Moret C, Briley M (1990) Serotonin autoreceptor subsensitivity and antidepressant activity, *Eur J Pharmacol* **180:**351–6.

Park SBG, Cowen PJ (1995) Effect of pindolol on the prolactin response to d-fenfluramine, *Psychopharmacology* **118:**471–4.

Park SBG, Williamson DJ, Cowen PJ (1996) 5-HT neuroendocrine function in major depression: prolactin and cortisol responses to d-fenfluramine, *Psychol Med* **26:**1191–6.

Power AC, Cowen PJ (1992) Neuroendocrine challenge tests: assessment of 5-HT function in anxiety and depression, *Mol Aspects Med* **13:** 205–20.

Price LH, Charney DS, Delgado PL et al (1989) Effects of desipramine and fluvoxamine treatment on the prolactin response to tryptophan: serotonergic function and the mechanism of antidepressant action, *Arch Gen Psychiatry* **46:**625–31.

Roy A, Virkkunen M, Linnoila M (1990) Serotonin in suicide, violence and alcoholism. In: Coccaro EF, Murphy DL, eds, *Serotonin in Major Psychiatric Disorders* (American Psychiatric Press: Washington DC) 187–208.

Seletti B, Benkelfat C, Blier P et al (1995) Serotonin$_{1A}$ receptor activation by flesinoxan in humans: body temperature and neuroendocrine responses, *Neuropsychopharmacology* **13:**93–104.

Shapira B, Cohen J, Newman ME et al (1993) Prolactin response to fenfluramine and placebo challenge following maintenance pharmacotherapy withdrawal in remitted depressed patients, *Biol Psychiatry* **33:**531–5.

Shopin P, Moret C, Briley M (1994) Neuropharmacology of 5-hydroxytryptamine$_{1B/D}$ receptor ligands, *Pharmacol Ther* **62:**385–405.

Smith KA, Fairburn CG, Cowen PJ (1997) Relapse of depression after rapid depletion of tryptophan. *Lancet* **349:**915–19

Sprouse JS, Aghajanian GK (1987) Electrophysiological responses of serotonergic dorsal raphe neurones to 5-HT$_{1A}$ and 5-HT$_{1B}$ agonists, *Synapse* **1:**3–9.

Upadhyaya AK, Pennell I, Cowen PJ et al (1991) Blunted growth hormone and prolactin responses to L-tryptophan in depression: a state-dependent abnormality, *J Affect Disord* **21:**213–18.

Van de Kar LD (1991) Neuroendocrine pharmacology of serotonergic (5-HT) neurones, *Annu Rev Pharmacol Toxicol* **31:**289–320.

Wing Y-K, Clifford EM, Sheehan BD et al (1996) Paroxetine treatment and the prolactin response to sumatriptan, *Psychopharmacology* **124:**377–9.

11
The prevalence of depression

Jules Angst

Introduction

Psychiatric epidemiology has developed in recent years into a major research discipline. The great advantage of the epidemiological method lies in its representativeness and in the presence of representative normal controls. I would propose to define psychiatric epidemiology purely in methodological terms as studies of representative populations, e.g. the general population or the population of subjects attending primary care. The subject of psychiatric epidemiological investigation can be any psychiatric question: health, health services, incidence and prevalence of symptoms and disorders, the validity of diagnoses, the associations between disorders (cross-sectional and longitudinal comorbidity), genetics, biology, course, personality, coping, and environmental and other risk factors for the development of a disorder (e.g. gender, social conditions and stressors).

This chapter will review the epidemiological literature on the incidence and prevalence of depression, including the prevalence of treated cases, because—as we know—only some depressives seek treatment. Using data from the Zurich cohort study, I will compare the prevalence rates and characteristics of treated major depressives versus untreated depressives in the normal population. The chapter ends with a brief discussion of the question whether there has really been an increase in depression in this century.

Incidence of depression

Incidence in this context is defined as the rate of first manifestation (new cases) of depression over 1 year. Incidence data are difficult to obtain, for their collection relies on prospective studies. From the Epidemiologic Catchment Area (ECA) study, incidence data were provided for four sites on the basis of a 1-year follow-up (Eaton et al, 1989) (Table 11.1). Across all age groups, the incidence rate was 1.56 per 100 person-years (males 1.1, females 1.98), providing powerful confirmation that females are at

Table 11.1   Incidence of major depressive disorder.[e]

	Instrument	N	M	F	M + F
Eaton et al (1989)[a]	DIS	10 861	1.4–0.9	2.0–1.48	1.72–1.25
Lewinsohn et al (1993)[b] Oregon	SADS-L	1 508			
First incidence			4.35	7.14	5.72
Total incidence			9.09	21.11	17.89
incl. recurrence			11.16	14.04	13.35[d]
Meller et al (1996)[c] Munich (1 year)	GMS-A	263			

[a] Adults.
[b] Adolescents.
[c] Age 85+.
[d] Depression, neurosis and psychosis.
[e] per 1000 per year.

higher risk for developing depression than males. Males up to the age of 44 showed higher incidence rates than those of 45 or older. By contrast, the incidence rate of females was shown to decline only slightly after the age of 65. This finding suggests that in the age group 45–64, females differ markedly from males, with about a three-fold higher incidence rate (females 2.02, males 0.64).

In a study of 1508 adolescents followed up over 1 year, Lewinsohn et al (1993) in Oregon reported an annual incidence for major depressive disorder of 4.35% for males and 7.14% for females (males and females together 5.72%). A recent 1-year follow-up study, this time in subjects aged 85 and over, carried out by Meller et al (1996) in Munich and providing data for a broader diagnosis of neurotic or psychotic depression, found the first incidence for males to be 11.16% and for females 14.04%.

All these studies establish that the female preponderance, which is familiar from prevalence studies, also applies to incidence data.

Point prevalence rates for major depression

Point prevalence rates are a far more reliable measure than period prevalence rates, since they are uncontaminated by memory artefacts. Most studies give 'current prevalence rates', which usually means presence over the past 4 weeks. Boyd and Weissman (1981) reviewed 16 studies, 15 of which reported rates between 1.0% and 10.8%. Something of an outlier was a study carried out in Uganda (Orley and Wing, 1979), which applied the Present State Examination (PSE) (Wing, 1970) and reported rates of 14.3% among males and 22.6% among females.

Since 1981 a number of new studies have been conducted (Table 11.2). Studies applying standard instruments (DIS, CIDI, SADS-L) have yielded rates between 2% and 5%. Some studies using other instruments (PSE) show slightly higher rates (Bebbington et al, 1989: 7%). In addition, two studies on adolescents (Lewinsohn et al, 1993; Reinherz et al, 1993) found rates within the same range, i.e. 3.8% and 2.9% respectively. The large ECA study ($N = 19\ 182$) reported by Weissman et al (1990) gave current prevalence rates for affective disorders (including bipolars) of 2.4% (males 1.7%, females 3.1%), whereas the National Comorbidity Survey in the USA (Blazer et al, 1994) identified a rate of 4.9% (males 3.8%, females 5.9%).

It is clear that the PSE gives higher rates: Abas and Broadhead (1997) reviewed comparative rates of their own study in Harare and studies carried out in Canberra, Camberwell and Uganda, all of which had applied the PSE-CATEGO classes and ICD-9 equivalents. The 1-month prevalence rate for ICD-9 depression (296.2 or 300.4) was lowest in Canberra (6.7%), followed by Camberwell (9.0%), Harare (12.2%) and Uganda (22.6%).

Table 11.2   Current prevalence rates of major depressive disorder.

		Instrument	N	M	F	M + F
Romanoski et al (1992)	Baltimore	DIS	810	0.9	1.4	1.1
Meltzer et al (1995)	UK	CIS-R	9 792	1.7	2.5	2.1
Roberts and Vernon (1982)	California	SADS-RDC	528			2.1
Regier et al (1993)	ECA	DIS	19 182	1.6	2.9	–
Weissman et al (1990)	USA, ECA	DIS	19 182	1.7	3.1	2.4
Lewinsohn et al (1993)	Oregon	SADS-L				
	T_1		1 710	1.7	3.4	2.6
	T_2		1 508	2.6	3.6	3.1
Reinherz et al (1993)	Boston, USA	DIS DSM-III-R	386[a]	–	–	2.9
Oliver and Simmons (1985)	St Louis	DIS	298	–	–	3.4
Faravelli and Incerpi (1985)	Florence	SADS-L	639	–	–	3.8
Weissman and Myers (1978)[b]	New Haven	SADS-L	720	3.2	5.2	4.3
Murphy et al (1988)	Stirling County, Canada	Quest/Int	1 003	–	–	5.3
		DPAX	1 094	–	–	5.6
Bebbington et al (1989)	London	PSE/CATEGO	310	–	–	7.0
Blazer et al (1994), age 15–54	USA, NCS	CIDI	8 098	3.8	5.9	4.9
Dean et al (1983)	Edinburgh	PSE/RDC	576	–	7.0	–
Orley and Wing (1979), age 18+	Uganda	PSE/Catego	221	14.3	22.6	–

[a] Adolescents.
[b] Primary unipolar depression.

It is worth emphasizing that the current prevalence rate for females was regularly reported to be higher than for males (usually nearly double); forgetting by males cannot in this case be a major interfering variable.

Six-month prevalence rates

Six-month prevalence rates should be higher than point prevalence rates if a proportion of the episodes recover within a few months. Reported rates for major depressive episodes range between 3.0% (Canino et al, 1987) and 6% (Oliver and Simmons, 1985; Reinherz et al, 1993). Again all studies found higher rates for females than for males (Table 11.3).

One-year prevalence rates

Low 1-year prevalence rates were found in Taiwan (0.8%) and Korea (2.3%) (Weissman et al, 1996) as well as in the ECA study (Weissman et al, 1990); the highest rate (10.3%) was reported in the National Comorbidity Survey (NCS) of Kessler et al (1993). Three other studies found rates ranging between 3.1% and 4.2% (Table 11.4). Again we find the preponderance of females confirmed. The differences in rates may partly be explained by the instruments applied (the CIDI used in the NCS may be more sensitive than the DIS); however, the study by Parikh et al (1996) in Ontario, Canada ($N = 9953$), which also used the CIDI, found much lower prevalence rates (urban population 4.2%; rural population 3.2%), a finding which contrasts with the figure of 10.3% provided by Kessler et al (1993) for the USA, which indicated no significant difference in rates between urban and rural populations.

Weissman et al (1996) compared the annual rates reported in studies applying the DIS, standardizing the figures to the US age and sex distribution. The annual rates varied between 0.8% (Taiwan) and 5.8% (New Zealand) among persons between the ages of 18 and 64.

Lifetime prevalence rates of major depression

Again, the ECA study (Weissman et al, 1990) found the relatively low overall lifetime prevalence rate of major depression of 4.9%; the five US sites investigated varied between 3.0% and 5.9%. Table 11.5 ranks a number of studies by the rates. The lowest rates, ranging between 0.9% and 1.7%, were reported in Taiwan, and the highest were 17.1% in the US NCS of Kessler et al (1993) and 18% in the New Haven study of Weissman and Myers (1978). The latter figures are close to some

Table 11.3   Six-month prevalence rates of major depressive disorder.

		Instrument	N	M	F	M + F
Weissman et al (1988)	USA, ECA, 5 sites	DIS	18 572	—	—	1.5–2.8
	New Haven		5 034	—	—	2.8
	Baltimore		3 481	—	—	1.7
	St Louis		3 004	—	—	2.3
	Piedmont		3 921	—	—	1.5
	Los Angeles		3 132	—	—	2.6
Canino et al (1987)	Puerto Rico	DIS	1 513	2.4	3.3	3.0
Bland et al (1988a)	Edmonton, Canada	DIS	3 258	2.5	3.9	3.2
Levav et al (1993)	Israel	SADS-I	2 741	3.8	4.5	4.1
Oakley-Browne et al (1989)	New Zealand	DIS	1 498	3.4	7.1	5.3
Reinherz et al (1993)	Boston, USA	DIS	386	—	—	6.0
Oliver and Simmons (1985), age 18+	St Louis, USA	DIS	298	5.2	6.6	6.0[a]
Lépine et al (1989)	Paris			1.5	3.6	6.9
Lépine (1995)	Europe (6 countries)	MINI	78 463	5.0	8.7	range (3.8–9.9)
Clayer et al (1995)	Australia	Questionnaire	991	6.9[b]	14.3[b]	10.8[b]

[a] +1.7% secondary.
[b] Including dysthymia.

Table 11.4   One-year prevalence rates of major depressive disorder.

		Instrument	N	M	F	M + F
Roberts and Vernon (1982)	California	SADS-RDC	528	–	–	4.7
Faravelli and Incerpi (1985)	Florence	SADS-L	639	–	–	5.2
Weissman et al (1990)	USA, ECA	DIS	19 182	1.4	4.0	2.7
Weissman et al (1996)[a]	Taiwan	DIS	11 004	–	–	0.8
	Korea	DIS	5 100	–	–	2.3
	USA, ECA	DIS	18 571	–	–	3.0
	Puerto Rico	DIS	1 513	–	–	3.0
	Paris	DIS	1 746	–	–	4.5
	West Germany	DIS	481	–	–	5.0
	Edmonton, Canada	DIS	3 258	–	–	5.2
	Christchurch, New Zealand	DIS	1 498	–	–	5.8
Brown et al (1995), age +18 year	USA[b]	DIS	865	2.8	3.2	3.1
Parikh et al (1996)						
Urban	Ontario, Canada	CIDI*	9 953	–	–	4.2
Rural						3.2
Lépine et al (1993)	Paris	DIS/CIDI	1 787	3.4	6.0	4.7
Kessler et al (1995)	NCS, USA	CIDI	8 098	7.7	12.9	10.3

[a] Figures standardized to US age and sex distribution.
[b] African-Americans.
* modified

Table 11.5   Lifetime prevalence rates of major depressive disorder.

		Instrument	N	M	F	M + F
Hwu et al (1985)	Taiwan (Metropolis)	DIS	5 005	0.7	1.0+	0.9
Hwu et al (1989)	Taiwan (small township)	DIS	3 004	0.9	2.5+	1.7
Chen et al (1993)	Hong Kong	DIS	7 229	1.3	2.4	–
Lee et al (1990a)	Korea	DIS	3 134	2.4	4.1	3.3
Lee et al (1990b)	Korea (rural)	DIS	2 995	2.9	4.1	3.5
Canino et al (1987)	Puerto Rico	DIS	1 513	3.5	5.5	4.6
Stefánsson et al (1991)	Iceland	DIS/DSM-III	862	2.9	7.8	5.3
Weissman et al (1990)	ECA, USA	DIS		5.2	10.2	4.9
	New Haven	DIS	5 063	–	–	5.9
	Baltimore	DIS	3 560	–	–	3.0
	St Louis	DIS	3 200	–	–	4.5
	Durham	DIS	4 101	–	–	3.5
	Los Angeles	DIS	3 436	–	–	5.6
Heun and Maier (1993)	Mainz (G)	SADS-L	80	–	–	7.7
Elliot et al (1985)	National Survey, USA					8.4
Bland et al (1988b)	Edmonton, Canada	DIS	3 258	5.9	11.4	8.6
Wittchen and von Zerssen (1987)	Munich, Germany	DIS	483	–	–	9.0
Reinherz et al (1993), adolescents	Boston, USA	DIS DSM-III-R	386	5.1	13.7	9.4
Carta et al (1995)	Sardinia	CIDI	552	11.6	14.8	13.3
Wells et al (1989)	Christchurch, New Zealand	DIS	1 498	8.8	16.3	12.6
Oliver and Simmons (1985[a])	St Louis, USA	DIS	298	12.8	23.8	14.8
Wacker (1995), Wacker et al (1992)	Basle, Switzerland	CIDI	470	11.0	19.5	15.7
Murphy (1980)	Stirling County, Canada	HDS (DPA)	1 003			16.0
Lépine et al (1993, personal communication)	Paris	DIS/CIDI	1 787	10.7	22.4	16.4
Kessler et al (1994) Blazer et al (1994)	NCS, USA	CIDI	8 098	F	F	17.1
Weissman and Myers (1978)	New Haven, USA	SADS-RDC		12.3	25.8	18.0
Lewinsohn et al (1993), adolescents	Oregon					
	T$_1$	SADS-L	1 508	11.6	24.8	18.5
	T$_2$			15.2	31.6	24.0
Lindahl and Stefánsson (1991)		DIS	862	2.0	7.8	–

[a] Primary unipolar depression.

European findings, e.g. 15.7% from Basle (Wacker et al, 1992) or 16.0% from Zurich. Only the Munich study by Wittchen and von Zerssen (1987), applying the DIS, gave a lower rate (9%).

A cross-national comparison of studies conducted using the DIS in 10 countries has published lifetime prevalence rates for the ages 18–65, standardized to US age and sex distribution (Weissman et al, 1996). The rates for males varied between 1.1% and 14.7%, and those for females between 1.8% and 23.1%. The lowest rates were found in Taiwan and the highest in Beirut/Lebanon. The F/M ratio ranged between 1.6 and 3.1. The mean age of onset was between 24.8 and 34.8 years.

While depressive disorders are rare in children between 7 and 11 (Costello and Shugart, 1992), their prevalence rises sharply in puberty, especially in girls (Cohen et al, 1993). Reinherz et al (1993) found a lifetime prevalence rate of 9.4% in adolescents, and Lewinsohn et al (1993) reported a rate of 18.5% and, in a follow-up 1 year later, 24.0%. Nevertheless, the studies on adolescents lend credence to the high adult lifetime rates.

Summarizing these conflicting findings, it should be noted that most studies applying the DIS tended to give rates lower than those using other instruments (CIDI, SADS-L, SPIKE). Differences in interview methodology may also explain the much higher adolescent rates found by Lewinsohn et al as compared to Reinherz et al (1993). Generally, lifetime prevalence rates are less reliable than point prevalence rates, a factor which has led child and adolescent psychiatric researchers to avoid using them (Angold and Costello, 1995).

The gender differences in lifetime prevalence rates are more marked than in 1-year and point prevalence rates; this may partly be attributable to the stronger male tendency to forget previous history.

On the whole, great caution is needed in interpreting lifetime prevalence rates, because of the certain shrinkage from forgetting (Ernst and Angst, 1992; Giuffra and Risch, 1994). A meta-analysis of the ECA study (Simon and von Korff, 1995) clearly demonstrated a systematic loss of information due to poor recall.

Minor depression

The literature on the epidemiology of minor depression has recently been reviewed by Tannock and Katona (1995). Although the first studies date back to Kay et al (1964), we shall restrict our review to the later studies using operationalized diagnoses. The definition of minor depression varies from study to study, making comparison of findings difficult. The highest lifetime risk was described in the study of Bebbington et al (1989) from London, applying the PSE-CATEGO methodology. The authors found rates of 26% in males and 50% in females. In the majority of

Table 11.6   Lifetime, 6-month and current prevalence rates of minor depression.

		Instrument	Age	N	M	F	M + F
Lifetime							
Copeland et al (1987)		GMS/AGECAT	Elderly	1 070	–	–	8.3
Gurland (1983)		CARE/ICD	Elderly	841	–	–	12.0
Beekman et al (1995)	Netherlands	DIS	55–85	660	9.8	15.7	12.9
Lindesay et al (1989)		CARE	Elderly	890	–	–	13.5
Bebbington et al (1989)	London	PSE/CATEGO	18–64	790	25.9	50.0	
Tannock and Katona (1995)	London		Review classic: no data				
Kay et al (1964)							
Six months							
Lépine (1995)	B, F, E, D, NL, UK	MINI		78 463	–	–	1.8
Point							
Dean et al (1983)	Ecinburgh	PSE/CAT/RDC	18–65 (F)	576	–	1.7	–
Weissman and Myers (1978)	New Haven, USA	SADS-RDC		720	5.9	17.4	9.2 (LT) 2.5 (current)
Roberts and Vernon (1982)	California	SADS-RDC		528		point	1.3

B = Belgium
F = France
E = Spain
D = Germany
NL = The Netherlands
UK = United Kingdom

LT = lifetime

studies, rates range from 8% to 13%; the early study of Weissman and Myers (1978), for instance, reported 9.2%. Several studies on the elderly also indicate rates within this range (Table 11.6), the most recent being the investigation by Beekman et al (1995) from The Netherlands, which found a rate of 12.9%. In the Zurich study we identified a lifetime rate for unipolar minor depression up to the age of 35 in 9.9% of subjects. The vast-scale European DEPRES study (Lépine, 1995) comprising 78 463 subjects from six European countries reported a 6-month prevalence rate for minor depression of only 1.8%. This figure is close to the 1.7% reported from Edinburgh by Dean et al (1983). These conflicting findings need further clarification.

Dysthymia

Dysthymia is defined as a chronic form of minor depression. In view of its chronicity, lifetime prevalence rates are of special interest (Table 11.7), but the accuracy of the reported rates of dysthymia is also affected by the phenomenon of forgetting. Moreover, the diagnosis itself may not be particularly reliable (Angst and Wicki, 1991). Published rates for dysthymia vary between 1% and 12%. Studies applying the DIS reported rates up to 6.4%, and those using the CIDI found rates between 6% and 7%. The highest rate (12%) was reported in Finland among elderly subjects examined by semi-structured interview (Pahkala et al, 1995). All studies found higher rates for females than males. There is some evidence that dysthymia and minor depression are more prevalent in the elderly, at the expense of major depression, which seems to be rarer in this age group (Blazer, 1994).

Recurrent brief depression (RBD)

RBD is highly prevalent in the normal population, but research on the disorder remains sparse. One-year prevalence rates for recurrent brief depression were found to be 5.8% (Maier, personal communication), 6.6% (Carta et al, 1994), and 4–8% (Angst, 1995). Longitudinally, up to the age of 35, 14.6% of the population investigated in the Zurich study received a diagnosis of recurrent brief depression. A high prevalence of RBD was confirmed worldwide by the WHO primary care study, which established a current prevalence rate of 5.2% for pure RBD and 4.8% for cases of RBD associated with other depression diagnoses (Weiller et al, 1994).

Table 11.7   Lifetime prevalence rates of dysthymia (DSM-III).

		Instrument	N	M	F	M + F
Yeh et al (1985)	Taipei (Taiwan)	DIS	5 005	0.7	1.1	0.9
	2 towns	DIS	3 004	1.4	1.6	1.5
Oliver and Simmons (1985)	St Louis, USA	DIS	298	–	–	1.7
Lee et al (1990a,b)	Seoul	DIS	3 134	1.8	3.0	2.4
	Rural Korea	DIS	2 995	1.3	2.5	1.9
Bland et al (1988b)	Edmonton, Canada	DIS	3 258	2.2	5.2	3.7
Chen et al (1993)	Hong Kong	DIS	7 229	1.1	2.8	–
Canino et al (1987)	Puerto Rico	DIS	1 551	1.6	7.6	4.7
Oakley-Browne et al (1989)	Christchurch, New Zealand	DIS	1 498	–	–	6.4
Wells et al (1989)	Christchurch, New Zealand	DIS	1 498	3.8	9.0	6.4
Stefànsson et al (1991)	Iceland	DIS	862[a]	2.3	10.7	6.4
Wacker et al (1992)	Basle, Switzerland	CIDI	470	–	–	7.2
Carta et al (1995)	Sardinia	CIDI	480	3.0	5.2	4.1
Kessler et al (1994)	NCS, USA	CIDI	8 098	4.8	8.0	6.4
Lépine et al (personal communication)	SOFRES survey, France	–	–	–	–	10.0
Pahkala et al (1995)	Finland	SSI[b]	1 225	9.3	13.6	11.9

[a] 55–57 years.
[b] Semi-structured interview.

Table 11.8   Longitudinal total and treatment prevalence rates up to age 35.

Unipolar[a]	Prevalence (%)	Treatment prevalence		
		M + F (%)	M (%)	F (%)
Major depression	16.0	6.9	2.8	10.8
Dysthymia	1.8	1.2	0.7	1.7
Recurrent brief depression	14.6	7.0	2.8	11.1
Minor depression	9.9	2.0	0.6	3.4
Total	33.1	11.7	5.7	17.5

[a] Categories not mutually exclusive.

Cumulative lifetime prevalence rates of depression

From the longitudinal Zurich study comprising five interviews from ages 20 to 35, Table 11.8 shows the cumulative rates of the population diagnosed as depressives. The rate for major depression was 16%; the cumulative rate for major depression plus dysthymia was 17.2%; adding RBD, the rate was 27.0%, and with the further addition of minor depression, it rose to 33.1% (Table 11.8). The preponderance of females was highest among major depressives, with a F/M ratio of 1.77; this fell to 1.5 when RBD and/or minor depression were included.

It is obvious from Table 11.8 that there is a considerable longitudinal overlap between depressive subgroups. Cases may change diagnoses longitudinally, e.g. from major depression to dysthymia (double depression) or from recurrent brief depression to major depression (combined depression).

Figure 11.1 illustrates this overlap and demonstrates clearly that the field is dominated by major, recurrent brief and minor depression, whereas pure dysthymia is relatively rare, and in most cases dysthymia overlaps with another diagnosis. Double depression was found in 0.8% of subjects and combined depression (the term given by Montgomery to a combination of RBD and major depression) in 4.8% of subjects (Merikangas et al, 1990). The ECA study identified double depression in 1.4% of subjects (Weissman et al, 1990).

Longitudinal treatment prevalence rates

We are interested not only in the prevalence rates but also in the treatment prevalence rates in the population. American community studies have reported unspecified treatment rates of between 30% and 40% for cases diagnosed for major depression (Weissman et al, 1981; Roberts

Dysthymia (1.8)

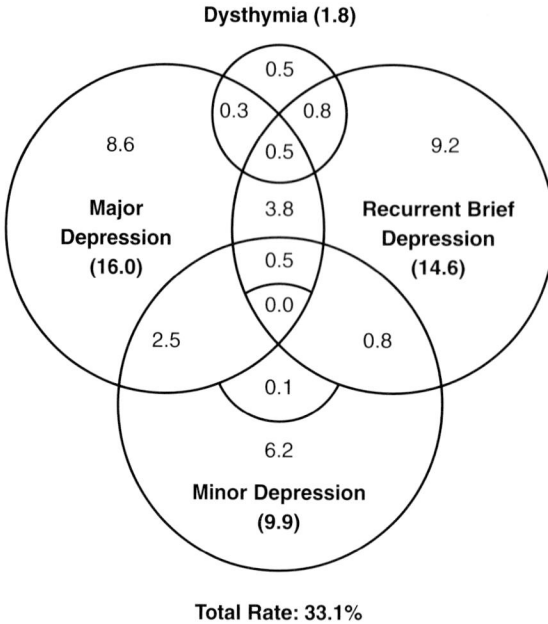

Total Rate: 33.1%

Figure 11.1

Longitudinal prevalence rates (%) of unipolar depressive subgroups.

and Vernon, 1982). Table 11.8 shows the treatment prevalence rates for unipolar depression identified by the Zurich study. As indicated earlier, over 15 years, 33.1% of all subjects received a diagnosis of depression. Weighted back to the normal population, 11.7% were treated for depression (males 5.7%, females 17.5%).

Again, account must be taken of the overlap between the depressive subgroups: Figure 11.2 shows the overlap of treatment prevalence rates. In treated cases we once more see the predominance of major depression, RBD and combined depression. The treatment prevalence rate for double depression was 0.5%, for combined depression 3.0%, for pure major depression 2.6% and for pure RBD 3.8%. Like pure dysthymia, with a prevalence of 0.4%, pure minor depression is a relatively small residual category, with a prevalence of 0.3%.

The European DEPRES study, which investigated 78 463 subjects from the normal population in Belgium, France, Germany, The Netherlands and the UK, established 6-month prevalence rates of 6.9% for major depression, 1.8% for minor depression and 8.3% for depressive symptoms. The study did not assess brief depression. Of the major depressives, 69% consulted health-care professionals, 41% received prescribed medication and 18% took antidepressants. In Switzerland, the Zurich study of subjects up to the age of 35 gave a longitudinal prevalence rate of 16% for major depression.

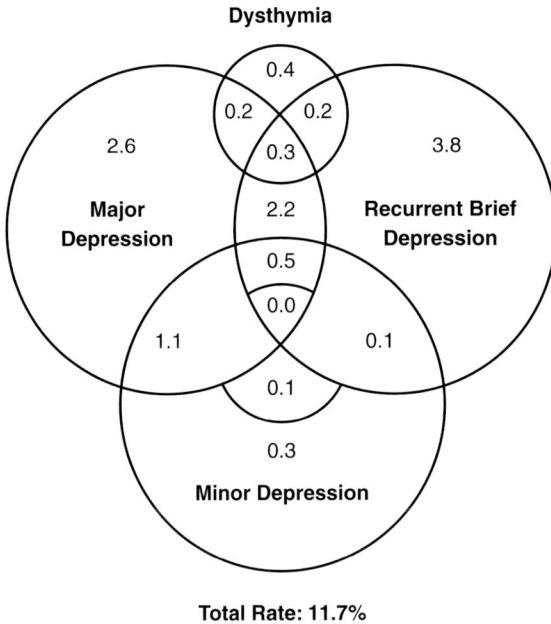

Total Rate: 11.7%

Figure 11.2

Longitudinal treatment prevalence rates (%) up to age 35: overlap.

Fifty-five per cent of major depressives sought treatment, but only 40% of them were prescribed medication, about half of them receiving antidepressants, and the other half benzodiazepines. Table 11.9 shows clearly that two-thirds of females and only one-third of males sought treatment. Only 11% of males were prescribed medication, which means that about 6% of depressed males took antidepressants, whereas this was the case in about 13% of females. In the Zurich study, the majority of treated major depressives received some form of psychotherapy without any drugs. By contrast, the European DEPRES study showed that two-thirds of the major depressives who consulted health-care professionals received prescribed medication; as in the Zurich study, only half of them were prescribed antidepressants.

Table 11.9   Treated major depressive disorder by sex.

	Prescribed medication (%)	Other treatment (%)	No treatment (%)
44 males	11.4	22.7	65.9
93 females	26.9	37.6	35.5
137 M + F	21.9	32.8	45.3

In an earlier paper (Angst, 1996), comparing treated and untreated major depressive episodes (including bipolars), we found that treated subjects were more severely ill; nevertheless, on the basis of prospective course data, they were, surprisingly, found to have a significantly better outcome than the untreated group.

The changing rate of major depression

Klerman and Weissman (1989) reviewed published data from community and family studies on the prevalence of major depression and concluded that there was an increase in the cumulative lifetime rates of major depression which could not be explained by retrospective recall or other artefacts. One of the crucial studies in this area is the Lundby study by Hagnell et al (1982), and their article 'Are we entering an age of melancholy?' The authors came to the conclusion that incidence rates had increased during the 1960s and 1970s. Among males aged 20 to 39 they found the rates to be ten times higher during the period 1957–1972 than in the period 1947–1957. However, a critical reading of the paper reveals a conspicuous absence of incidence of depression in the first ten year period (1947–1957) of the Lundby study. In the age group 0 to 19 there was not a single male case of depression (not even a mild one). In female children and in adolescents there were only three cases in each of the two periods 1947–1957 and 1957–1972. In the first ten year period, 1947–1957, only one male case (in the male age group 20–39) with severe and medium impairment and five cases if mild impairment is included. Given these small baseline numbers, one should be very cautious about generalisations.

In 1988 Weissman et al published the findings of a large group of investigators with an impressive cross-national comparison. This again showed an increase in the cumulative lifetime rates of major depression in each successive birth cohort at all sites with the exception of one (a Hispanic sample). The conclusion was reiterated that the more recent birth cohorts run a higher risk of developing major depression. In addition, the large National Comorbidity Survey (Kessler et al, 1994) confirmed increasing lifetime prevalence rates for major depressive episodes for both women and men in more recent cohorts. They also found stable female/male risk ratios between the ages 24 and 54.

The issue neverthless remains highly controversial. There is a growing body of evidence against the argument that depression is on the increase. Giuffra and Risch (1994) showed by a simulation study that lifetime prevalence rates based on recall may vastly underestimate earlier experiences: forgetting at a rate of 3–5% per year would explain the findings. Another strong counter-argument is that cohort differences are not confined to major depression but apply to a wide range of psychopathology, suggesting that there are methodological problems in data collection. This hypothesis was borne out by the large WHO study of primary care (Simon et al, 1995). Investigating 26 421 subjects, the authors again confirmed a global increase in depressive cases in different cohorts over recent years. However, the cohort effect was found not only in different countries but also for different diagnoses (depression, panic disorder and agoraphobia). If pure recall plays a major role in determining the findings, the reported time-span since first onset of depression would cluster into more recent years; this was indeed the case. The majority of onsets dated from the past 5 years, and this was true across all diagnoses.

The WHO data seriously undermine the argument that there has been a true increase in depression and provide evidence of the role played by memory artefacts. With the exception of the Lundby study, all studies suggesting an increase in depression have in fact been retrospective. In the present state of our knowledge, there are no true prospective data proving a dramatic worldwide increase of depression. Helgason's (1996) recent review of research in Iceland confirmed this negative conclusion: there was no increase, either in mental disorder or in depression, on the basis of incidence and lifetime prevalence rates.

Discussion

All modern community studies clearly indicate high prevalence rates for major depression up to the age of 65 and of RBD up to 35; dysthymia and minor depression, on the other hand, seem to be frequent problems in the elderly. There is no conclusive evidence as to whether dysthymia in adolescents and young adults is the same as in the elderly; major depression is certainly relatively rare in the elderly.

Conclusive lifetime prevalence rates based on prospective data are not yet available, but there is no doubt that prospective studies conducted through repeated interviews yield cumulatively much higher lifetime prevalence rates than the usual studies published, in which data have been collected retrospectively. It is therefore probable that the lifetime prevalence rates currently available still underestimate the extent of the problem in the normal population.

The so-called cohort effect, which postulated an increasing incidence of depression in the population that has grown up in recent decades, is a subject of considerable controversy; it may well turn out to be no more than an artefact of recall, which has been shown to be poor.

Most of the epidemiological studies applied instruments which did not specifically assess the treatment rates of depressive patients but restricted themselves to 'utilisation of health services based on any kind of morbidity' (this is true, for instance, of the Diagnostic Interview Schedule used in the ECA and many other studies). The European DEPRES study suggests that almost 70% of patients with major depression sought treatment but that only 18% took antidepressants. The arguably even more reliable data collected by the Zurich study paint an even gloomier picture, showing that two-third of males and one-third of females with unipolar major depression sought no treatment at all. Of the total population, 9.1% suffered from untreated major depression and 6.9% from treated major depression. There is no reason to assume that treatment rates in the elderly would be higher; on the contrary, many findings suggest that these rates are lower in this group because their depression is underdiagnosed and the subjects themselves fail to seek treatment. The European DEPRES study and the Zurich study both agree upon the fact that only about half of the medications prescribed for depressives consist of antidepressants.

To sum up, we conclude that depression is highly prevalent but that it is very often insufficiently or inadequately treated or simply not treated at all.

References

Abas MA, Broadhead JC (1997) Depression and anxiety among women in an urban setting in Zimbabwe, *Psychol Med* **27**:59–71

Angold A, Costello EJ (1995) Developmental epidemiology, *Epidemiol Rev* **17**:74–82.

Angst J (1995) Dépressions brèves récurrentes. In: Olié JP, Poirier MF, Lôo H, eds, *Les Maladies Dépressives* (Médecine Sciences Flammarion: Paris) 223–33.

Angst J (1996) Outcome of treated vs. non-treated depressive episodes. *Psychopathology* (in press).

Angst J, Wicki W (1991) The Zurich Study XI. Is dysthymia a separate form of depression? Results of the Zurich cohort study, *Eur Arch Psychiatry Clin Neurosci* **240**:349–54.

Bebbington P, Katz R, Mcguffin P et al (1989) The risk of minor depression before age 65: results from a community survey, *Psychol Med* **19**: 393–400.

Beekman ATF, Deeg DJH, van Tilburg T et al (1995) Major and minor depression in later life: a study of prevalence and risk factors, *J Affect Disord* **36**:65–75.

Bland RC, Newman SC, Orn H (1988a) Period prevalence of psychiatric disorders in Edmonton, *Acta Psychiatr Scand* **77**(suppl 338):33–42.

Bland RC, Orn H, Newman SC (1988b) Lifetime prevalence of psychiatric disorders in Edmonton, *Acta Psychiatr Scand* **77**(suppl 338):24–32.

Blazer DG (1994) Dysthymia in community and clinical samples of older adults, *Am J Psychiatry* **151**:1567–9.

Blazer DG, Kessler RC, McGonagle KA, Swartz MS (1994) The prevalence and distribution of major depression in a national community sample: the National Comorbidity Survey, *Am J Psychiatry* **151**:979–86.

Boyd JH, Weissman MM (1981) Epidemiology of affective disorders. A reexamination and future directions, *Arch Gen Psychiatry* **38**:1039–46.

Brown DR, Ahmed F, Gary LE et al (1995) Major depression in a community sample of African Americans, *Am J Psychiatry* **152:**373–8.

Canino GJ, Bird HR, Shrout PE et al (1987) The prevalence of specific psychiatric disorders in Puerto Rico, *Arch Gen Psychiatry* **44:**727–35.

Carta MG, Carpiniello B, Piras A et al (1994) Brief recurrent depression in a sample of urban population in Sardinia, *Neuropsychopharmacology* **1775:**117–94.

Carta MG, Carpiniello B, Porcedda R (1995) Lifetime prevalence of major depression and dysthymia: results of a community survey in Sardinia, *Eur Neuropsychopharmacol* suppl:103–7.

Chen C-N, Wong J, Lee N et al (1993) The Shatin community mental health survey in Hong Kong. II. Major findings, *Arch Gen Psychiatry* **50:**125–33.

Clayer JR, McFarlane AC, Bookless CL et al (1995) Prevalence of psychiatric disorders in rural South Australia, *Med J Aust* **163:**124–9.

Cohen P, Cohen J, Kasen S et al (1993) An epidemiological study of disorders in late childhood and adolescence—I. Age- and gender-specific prevalence, *J Child Psychol Psychiatry* **34:**851–67.

Copeland JRM, Dewey ME, Wood N et al (1987) Range of mental illness among the elderly in the community, *Br J Psychiatry* **150:**815–23.

Costello EJ, Shugart MA (1992) Above and below the threshold: severity of psychiatric symptoms and functional impairment in a pediatric sample, *Pediatrics* **90:**359–68.

Dean C, Surtees PG, Sashidharan SP (1983) Comparison of research diagnostic systems in an Edinburgh community sample, *Br J Psychiatry* **142:**247–56.

Eaton WW, Kramer M, Anthony JC et al (1989) The incidence of specific DIS/DSM-III mental disorders: data from the NIMH Epidemiologic Catchment Area Program, *Acta Psychiatr Scand* **79:**163–78.

Elliot D, Huizinger D, Morse BJ (1985) *The dynamics of deviant behaviour. A National Survey: Progress Report* (Behavioural Research Institute: Boulder, CO).

Ernst C, Angst J (1992) The Zurich Study XII. Sex differences in depression. Evidence from longitudinal epidemiological data, *Eur Arch Psychiatry Clin Neurosci* **241:**222–30.

Faravelli C, Incerpi G (1985) Epidemiology of affective disorders in Florence. Preliminary results, *Acta Psychiatr Scand* **72:**331–3.

Giuffra LA, Risch N (1994) Diminished recall and the cohort effect of major depression: a simulation study, *Psychol Med* **24:**375–83.

Gurland BJ (1983) *The Mind and the Mood of Aging* (Haworth Press: New York, NY).

Hagnell O, Lanke J, Rorsman B et al (1982) Are we entering an age of melancholy? Depressive illnesses in a prospective epidemiological study over 25 years: the Lundby Study, Sweden, *Psychol Med* **12:**279–89.

Helgason T (1996) Epidemiology of psychiatric disorders in Iceland, *Nord J Psychiatry* **50**(suppl 36):31–8.

Heun R, Maier W (1993) The distinction of bipolar II disorder from bipolar I and recurrent unipolar depression: results of a controlled family study, *Acta Psychiatr Scand* **87:**279–84.

Hwu EK, Hwu HG, Chang LY et al (1985) Lifetime prevalence of mental disorders in a Chinese metropolis and 2 townships. In: *Proceedings, International Symposium in Psychiatric Epidemiology*, Taipei City.

Hwu HG, Yeh EK, Chang LY (1989) Prevalence of psychiatric disorders in Taiwan defined by the Chinese Diagnostic Interview Schedule, *Acta Psychiatr Scand* **79:**136–47.

Kay DWK, Beamish P, Roth M (1964) Old age mental disorders in Newcastle upon Tyne. Part I: a study of prevalence, *Br J Psychiatry* **110:** 146–58.

Kessler RC, McGonagle KA, Swartz M et al (1993) Sex and depression in the National Comorbidity Survey. I: lifetime prevalence, chronicity and recurrence, *J Affect Disord* **29:**85–96.

Kessler RC, McGonagle KA, Nelson CB (1994) Sex and depression in the National Comorbidity Survey. II: cohort effects, *J Affect Disord* **30:**15–26.

Kessler RC, Foster CL, Saunders WB et al (1995) Social consequences of psychiatric disorders. I. Educational attainment, *Am J Psychiatry* **152:** 1026–32.

Klerman GL, Weissman MM (1989) Increasing rates of depression, *JAMA* **261:**2229–35.

Lee CK, Kwak YS, Yamamoto J et al (1990a) Psychiatric epidemiology in Korea. Part I: Gender and age differences in Seoul, *J Nerv Ment Dis* **178:**242–6.

Lee CK, Kwak YS, Yamamoto J et al (1990b) Psychiatric epidemiology in Korea. Part II: Urban and rural differences, *J Nerv Ment Dis* **178:**247–52.

Lépine JP (1994) Personal communication.

Lépine JP (1995) European perspective on depression: the patient's view. In: *Patients in Mind*, 8th ECNP Congress, Venice, 1–2 (abstract).

Lépine JP, Lellouch J, Lovell A et al (1989) Anxiety and depressive disorders in a French population: methodology and preliminary results, *Psychiatr Psychobiol* **4:**267–74.

Lépine JP, Lellouch J, Lovell A et al (1993) L'épidémiologie des troubles anxieux et dépressifs dans une population générale française, *Confront Psychiatr*, **No. 35:**139–61.

Levav I, Kohn R, Dohrenwend BP et al (1993) An epidemiological study of mental disorders in a 10-year cohort of young adults in Israel, *Psychol Med* **23:**691–707.

Lewinsohn PM, Hops H, Roberts RE et al (1993) Adolescent psychopathology: I. prevalence and incidence of depression and other DSM-III-R disorders in high school students, *J Abnorm Psychol* **102:**133–44.

Lindal E, Stefansson JG (1991) The frequency of depressive symptoms in a general population with reference to DSM-111, *Int J Soc Psychiatry* **37:**233–41.

Lindesay J, Briggs K, Murphy E (1989) The Guy's age concern survey: prevalence rates of cognitive impairment, depression and anxiety in an urban elderly community, *Br J Psychiatry* **155:**317–29.

Maier W (1993) Personal communication.

Meller I, Fichter M, Schröppel H (1996) Incidence of depression in octo- and nonagenerians: results of an epidemiological follow-up community study, *Eur Arch Psychiatr Clin Neurosci* **246:**93–9.

Meltzer H, Gill B, Petticrew M et al (1995) *The Prevalence of Psychiatric Morbidity Among Adults Living in Private Household*. OPCS Surveys of Psychiatric Morbidity in Great Britain, Report 1. London: HMSO.

Merikangas KR, Wicki W, Angst J (1990) Combined depression. The Royal College of Psychiatrists, Annual Meeting, Birmingham, abstract.

Murphy JM (1980) Continuities in community-based psychiatric epidemiology, *Arch Gen Psychiatry* **37:**1215–23.

Murphy JM, Olivier DC, Monson RR et al (1988) Incidence of depression and anxiety: the Stirling County Study, *Am J Public Health* **78:**534–40.

Oakley-Browne MA, Joyce PR, Wells JE et al (1989) Christchurch psychiatric epidemiology study, part II: six month and other period prevalences of specific psychiatric disorders, *Aust NZ J Psychiatry* **23:**327–40.

O'Hara MW, Kohout FJ, Wallace RB (1985) Depression among the rural elderly, *J Nerv Ment Dis* **173:** 582–9.

Oliver JM, Simmons ME (1985) Affective disorders and depression as measured by the Diagnostic Interview Schedule and the Beck Depression Inventory in an unselected adult population, *J Clin Psychol* **41**:469–76.

Orley J, Wing JK (1979) Psychiatric disorders in two African villages, *Arch Gen Psychiatry* **36**:513–20.

Pahkala K, Kesti E, Köngäs-Saviaro P et al (1995) Prevalence of depression in an aged population in Finland, *Soc Psychiatry Psychiatr Epidemiol* **30**:99–106.

Parikh SV, Wasylenki D, Goering P et al (1996) Mood disorders: rural/urban differences in prevalence, health care utilization, and disability in Ontario, *J Affect Disord* **38**:57–65.

Regier DA, Farmer ME, Rae DS et al (1993) One-month prevalence of mental disorders in the United States and sociodemographic characteristics: the Epidemiologic Catchment Area Study, *Acta Psychiatr Scand* **88**:35–47.

Reinherz HZ, Giaconia RM, Lefkowitz ES et al (1993) Prevalence of psychiatric disorders in a community population of older adolescents, *J Am Acad Child Adolesc Psychiatry* **32**:369–77.

Roberts RE, Vernon SW (1982) Depression in the community. Prevalence and treatment, *Arch Gen Psychiatry* **39**:1407–9.

Robins LN, Helzer JE, Croughan J et al (1981) National Institute of Mental Health Diagnostic Interview Schedule. Its history, characteristics, and validity, *Arch Gen Psychiatry* **38**:381–9.

Romanoski AJ, Folstein MF, Nestadt G et al (1992) The epidemiology of psychiatrist-ascertained depression and DSM-III depressive disorders. Results from the Eastern Baltimore Mental Health Survey clinical reappraisal, *Psychol Med* **22**:629–55.

Simon GE, von Korff M (1992) Reevaluation of secular trends in depression rates, *Am J Epidemiol* **135**:1411–22.

Simon GE, von Korff M, Üstün B et al (1995) Is the lifetime risk of depression actually increasing? *J Clin Epidemiol* **48**:1109–18.

Stefànsson JG, Lindal E, Bjönsson JK et al (1991) Lifetime prevalence of specific mental disorders among people born in Iceland, *Acta Psychiatr Scand* **84**:142–9.

Tannock C, Katona C (1995) Minor depression in the aged. Concepts, prevalence and optimal management, *Drugs Aging* **6**:278–92.

Wacker HR (1995) *Angst und Depression. Eine Epidemiologische Untersuchung* (Hans Huber: Bern, Göttingen, Toronto).

Wacker HR, Müllejahns R, Klein KH et al (1992) Identification of cases of anxiety disorders and affective disorders in the community according to ICD-10 and DSM-III-R by using the Composite International Diagnostic Interview (CIDI), *Int J Meth Psychiatr Res* **2**:91–100.

Weiller E, Boyer P, Lépine JP et al (1994) Prevalence of recurrent brief depression in primary care, *Eur Arch Psychiatry Clin Neurosci* **244**:174–81.

Weissman MM, Myers JK (1978) Affective disorders in a US urban community. The use of Research Diagnostic Criteria in an epidemiological survey, *Arch Gen Psychiatry* **35**:1304–11.

Weissman MM, Myers JK, Thompson ED (1981) Depression and its treatment in a US urban community— 1975–1976, *Arch Gen Psychiatry* **38**:417–21.

Weissman MM, Leaf PJ, Tischler GL et al (1988) Affective disorders in five United States communities, *Psychol Med* **18**:141–53.

Weissman MM, Bruce LM, Leaf PJ et al (1990) Affective disorders. In: Robins LN, Regier DA, eds, *Psychiatric Disorders in America. The Epidemiologic Catchment Area Study* (The Free Press: New York) 53–80.

Weissman MM, Bland RC, Canino GJ

et al (1996) Cross-national epidemiology of major depression and bipolar disorder, *JAMA* **276**:293–9.

Wells KB, Stewart A, Hays RD et al (1989) The functioning and well-being of depressed patients. Results from the medical outcomes study, *JAMA* **262**:914–19.

Wing JK (1970) A standard form of psychiatric present state examination (PSEE and a method for standardising the classification of symptoms. In: Hare EH, Wing JK, eds, *Psychiatric Epidemiology: an International Sympo-* sium (Oxford University Press: London). 93–108.

Wittchen HU, von Zerssen D (1987) *Verläufe behandelter und unbehandelter Depressionen und Angstsörungen. Eine Klinisch-psychiatrische und epidemiologische Verlaufsuntersuchung* (Springer: Berlin, Heidelberg, New York).

Yeh E-K, Hwu H-G, Chang L-Y et al (1985) Lifetime prevalence of mental disorders in a Chinese metropolis and 2 townships In: *Proceedings, International Symposium on Psychiatric Epidemiology*, Taipei City, 175–97.

12

Existing therapies with newer antidepressants—their strengths and weaknesses

Otto Benkert, Martin Burkart and Hermann Wetzel

Introduction

Generally accepted groups of antidepressants with well-established antidepressive efficacy comprise tricyclic and tetracyclic compounds (TCAs), irreversible monoamine oxidase inhibitors (MAOIs), and selective serotonin reuptake inhibitors (SSRIs). However, potential toxicity, drug interactions and side effects may reduce these substances' safety and tolerability, thus limiting use in certain populations at risk. For example, overdose toxicity of TCAs and MAOIs can cause problems in outpatient treatment, because suicidal intoxication with antidepressants is a typical complication of depressive illness (Crome, 1993). Significant drug interactions with various groups of drugs that complicate treatment of comorbid patients occur with TCAs and also with some SSRIs (Breyer-Pfaff and Brinschulte, 1989; Gibaldi, 1992; Härtter et al, 1993; Riesenman, 1995; Hiemke et al, 1997). Specific side effects that frequently accompany treatment with TCAs are weight gain and sexual dysfunction (Gitlin, 1994; Fernstrom, 1995), and abnormal orgasm is found with SSRIs (Preskorn, 1995).

Moreover, the above-mentioned antidepressants do not satisfactorily meet the major requirements for efficacy of antidepressive therapy. These are: (1) early onset of action; (2) high response rate; (3) optimal relapse prevention; and (4) early and reliable suppression of suicidality. Early onset of action is desirable to offer patients rapid relief from their burden and to shorten hospital stay. However, the response latency of established therapies amounts to at least 2 weeks (e.g. Stassen et al, 1993; Benkert et al, 1996a). High response rate is a major demand for a first-choice antidepressant. By contrast, non-response rates in acute treatment with any available substance range from 20% to 50% (e.g. Laux, 1994). Optimal relapse prevention is required for maintenance treatment. However, relapse rates of 10% to 20% within 1 year of maintenance treatment are found with TCAs and SSRIs in major depression (Hirschfeld, 1994). Finally, early and reliable suppression of suicidality is most important for antidepressive therapy. However, non-sedating antidepressants have been suspected to provoke suicidality. Fluoxetine in particular was reported to aggravate suicidality (Teicher et al, 1990), although this supposition could not be verified by systematic studies (Jick et al, 1995; Warshaw and Keller, 1996).

Because of the shortcomings of established antidepressive drugs listed above, further progress is required in antidepressive pharmacotherapy. A number of novel antidepressive substances have recently been developed and approved by drug registration authorities. The strengths and weaknesses of these novel antidepressants will be reviewed and compared to those of established drugs: selective serotonin and noradrenaline reuptake inhibitors (SNRIs: milnacipran, venlafaxine), reversible selective MAO-A inhibitors (RIMAs: befloxatone, moclobemide), the serotonin reuptake enhancer tianeptine, the dopamine reuptake inhibitor amineptine, the α_2, 5-HT_2 and 5-HT_3 antagonist mirtazapine, and the SSRI and 5-HT_2 antagonist nefazodone.

Efficacy

Acute treatment

Most studies found no significant differences between novel antidepressants and comparator substances (TCAs, MAOIs and SSRIs) in response rates and mean reduction of symptomatology (reviews: by Laux 1994; Mendlewicz, 1995; Wilde and Benfield, 1995; Kasper, 1996; Kasper et al, 1996; Montgomery, 1996). However, this does not necessarily imply that the novel substances are equipotent with established antidepressants. The failure to detect differences in efficacy between novel antidepressants and comparator substances might in part also be attributed to the methodological shortcomings of many studies. One major flaw of most studies that used TCAs or MAOIs as reference drugs was the reference drugs' suboptimal dosing (Bruijn et al, 1996). Suboptimal dosing resulted in part from free dosing schedules that allowed the investigators to select doses within a predefined range, guided by effect and side effects. The frequent side effects of TCAs and MAOIs might have biased the investigators to use suboptimal doses. Although the free dosing design corresponds to clinical routine, where TCAs often cannot be given in adequate doses due to side effects, it confounds efficacy and tolerability. Therefore, rigorous assessment of efficacy is difficult with free dosing designs.

Some studies tried to eliminate this bias by applying fixed doses or blood levels of TCAs: milnacipran (200 mg/day) proved to be equipotent with 150 mg of amitriptyline in 4 weeks' treatment of severely endogeneous depressed inpatients (von Frenckell et al, 1990). Seven other studies including 842 patients with major depression compared 100 mg milnacipran with 150 mg imipramine or clomipramine and found no significant differences between the two treatments, either in individual analyses of each study or in a meta-analysis of pooled data (Kasper et al, 1996).

Venlafaxine was at least equivalent to 200 mg imipramine in 6 weeks' treatment of 167 severely depressed inpatients with melancholia (Benkert et al, 1996a).

Moclobemide was reported to be inferior to a fixed dose of clomipramine in three different settings: treatment response (Hamilton Depression Rating Scale <9 points) was reported in 65% of 20 patients with reactive depression taking 150 mg clomipramine, in 35% of 22 patients treated with 300 mg moclobemide and in 29% of 18 patients taking placebo (Larsen et al, 1989). However, this difference did not reach significance, due to the small sample size. In 167 depressed outpatients, improvement was more pronounced with 150 mg clomipramine or 30 mg isocarboxazide than with 300 mg moclobemide (Larsen et al, 1991). Finally, a multicenter study of 400 mg moclobemide versus 150 mg clomipramine in 115 inpatients with major depression demonstrated weaker efficacy of moclobemide versus clomipramine and a higher rate of drop-outs due to worsening with moclobemide (Danish University Antidepressant Group, 1993). However, the doses of moclobemide were probably too low in these three studies. It remains to be determined whether higher doses of moclobemide are equipotent with fixed doses of TCAs.

A single-center study applying predefined fixed blood levels of mirtazapine (50–100 ng/ml) or imipramine (200–300 ng/ml) in 107 inpatients with severe depression for 4 weeks reported 22% responders in the mirtazapine group and a response rate of 50% in the imipramine group (Bruijn et al, 1996). The authors attributed this significant difference to optimization of imipramine treatment, exclusion of non-compliance, reduction of concomitant medication, and a low drop-out rate. However, therapeutic blood levels are not known for mirtazapine and it remains open to question whether the optimal effective dose of mirtazapine was given in this study (Pinder and Zivkov, 1997).

In summary, these few studies suggest that the SNRIs venlafaxine and milnacipran are equipotent with TCAs. By contrast, moclobemide and mirtazapine might possibly be inferior to TCAs in the treatment of severe depression. Studies with sufficient fixed doses of TCAs as comparators have not been published for nefazodone and befloxatone. More and larger studies with optimal fixed doses of both new antidepressants and comparators are needed to clarify whether there are real differences in efficacy.

Onset of action

Some authors reported a slightly earlier onset of action of moclobemide versus TCAs (e.g. Casacchia and Rossi, 1989; Lecrubier and Guelfi, 1990; Philipp et al, 1993). However, a shorter response latency was not reported with moclobemide in more than 30 other controlled studies (review: Laux, 1994). Therefore, the validity and clinical significance of this finding remain to be determined by studies specifically approaching this issue with adequate methodology (Gachoud et al, 1992).

Venlafaxine treatment was reported to be superior to placebo as early as day 4 in inpatients with melancholic depression (Guelfi et al, 1995) and at week 1 in an outpatient study (Rudolph et al, 1991). A rapid escalating-dose scheme of venlafaxine (escalating dose to 375 mg within 5 days) resulted in more rapid relief of depression, when compared to imipramine increased to 200 mg over 5 days (Benkert et al, 1996a; Figure 12.1).

Venlafaxine's early onset of action has been attributed to the double mode of action—serotonin and noradrenaline reuptake inhibition (Derivan et al, 1995; Romero et al, 1996). However, an alternative explanation is that early onset of action resulted from the rapid escalating schedule, not from the drug's pharmacodynamic profile. Early onset of action might also be found if imipramine was given according to the same schedule

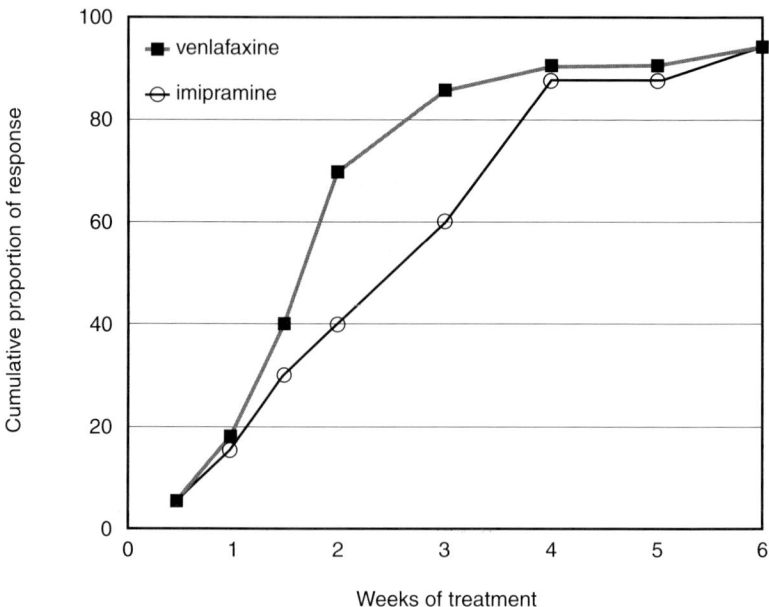

Figure 12.1
Life table analysis of the cumulative proportion of responders to venlafaxine or imipramine among Ham-D responders only.

as venlafaxine (Benkert et al, 1996a; Malhotra and Santosh, 1996), but this has not yet been tested. Therefore, it remains unclear whether early onset of action can be attributed to combined noradrenaline and serotonin reuptake inhibition. Moreover, early response has not yet been found with the SNRI milnacipran: the difference in improvement between milnacipran and placebo reached statistical significance not before day 14 (Macher et al, 1989). A loading dose of 300 mg milnacipran given from the first day of the study for 2 weeks did not result in more rapid response than 200 mg milnacipran or 200 mg fluvoxamine in 120 endogenous depressed inpatients (Ansseau et al, 1991). However, due to small sample sizes, these trials had low statistical power and milnacipran's onset of action deserves further study.

Continuation treatment

In continuation treatment for at least 6 months, all novel substances that were tested showed efficacy against placebo (Anton et al, 1994; Bremner and Smith, 1996; Entsuah et al, 1996). Comparisons of novel drugs with established antidepressants in continuation treatment found no significant differences: nefazodone was equivalent to imipramine (Anton et al, 1994), mirtazapine to amitriptyline (Bremner and Smith, 1996), and moclobemide to TCAs (Laux, 1994). A trend in favor of venlafaxine versus imipramine was reported when analyzing response rates and compliance (Shrivastava et al, 1994a). Studies assessing prevention of recurrence (onset of a new episode after 6 months' remission) by maintenance treatment with novel antidepressants have not yet been published.

Safety

Fatal overdose

Fatal overdose is the most serious complication of TCA therapy: TCAs have a fatal toxicity index of about 40 deaths per million prescriptions; MAOIs and tetracyclics also bear a substantial risk for fatal overdose (fatal toxicity index 13–27 deaths per million prescriptions) (Crome, 1993). By contrast, SSRIs are much safer and intoxications usually resolve without serious complication (Lader, 1996). Nevertheless, single cases with fatal overdose have been reported for all members of this group except paroxetine and sertraline (Kincaid et al, 1990; Henry and Antao, 1992; Ostrom et al, 1996). Case reports on overdoses are available for most novel substances (Lasnier et al, 1991; Loo et al, 1992; Hilton et al, 1995; Hoes and Zeijpveld, 1996; Marcus, 1996; Montgomery et al, 1996). Symptoms are generally mild and no intoxication has been fatal so far. However, in a case of ingestion of 4.5 g venlafaxine plus minor doses of sedatives, intensive care and intubation was necessary for several hours (Fantaskey and Burkhart, 1995).

Central serotonin syndrome

Central serotonin syndrome is a rare but serious and potentially fatal complication of antidepressive treatment (Sternbach, 1991). Central serotonin syndrome has been reported for combination treatment of an MAOI and an SSRI (Graber et al, 1994) as well as an MAOI and the SNRI venlafaxine (Klysner et al, 1995; Phillips and Ringo, 1995). Although many patients tolerate the combination of the RIMA moclobemide and an SSRI (Joffe and Bakish, 1994; Ebert et al, 1995), this combination may also produce a toxic serotonin syndrome (Neuvonen et al, 1993). There are no reports of a serotonin syndrome with combination treatment with a RIMA and an SNRI so far, but this serious complication has to be expected.

Mirtazapine might offer a valuable treatment approach to serotonin syndrome by blocking 5-HT_2 and 5-HT_3 receptors: two cases of suspected mild serotonin syndrome were reported to resolve rapidly after oral doses of 15 mg and 37.5 mg mirtazapine (Hoes, 1996).

Drug interactions

Another important aspect of safety concerns drug interactions. Multiple significant drug interactions are found with TCAs (Breyer-Pfaff and Brinschulte, 1989; Gibaldi, 1992). Drug interactions are less frequent with SSRIs, but important interactions occur because of inhibition of cytochrome P450 isoenzymes with fluoxetine, fluvoxamine and paroxetine (Riesenman, 1995). The drug interaction potential of novel substances is generally low (Zimmer et al, 1990; Puozzo and Leonard, 1996). However, a few exceptions need to be mentioned: tianeptin has a substantial interaction potential because of inhibition of cytochrome P450 III A 3 (Larrey et al, 1990). Significant drug interactions are also found with nefazodone, due to inhibition of cytochrome P450 III A 4 (Marcus, 1996). Venlafaxine and mirtazapine are weak inhibitors of cytochrome P450 I A 2, II D 6 and III A 4, but clinically significant drug interactions have not been reported (Ereshefsky, 1996; N.V. Organon, 1996).

Tolerability

Weight gain

Weight gain is a frequent and inconvenient side effect of TCAs, possibly related to 5-HT_2 and histamine receptor antagonism (Bernstein, 1988; Garland et al, 1988; Fernstrom, 1995). By contrast, some SSRIs can reduce body weight (Silverstone, 1992). Increased appetite and weight gain have also been reported in 10% of patients taking mirtazapine, which is a potent 5-HT_2 and histamine H_1 receptor antagonist (Montgomery, 1995). No other novel antidepressant has been observed to increase body weight.

Sexual dysfunctions

Erectile dysfunction and decreased libido are frequent side effects of TCAs, while abnormal ejaculation/orgasm is found with SSRIs (Gitlin, 1994; Preskorn, 1995). These sexual dysfunctions have been attributed to antiadrenergic and 5-HT_2-mediated mechanisms (Segraves, 1989). According to this theoretical framework, sexual dysfunction is expected with SNRIs, but not with RIMAs and substances showing 5-HT_2 antagonism.

The SNRI venlafaxine produced sexual dysfunction significantly more often than placebo in 12% of male patients (Preskorn, 1995). By contrast, sexual dysfunction has not yet been reported in association with the SNRI milnacipran (Montgomery et al, 1996). However, only spontaneous reports were recorded and patients were not systematically screened for this side effect. In the studies comparing milnacipran and SSRIs, there were no spontaneous complaints about sexual dysfunction with either treatment. Therefore, milnacipran's potential to induce sexual dysfunction has still to be determined in more detail. As expected, the RIMA moclobemide and the 5-HT_2 antagonists nefazodone and mirtazapine were not associated with sexual disturbances (Stabl et al, 1989; Baier and Philipp, 1994; Segraves, 1995; Klint et al, 1996).

Priapism, a side effect reported especially in association with trazodone (Thompson et al, 1990), has not yet been reported during treatment with any novel antidepressant. However, another sexual dysfunction, spontaneous ejaculation, was described with nefazodone in a case report (Michael and Ramana, 1996).

Gaps in knowledge

Induction of mania or cycling

Induction of mania has been reported with TCAs, MAOIs and SSRIs in patients with and without previous manic or hypomanic episodes (Stoll et al, 1994; Altshuler et al, 1995; Howland, 1996). Bipolar patients in particular are at a certain risk of developing mania under therapy. Therefore, antidepressive treatment in these patients requires drugs that are not likely to induce mania. Switch to mania was spontaneously reported in 0.25% of patients during mirtazapine treatment (Montgomery, 1995), in 0.5% of patients taking venlafaxine (Rudolph and Derivan, 1996), in 1 of

189 (0.5%) moclobemide-treated patients in an outpatient study (Baumhackl et al, 1989), and in 2 of 150 (1.3%) outpatients taking tianeptine (Invernizzi et al, 1994). Mania or hypomania emerged in 0.4% of unipolar and in 1.6% of bipolar patients treated with nefazodone, whereas 5.1% of TCA-treated bipolar patients developed mania in studies comparing nefazodone with TCAs (Robinson et al, 1996). However, this difference was not statistically significant, due to the low numbers. Interestingly, one patient with treatment-resistant dysphoric mania markedly improved during nefazodone treatment (Worthington and Pollack, 1996). Mania has not been reported in association with milnacipran, but only unipolar patients have been included in clinical trials so far.

Moreover, cycle acceleration and bipolar rapid cycling have been associated with TCAs and MAOIs in a substantial proportion of bipolar patients, although there remains some controversy (Wehr et al, 1988; Bräunig, 1990; Coryell et al, 1992; Hurowitz and Liebowitz, 1993; Murdock, 1993; Persad, 1993; Wehr, 1993; Altshuler et al, 1995). Unipolar rapid cycling and cycle acceleration are also suspected to occur in relation to antidepressive treatment. However, these conditions are only rarely reported in the literature, so conclusive data are missing (Coryell et al, 1992; Altshuler et al, 1995). There are no reports of cycle acceleration or rapid cycling induced by any of the novel substances. However, cycle length and frequency have not yet been systematically assessed. Therefore, there is an urgent need for studies analyzing the effects of novel antidepressants on cycle length and frequency. From a strict methodological point of view, every novel drug should be tested in bipolar depression before being approved for this indication.

Efficacy in subtypes of depression

Differential efficacy of TCAs, MAOIs, SSRIs and novel substances in subtypes of depression is an ill-studied field. We would like to draw attention to two subtypes of depression that are quite important from an epidemiologic point of view, but that have been neglected in treatment research: brief, recurrent brief or fluctuating depression and minor depression.

Brief depression or 'fluctuating depression'
This describes depressive episodes that are as severe as major depression, but last less than 2 weeks, and recur frequently. A narrow definition of recurrent brief depression requires monthly episodes over 1 year (Angst et al, 1990). However, this might be a somewhat artificially defined subtype, out of a spectrum of fluctuating brief depressions (Benkert et al, 1995). Effective treatments for brief depression are urgently needed, because this disorder appears to be characterized by high suicidality (Montgomery et al, 1989), and the only controlled trial has been negative (Montgomery et al, 1995).

% of patients

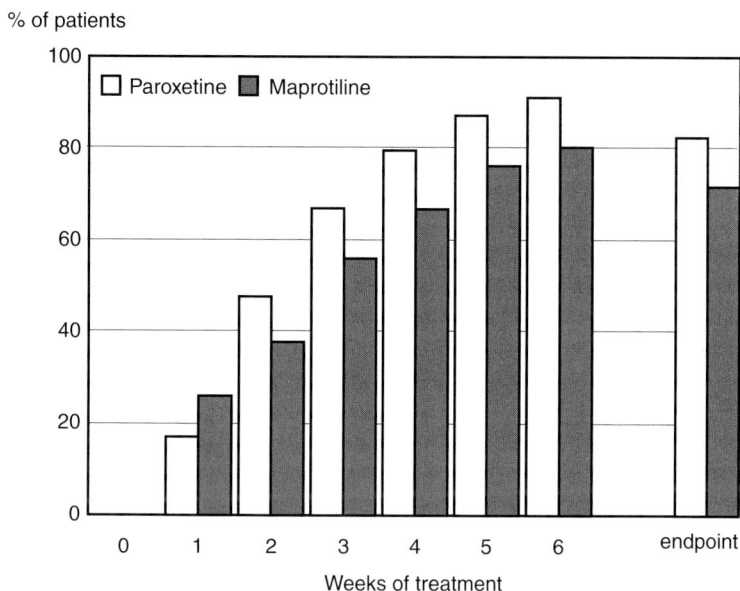

Figure 12.2

Percentage of patients with minor depression responding to treatment with a reduction of 50% or more of initial Ham-D-17 score by treatment group (20 mg paroxetine versus 100 mg maprotiline) and duration.

Minor depression

This is defined as a depressive episode of at least 2 weeks' duration that is similar to major depression in symptomatology, but presenting with less symptoms (e.g. 3–4 from the RDC symptom list) (Szegedi et al, 1997). Minor depression is a frequent disorder (Skodol et al, 1994) that causes substantial disablement and suffering (Jaffe et al, 1994; Tannock and Katona, 1995). Nevertheless, well-established treatment guidelines are not available. In a multicenter outpatient study, we observed that high rates of 82% of 126 patients with minor depression responded to 20 mg paroxetine and 71% of 119 patients to 100 mg maprotiline (Szegedi et al, 1997; Figure 12.2). This encouraging result justifies further research into this area.

The novel antidepressants might be promising for the treatment of fluctuating and minor depression, because they are safe and well tolerated: safety is an important requirement for the long-term outpatient treatment of patients with fluctuating and therefore hardly predictable suicidality. Tolerability is a prerequisite for compliant long-term treatment of patients with only mild symptomatology.

Indications

'Antidepressants' are no longer just drugs for depression. A spectrum of psychiatric disorders responds to treatment with some antidepressants which might functionally be classified as serotonin dysfunction syndromes (Benkert et al, 1993): depression, obsessive-compulsive disorder, anxiety disorders, eating disorders, migraine, and disorders of impulse control are syndromes for which serotonergic dysfunction is probable. Moreover, there is some evidence of serotonergic dysfunction in chronic pain, substance abuse, sleep disturbances, disorders of sexual behavior, chronic fatigue syndrome, late luteal phase dysphoric mood disorder, and some personality disorders.

Promising case reports indicate that novel antidepressants might be efficacious in many of these conditions (Grivois et al, 1992; Ananth et al, 1995; Geracioti, 1995; Goodnick, 1996; Greist, 1996; Grossman and Hollander, 1996; Priest et al, 1995; Yaryura Tobias and Neziroglu, 1996). However, positive multiply replicated controlled trials are lacking. Systematic evaluation of the novel substances in this spectrum of disorders will both enrich treatment options and hopefully increase our understanding of the mechanisms underlying these conditions.

Methodological considerations for future developments

For approval of an antidepressant, the US Food and Drug Administration, like many other government regulatory agencies, requires that superior efficacy versus placebo, a minimal effective dose and a dose–response relationship are demonstrated. We question the justification of all three requirements and propose reformulations of antidepressant approval conditions.

Placebo-controlled trials

The need for and justification of placebo-controlled trials in moderate and severe depression with substances emerging in the future are questionable. There are enough equipotent antidepressants and a number of safe substances with low rates of side effects. Evaluation of further substances that are superior to placebo in the treatment of moderate and severe depression represents no progress in psychiatric treatment. Moreover, placebo-controlled trials consume large amounts of manpower, financial resources and samples of patients willing to participate in treatment trial, without substantially improving treatment options. Finally, it may cause ethical concerns to treat large numbers of depressed patients with placebo, while several efficacious, safe and well-tolerated treatments are available. Instead, we propose that superior efficacy versus a standard drug (TCA, SSRI, SNRI, RIMA, MAOI) in acute and continuation treatment of moderate and severe depression should be required for approval of future antidepressants.

Minimal effective dose

The rationale for establishing a minimal effective dose is to avoid the use of unnecessarily high doses that might be dangerous, ill-tolerated and expensive. However, with safe and well-tolerated drugs, the need to define a minimal effective dose is less straightforward. Moreover, establishing a minimum effective dose is complicated, because such a dose might vary with subtype and severity of depression and might be confounded by duration of the study, pharmacokinetic variability between probands, age, sex, comorbidity and treatment setting. The need to define a minimal effective dose is, furthermore, questioned by the fact that such a dose has never been established for a number of well-accepted antidepressants, e.g. imipramine, amitriptyline, tranyl-cypromine or some SSRIs. Moreover, from an ethical point of view it is problematic to treat large numbers of depressed patients with placebo or presumably ineffective doses, which is necessary to show superiority of the minimal effective dose versus placebo and lower doses' equipotency with placebo (Benkert et al, 1996b).

A number of treatment results with SSRIs suggest that, besides a minimum effective dose, a maximum effective dose also exists: 60 mg fluoxetine were less effective than lower doses in the treatment of depression (Beasley et al, 1990). Similar results have been reported for citalopram (Montgomery et al, 1994). A meta-analysis of trials with nefazodone revealed that 300–500 mg were superior to lower doses, but 600 mg was less effective (Robinson et al, 1996). Because fixed-dose nefazodone trials have not been performed, it remains open whether the highest dose of nefazodone is less efficacious or whether dose was maximally raised in non-responders. When fluvoxamine plasma levels were compared between responders and non-responders in a fixed-dose study of 20 depressed inpatients, responders had lower plasma levels, below a threshold of 85 µg/l after 2 weeks on 100 mg and below 310 µg/l after 2 weeks on 200 mg (Härtter et al, 1997).

For the reasons discussed, the requirement for establishing a minimal effective dose should be questioned. Instead, identification of a therapeutic dose range, established in fixed-dose or fixed-blood-level studies, is a reasonable requirement for antidepressive drug approval. Clinical trials could be further improved by incorporation of therapeutic drug monitoring. This would facilitate interpretation of the results and yield therapeutic blood levels as guidelines for therapeutic drug monitoring in clinical routine. Therefore, incorporation of therapeutic drug monitoring in clinical trials is another desirable requirement for future antidepressant approval.

Dose–response relationship

Dose–response relationships are well established for TCAs. They are also found with the RIMA moclobemide and SNRIs (Rudolph et al, 1991; Fitton et al, 1992; Mendels et al, 1993; Shrivastava et al, 1994b; Lecrubier et al, 1996). The rationale for requiring dose–response relationships for novel antidepressants is that such a relationship clearly demonstrates a substance's efficacy in depression. Nevertheless, the well-accepted antidepressants paroxetine, sertraline, citalopram and fluoxetine failed to exhibit clear dose–response or blood-level–response relationships for the treatment of depression (Beasley et al, 1990; Jenner, 1992; Montgomery et al, 1994; Thompson and Lane, 1994). Some results cited above suggest curvilinear dose–response relationships for some SSRIs, but this issue needs further clarification. Dose–response relationships have not yet been investigated with fixed-dose studies for mirtazapine and nefazodone.

The failure to demonstrate linear dose–response relationships with SSRIs suggests that the antidepressive effect is not mediated by maximal inhibition of serotonin reuptake. Instead, some regulation or normalization of serotonergic function might underlie the SSRIs' clinical effect. This is further supported by the observation that the serotonin reuptake *enhancer* tianeptine is an efficacious antidepressant (e.g. Invernizzi et al, 1994; Costa e Silva et al, 1997). Therefore, establishment of a dose–response relationship might not be an obligatory requirement for a future antidepressant mainly acting on the serotonergic system.

Conclusions

The novel antidepressants are comparable to established drugs with respect to efficacy. A number of results suggest that TCAs might be superior to some of the novel substances in the treatment of severe depression, but this issue needs further research. The differential efficacy of antidepressants in subtypes of depression has not been sufficiently analyzed. Because of safety in overdose, low drug interaction potential, and low rates of side effects, the novel substances might be preferable to TCAs, MAOIs and SSRIs in certain situations.

However, the main requirement for antidepressive therapy, substantial improvement of efficacy, has not been achieved by the novel antidepressants.

References

Altshuler LL, Post RM, Leverich GS, Mikalauskas K, Rosoff A, Ackerman L (1995) Antidepressant-induced mania and cycle acceleration: a controversy revisited, *Am J Psychiatry* **152:** 1130–8.

Ananth J, Burgoyne K, Smith M, Swartz R (1995) Venlafaxine for treatment of obsessive-compulsive disorder, *Am J Psychiatry* **152:**1832.

Angst J, Merikangas K, Scheidegger P, Wicki W (1990) Recurrent brief discussion: a new subtype of affective disorder, *J Affect Disord* **19:**87–98.

Ansseau M, von Frenckell R, Gerard MA et al (1991) Interest of a loading dose of milnacipran in endogenous depressive inpatients. Comparison with the standard regimen and with fluvoxamine, *Eur Neuropsychopharmacol* **1:**113–21.

Anton SF, Robinson DS, Roberts DL, Kenster TT, English PA, Archibald DG (1994) Long-term treatment of depression with nefazodone, *Psychopharmacol Bull* **30:**165–9.

Baier D, Philipp M (1994) Modification of sexual functions by antidepressants, *Fortschr Neurol Psychiatr* **62:**14–21.

Baumhackl U, Bizière K, Fischbach R et al (1989) Efficacy and tolerability of moclobemide compared with imipramine in depressive disorder (DSM-III): an Austrian double-blind, multicentre study, *Br J Psychiatry* **155**(suppl 6):78–83.

Beasley CM Jr, Bosomworth JC, Wernicke JF (1990) Fluoxetine: relationship among dose, response, adverse events, and plasma concentrations in the treatment of depression, *Psychopharmacol Bull* **26:**18–24.

Benkert O, Wetzel H, Szegedi A (1993) Serotonin dysfunction syndromes: a functional common denominator for classification of depression, anxiety, and obsessive-compulsive disorder, *Int Clin Psychopharmacol*

8(suppl 1):3–14.

Benkert O, Fickinger MP, Philipp M, Heun R (1995) Distinction of recurrent brief depression from other fluctuating brief depressions. Consequences for therapy evaluation (short communication), *Eur Neuropsychopharmacol* **3:**229–30.

Benkert O, Gründer G, Wetzel H, Hackett D (1996a) A randomized, double-blind comparison of a rapidly escalating dose of venlafaxine and imipramine in inpatients with major depression and melancholia, *J Psychiatr Res* **30:**441–51.

Benkert O, Szegedi A, Wetzel H (1996b) Minimum effective dose for antidepressants—an obligatory requirement for antidepressant drug evaluation? *Int Clin Psychopharmacol* **11:**177–85.

Bernstein JG (1988) Psychotropic drug induced weight gain: mechanisms and management, *Clin Neuropharmacol* **11**(suppl 1):S194–206.

Bräunig P (1990) Passageres 'rapid cycling' bei einer bipolaren affektiven Psychose, *Nervenarzt* **61:**569–72.

Bremner JD, Smith WT (1996) Org 3770 vs amitriptylin in the continuation treatment of depression: a placebo-controlled trial, *Eur J Psychiatry* **10:** 5–15.

Breyer-Pfaff U, Brinkschulte M (1989) Binding of tricyclic psychoactive drugs in plasma: contribution of individual proteins and drug interactions, *Prog Clin Biol Res* **300:**351–61.

Bruijn JA, Moleman P, Mulder PGH et al (1996) A double blind, fixed blood-level study comparing mirtazapine with imipramine in depressed patients, *Psychopharmacology* **127:**231–7.

Casacchia M, Rossi A (1989) A comparison of moclobemide and imipramine in treatment of depression, *Pharmacopsychiatry* **22:**152–5.

Coryell W, Endicott J, Keller M (1992)

Rapid cycling affective disorder. Demographics, diagnosis, family history, and course, *Arch Gen Psychiatry* **49:**126–31.

Costa e Silva JA, Ruschel SI, Caetano D et al (1997) Placebo-controlled study of tianeptine in major depressive episodes, *Neuropsychobiology* **35:** 24–9.

Crome P (1993) The toxicity of drugs used for suicide, *Acta Psychiatr Scand Suppl* **371:**33–7.

Dalery J, Rochat C, Peyron E, Bernard G (1992) Comparative study of the efficacy and acceptability of amineptine and fluoxetine in patients with major depression, *Encephale* **18:** 257–62.

Danish University Antidepressant Group (1993) Moclobemide: a reversible MAO-A-inhibitor showing weaker antidepressant effect than clomipramine in a controlled multicenter study, *J Affect Disord* **28:**105–16.

Derivan A, Entsuah R, Kikta D (1995) Venlafaxine: measuring the onset of antidepressant action, *Psychopharmacol Bull* **31:**439–47.

Ebert D, Albert R, May A, Stosiek I, Kaschka W (1995) Combined SSRI-RIMA treatment in refractory depression. Safety data and efficacy, *Psychopharmacol (Berl)* **119:**342–4.

Entsuah AR, Rudolph RL, Hackett D, Miska S (1996) Efficacy of venlafaxine and placebo during long-term treatment of depression: a pooled analysis of relapse rates, *Int Clin Psychopharmacol* **11:**137–45.

Ereshefsky L (1996) Drug–drug interactions involving antidepressants: focus on venlafaxine, *J Clin Psychopharmacol* **16**(suppl 2):S37–50.

Fantaskey A, Burkhart KK (1995) A case report of venlafaxine toxicity, *J Toxicol Clin Toxicol* **33:**359–61.

Fernstrom MH (1995) Drugs that cause weight gain, *Obesity Res* **3**(suppl 4):435S–9S.

Fitton A, Faulds D, Goa KL (1992)

Moclobemide. A review of its pharmacological properties and therapeutic use in depressive illness, *Drugs* **4:**561–96.

Gachoud JP, Mikkelsen H, Ammar S, Widlöcher D, Jouvent R (1992) Theoretical considerations and perspectives on the onset of action of moclobemide, *Psychopharmacology* **106:**S96–7.

Garland EJ, Remick RA, Zis AP (1988) Weight gain with antidepressants and lithium, *J Clin Psychopharmacol* **8:** 323–30.

Geracioti TD Jr (1995) Venlafaxine treatment of panic disorder: a case series, *J Clin Psychiatry* **56:**408–10.

Gibaldi M (1992) Drug interactions: Part I, *Ann Pharmacother* **26:**709–13.

Gitlin MJ (1994) Psychotropic medications and their effects on sexual function: diagnosis, biology, and treatment approaches, *J Clin Psychiatry* **55:** 406–13.

Goodnick PJ (1996) Treatment of chronic fatigue syndrome with venlafaxine, *Am J Psychiatry* **153:**294.

Graber MA, Hoehns TB, Perry PJ (1994) Sertraline–phenelzine drug interaction: a serotonin syndrome reaction, *Ann Pharmacother* **28:**732–5.

Greist JH (1996) Venlafaxine in obsessive-compulsive disorder, *Arch Gen Psychiatry* **53:**654–5.

Grivois H, Deniker P, Ganry H (1992) Efficacy of tianeptine in the treatment of psychasthenia. A study versus placebo, *Encephale* **18:**591–9.

Grossman R, Hollander E (1996) Treatment of obsessive-compulsive disorder with venlafaxine, *Am J Psychiatry* **153:**576–7.

Guelfi JD, White C, Hackett D, Guichoux JY, Magni G (1995) Effectiveness of venlafaxine in patients hospitalized for major depression and melancholia, *J Clin Psychiatry* **56:** 450–8.

Härtter S, Wetzel H, Hammes E, Hiemke C (1993) Inhibition of antidepressant demethylation and hydroxylation by fluvoxamine in depressed patients, *Psychopharmacology* **110:** 302–8.

Härtter S, Wetzel H, Hammes E, Torkzadeh M, Hiemke C (1997) Steady state blood levels of fluvoxamine and clinical effects. A prospective fixed dose study, *Pharmaco-psychiatry* (submitted).

Henry JA, Antao CA (1992) Suicide and fatal antidepressant poisoning, *Eur J Med* **1:**343–8.

Hiemke C, Szegedi A, Anghelescu I et al (1997) Drug interactions between clozapine and selective serotonin reuptake inhibitors. In: *IBC's Recent Advances in Drug-Drug Interactions* eds Ferrero J, Levy RH, Rodrigues AD (Southborough, MA: International Business Communications).

Hilton S, Jaber B, Ruch R (1995) Moclobemide safety: monitoring a newly developed product in the 1990s, *J Clin Psychopharmacol* **15**(suppl 2):76S–83S.

Hirschfeld RM (1994) Guidelines for the long-term treatment of depression, *J Clin Psychiatry* **55**(suppl):61–9.

Hoes MJAJM (1996) Mirtazapine as treatment for serotonin syndrome *Pharmacopsychiatry* **29:**81

Hoes MJAJM, Zeijpveld JHB (1996) First report of mirtazapine overdose, *Int Clin Psychopharmacol* **11:**147.

Howland RH (1996) Induction of mania with serotonin reuptake inhibitors, *J Clin Psychopharmacol* **16:**425–7.

Hurowitz GI, Liebowitz MR (1993) Antidepressant-induced rapid cycling: six case reports, *J Clin Psychopharmacol* **13:**52–6.

Invernizzi G, Aguglia E, Bertolino A et al (1994) The efficacy and safety of tianeptine in the treatment of depressive disorder: results of a double-blind multicentre study vs. amitriptylin, *Neuropsychobiology* **30:**85–93.

Jaffe A, Froom J, Galambos N (1994)

Minor depression and functional impairment, *Arch Family Med* **3:** 1081–6.

Jenner PN (1992) Paroxetine: an overview of dosage, tolerability and safety, *Int Clin Psychopharmacol* **6:** 69–80.

Jick SS, Dean AD, Jick H (1995) Antidepressants and suicide, *Br Med J* **310:**215–18.

Joffe RT, Bakish D (1994) Combined SSRI–moclobemide treatment of psychiatric illness, *J Clin Psychiatry* **55:**24–5.

Kasper S (1996) Klinische Wirksamkeit von mirtazapin: übersicht der gerpoolen Daten aus metaanalyseis, *Jatros Neuro* **12:**60–8.

Kasper S, Pletan Y, Solles A, Tournoux A (1996) Comparative studies with milnacipran and tricyclic antidepressants in the treatment of patients with major depression: a summary of clinical trial results, *Int Clin Psychopharmacol* **11**(suppl 4):35–9.

Kincaid RL, McMullin MM, Crookham SB, Rieders F (1990) Report of a fluoxetine fatality, *J Anal Toxicol* **14:** 327–9.

Klint T, Helsdingen JT, (1996) The lack of typical SSRI-related adverse effects and sexual dysfunction with mirtazapine is related to its specific blockade of 5-HT$_2$ and 5-HT$_3$ receptors. *European Psychiatry* **11:**347s.

Klysner R, Larsen JK, Sorensen P, Hyllested M, Pedersen BD (1995) Toxic interaction of venlafaxine and isocarboxazide, *Lancet* **346:**1298–9.

Lader MH (1996) Tolerability and safety: essentials in antidepressant pharmacotherapy, *J Clin Psychiatry* **57**(suppl 2):39–44.

Larrey D, Tinel M, Letteron P et al (1990) Metabolic activation of the new tricyclic antidepressant tianeptine by human liver cytochrome P450, *Biochem Pharmacol* **40:**545–50.

Larsen JK, Holm P, Hoyer E et al (1989) Moclobemide and clomipramine in reactive depression. A placebo-controlled randomized clinical trial, *Acta Psychiatr Scand* **79:**530–6.

Larsen JK, Gjerris A, Holm P et al (1991) Moclobemide in depression: a randomized, multicentre trial against isocarboxazide and clomipramine emphasizing atypical depression, *Acta Psychiatr Scand* **84:**564–70.

Lasnier C, Marey C, Lapeyre G, Delalleau B, Ganry H (1991) Cardiovascular tolerance to tianeptine, *Presse Med* **20:**1858–63.

Laux G (1994) Kontrollierte Vergleichsstudien mit Moclobemide in der Depressionsbehandlung, *Psychopharmakotherapie* **4:**9–18.

Lecrubier Y, Guelfi JD (1990) Efficacy of reversible inhibitors of monoamine oxidase-A in various forms of depression, *Acta Psychiatr Scand Suppl* **360:**18–23.

Lecrubier Y, Pletan Y, Solles A, Tournoux A, Magne V (1996) Clinical efficacy of milnacipran: placebo-controlled trials, *Int Clin Psychopharmacol* **11**(suppl 4):29–33.

Loo H, Ganry H, Dufour H et al (1992) Long-term use of tianeptine in 380 depressed patients, *Br J Psychiatry* **160:**61–5.

Macher JP, Sichel JP, Serre C, Von Frenckell R, Huck JC, Demarez JP (1989) Double-blind placebo-controlled study of milnacipran in hospitalized patients with major depressive disorders, *Neuropsychobiology* **22:** 77–82.

Malhotra S, Santosh PJ (1996) Loading dose imipramine—new approach to pharmacotherapy of melancholic depression, *J Psychiatr Res* **30:**51–8.

Marcus RN (1996) Safety and tolerability profile of nefazodone, *J Psychopharmacol* **10**(suppl 1):11–17.

Mendels J, Johnston R, Mattes J, Reisenberg R (1993) Efficacy and safety of b.i.d. doses of venlafaxine in a dose–response study, *Psychopharmacol Bull* **29:**169–74.

Mendlewicz J (1995) Pharmacologic profile and efficacy of venlafaxine, *Int Clin Psychopharmacol* **10**(suppl 2): 5–13.

Michael A, Ramana R (1996) Nefazodone-induced spontaneous ejaculation, *Br J Psychiatry* **169:**672–3.

Montgomery DB, Montgomery D, Baldwin D, Green M (1989) Intermittent 3-day depressions and suicidal behaviour, *Neuropsychobiology* **22:** 128–34.

Montgomery DB, Pedersen V, Tanghoj P, Rasmussen C, Rioux P (1994) The optimal dosing regimen for citalopram—a meta-analysis of nine placebo-controlled studies, *Int Clin Psychopharmacol* **9**(suppl 1):35–40.

Montgomery DB, Roberts A, Green M, Bullock T, Baldwin D, Montgomery SA (1995) Lack of efficacy of fluoxetine in recurrent brief depression and suicidal attempts, *Eur Arch Psychiatry Clin Neurosci* **244:**211–15.

Montgomery SA (1995) Safety of mirtazapine: a review, *Int Clin Psychopharmacol* **10**(suppl 4):38–48.

Montgomery SA (1996) Efficacy of nefazodone in the treatment of depression, *J Psychopharmacol* **10**(suppl 1):5–10.

Montgomery SA, Prost JF, Solles A, Briley M (1996) Efficacy and tolerability of milnacipran: an overview, *Int Clin Psychopharmacol* **11**(suppl 4):47–51.

Murdock R (1993) *Arch Gen Psychiatry* **50:**496.

Neuvonen PJ, Pohjola Sintonen S, Tacke U, Vuori E (1993) Five fatal cases of serotonin syndrome after moclobemide–citalopram or moclobemide–clomipramine overdoses, *Lancet* **342:**1419.

N.V. Organon (1996) *Remeron Scientific Information* (N.V. Organon: BH Oss, The Netherlands).

Ostrom M, Eriksson A, Thorson J, Spigset O (1996) Fatal overdose with citalopram, *Lancet* **348:**339–40.

Persad E (1993) *Arch Gen Psychiatry* **50:**497.

Philipp M, Kohnen R, Benkert O (1993) A comparison study of moclobemide and doxepin in major depression with special reference to effects on sexual dysfunction, *Int Clin Psychopharmacol* **7:**149–53.

Phillips SD, Ringo P (1995) Phenelzine and venlafaxine interaction, *Am J Psychiatry* **152:**1400–1.

Pinder RM, Zivkov M (1997) Imipramine and mirtazapine are less effective than expected, *Psychopharmacology* **129:**297–8.

Preskorn SH (1995) Comparison of the tolerability of bupropion, fluoxetine, imipramine, nefazodone, paroxetine, sertraline, and venlafaxine, *J Clin Psychiatry* **56:**12–21.

Priest RG, Gimbrett R, Roberts M, Steinert J (1995) Reversible and selective inhibitors of monoamine oxidase A in mental and other disorders, *Acta Psychiatr Scand Suppl* **386:**40–3.

Puozzo C, Leonard BE (1996) Pharmacokinetics of milnacipran in comparison with other antidepressants, *Int Clin Psychopharmacol* **11**(suppl 4): 15–27.

Riesenman C (1995) Antidepressant drug interactions and the cytochrome P450 system: a critical appraisal, *Pharmacotherapy* **15:**84S–99S.

Robinson DS, Marcus RN, Archibald DG, Sterling AH (1996) Therapeutic dose ranges of nefazodone in the treatment of depression, *J Clin Psychiatry* **57**(suppl 2):6–9.

Romero L, Bel N, Casanovas JM, Artigas F (1996) Two actions are better than one: avoiding self-inhibition of serotonergic neurones enhances the effects of serotonin uptake inhibitors, *Int Clin Psychopharmacol* **11**(suppl 4): 1–8.

Rudolph RL, Derivan AT (1996) The safety and tolerability of venlafaxine hydrochloride: analysis of the clinical trials database, *J Clin Psychopharmacol* **16**(suppl 2):S54–9.

Rudolph R, Entsuah R, Derivan A (1991) Early clinical response in depression to venlafaxine hydrochloride, *Biol Psychiatry* **29:**630S (abstract).

Segraves RT (1989) Effects of psychotropic drugs on human erection and ejaculation, *Arch Gen Psychiatry* **46:**275–84.

Segraves RT (1995) Antidepressant-induced orgasm disorder, *J Sexual Marital Ther* **21:**192–201.

Shrivastava RK, Cohn C, Crowder J et al (1994a) Long-term safety and clinical acceptability of venlafaxine and imipramine in outpatients with major depression, *J Clin Psychopharmacol* **14:**322–9.

Shrivastava RK, Patrick R, Scherer N, Upton GV (1994b) A dose–response study of venlafaxine, *Neuropsychopharmacology* **10**(suppl):221 (abstract).

Silverstone T (1992) Appetite suppressants. A review, *Drugs* **43:**820–36.

Skodol AE, Schwartz S, Dohrenwend BP, Levav I, Shrout PE (1994) Minor depression in a cohort of young adults in Israel, *Arch Gen Psychiatry* **51:**542–51.

Stabl M, Biziere K, Schmid Burgk W, Amrein R (1989) Review of comparative clinical trials. Moclobemide vs tricyclic antidepressants and vs placebo in depressive states, *J Neural Trans* **28**(suppl):77–89.

Stassen HH, Delini-Stula A, Angst J (1993) Time course of improvement under antidepressant treatment: a survival-analytic approach, *Eur Neuropsychopharmacol* **3:**127–35.

Sternbach H (1991) The serotonin syndrome, *Am J Psychiatry* **148:**705–13.

Stoll AL, Mayer PV, Kolbrener M et al (1994) Antidepressant-associated mania: a controlled comparison with spontaneous mania, *Am J Psychiatry* **151:**1642–5.

Szegedi A, Wetzel H, Angersbach D, Philipp M, Benkert O (1997) Response to treatment in minor and major depression: results of a double-blind comparative study with paroxetine and maprotiline, *J Affect Disord* (in press).

Tannock C, Katona C (1995) Minor depression in the aged. Concepts, prevalence and optimal management, *Drugs Ageing* **6:**278–92.

Teicher MG, Clod C, Cole JO (1990) Emergence of intense suicidal preoccupating during fluoxetine treatment, *Am J Psychiatry* **147:**207–10.

Thompson JW Jr, Ware MR, Blashfield RK (1990) Psychotropic medication and priapism: a comprehensive review, *J Clin Psychiatry* **51:**430–3.

Thompson C, Lane R (1994) Sertraline 50mg: optimal daily dose in depression, *Neuropsychopharmacology* **10:**2225.

von Frenckell R, Ansseau M, Serre C, Sutet P (1990) Pooling two controlled comparisons of milnacipran (F2207) and amitriptyline in endogenous inpatients. A new approach in dose ranging studies, *Int Clin Psychopharmacol* **5:**49–56.

Warshaw MG, Keller MB (1996) The relationship between fluoxetine use and suicidal behavior in 654 subjects with anxiety disorders, J Clin Psychiatry **57:**158–66.

Wehr TA (1993) Can antidepressants induce rapid cycling? *Arch Gen Psychiatry* **50:**495–6.

Wehr TA, Sack DA, Rosenthal NE, Cowdry RW (1988) Rapid cycling affective disorder: contributing factors and treatment response in 51 patients, *Am J Psychiatry* **145:**179–84.

Wilde MI, Benfield P (1995) Tianeptine. A review of its pharmacodynamic and pharmacokinetic properties, and therapeutic efficacy in depression and coexisting anxiety and depression, *Drugs* **49:**411–39.

Worthington JJ, Pollack MH (1996) Treatment of dysphoric mania with nefazodone, *Am J Psychiatry* **153:** 732–3.

Yaryura Tobias JA, Neziroglu FA (1996) Venlafaxine in obsessive-compulsive disorder, *Arch Gen Psychiatry* **53:**653–4.

Zimmer R, Gieschke R, Fischbach R, Gasic S (1990) Interaction studies with moclobemide, *Acta Psychiatr Scand Suppl* **360:**84–96.

13

Antidepressant drugs and sexual function: improving the recognition and management of sexual dysfunction in depressed patients

David S Baldwin and Jon Birtwistle

Introduction

The sexual health of depressed patients is often poor. In some, this is due to the effects of depression on the individual, while in others it results from untoward consequences of depression on interpersonal relationships. In many depressed patients, the loss of sexual interest and function either arises from or is worsened by side effects of antidepressant drugs. However, before ascribing problems to a particular drug, many other causes of sexual dysfunction need to be considered, including the depression itself, the presence of comorbid psychiatric or physical illness, and the use of other drug treatments (Baldwin, 1996).

There have been rather few epidemiological investigations that are of sufficient rigour to allow accurate estimation of the prevalence of sexual difficulties within the general population. This relative lack of 'normative' data must be remembered when considering the incidence of sexual dysfunction in depressed patients. Perhaps the most detailed assessment of the incidence of sexual difficulties in the general population comes from the Zurich study, a prospective epidemiological investigation of depressive, anxiety and psychosomatic syndromes among young adults from the canton of Zurich in Switzerland. In this study, a minimum of 27% of men and 46% of women reported sexual problems before the age of 35 years. Low sexual desire was found to be associated with depression, generalized anxiety disorder, alcohol abuse and cannabis abuse, but not with panic attacks, phobic disorders or cigarette smoking (J Angst, personal communication).

Depression is often associated with impairments of sexual function and satisfaction. Because most depressed patients are troubled by a general reduction in interest, loss of energy, and inability to gain pleasure, depression should be expected to lead to sexual difficulties. Further-more, depression is linked to reduced self-esteem, irritability and social withdrawal, all of which can cause problems in forming and maintaining intimate relationships.

Most depressed patients describe a reduction in sexual interest and activity. This complaint is usually associated with other depressive symp-toms, including 'biological' features such as weight loss, reduced energy and disturbed sleep. The results of a Finnish epidemiological study sug-gest that reduction in sexual interest is associated with depression in all groups, other than in women older than 70 years. For older women a decline in libido appeared to be a normal part of ageing (Kivela and Pahkala, 1988). In some investigations, a minority of depressed patients describe an increase in sexual interest and activity. This may be due to the search for reassurance and intimacy, rather than resulting from a genuine increase in sexual desire (Matthew and Weinman, 1982).

Although loss of desire is the most common sexual difficulty experi-enced by depressed patients, other forms of dysfunction are also com-mon. For example, in a comparative study of the sexual function of depressed patients with that of age- and sex-matched controls, erectile dysfunction was present in up to 35% of the depressed men, but in none of the control subjects. Furthermore, premature or delayed ejaculation were described by 38% and 47% of the depressed patients, compared to 0% and 6% of the controls, respectively (Matthew and Weinman, 1982).

Loss of sexual interest may be the presenting complaint of some patients, many of whom will be found to be suffering from depression. Even when not currently depressed, patients with reduced sexual desire have often suffered from depression in their past (Schreiner-Engel and Schiavi, 1986). As loss of sexual desire may have been a feature of ear-lier depressive episodes, it makes sense to follow up patients who com-plain of low sexual desire, particularly when there is a history of depressive illness.

Of course, many patients have both a mental disorder and a disorder of sexual function. For example, in an early study of psychiatric outpa-tients, sexual and marital difficulties were reported by 25%, and sexual or marital therapy was considered to be suitable in approximately half of the patients (Swan and Wilson, 1979). A recent comparative study found that sexual dysfunction was present in 35% of outpatients with severe affec-tive illness, 49% of outpatients with schizophrenia, and 13% of patients receiving treatment for a range of dermatological conditions (Kockott and Pfeiffer, 1996). Finally, an investigation of the comorbidity of sexual prob-lems and mental disorder among patients with a primary diagnosis of sexual dysfunction found that a dual diagnosis was present in 30% of men and 31% of women, affective illness being found in 16% of men and 30% of women (Fagan et al, 1988).

Table 13.1   Neurotransmitters with effects on sexual behaviour
(Segraves, 1989; Wilson, 1993).

Dopamine	Oxytocin
Noradrenaline	Arg-vasopressin
Serotonin	Angiotensin II
Acetylcholine	Gonadotrophin-releasing hormone
GABA	Substance P
	Neuropeptide Y
	Cholecystokinin-8
	Nitric oxide

Neurotransmitters and sexual behaviour

Many aspects of the neurophysiological basis of the human sexual response remain unclear. Research in animal models can provide some insight into human sexual behaviour, but the findings of such studies are often not applicable to other species. However, it is clear that male and female sexual behaviour is affected by many neurotransmitters (Table 13.1). The following account is only a brief description: further details can be found elsewhere (Segraves, 1989; Wilson, 1993; Dunsmuir and Emberton, 1997).

In general terms, dopamine facilitates sexual activity, probably through actions within the central nervous system. It increases sexual behaviour in experimental male animals, this effect being blocked by central but not peripheral dopamine antagonists. The effects of dopamine on female sexual behaviour in animal models vary, according to whether the animal is in a receptive or non-receptive state. In clinical practice, dopamine antagonists such as conventional antipsychotic drugs are often linked to the development of sexual dysfunction (Wilson, 1993). Like dopamine, noradrenaline has a significant role in sexual behaviour, with both central and peripheral actions. In animal models of male sexual behaviour, enhancing central noradrenergic neurotransmission often results in increased sexual arousal. However, its peripheral actions can impair sexual performance, through the inhibition of penile reflexes. Any effect on copulatory behaviour is probably indirect (Wilson, 1993).

The role of serotonin (5-hydroxytryptamine, 5-HT) in sexual behaviour is not understood fully. Studies in experimental animals have produced inconsistent findings, but suggest that 5-HT has different effects in females and males. Increased transmission within central serotonergic pathways produces a reduction in sexual arousal and activity. In animal models, these inhibitory actions are mediated by $5-HT_2$ receptors. Peripheral serotonergic fibres probably inhibit penile sensation and ejaculation (Wilson, 1993). These findings correspond with the clinical observation that sexual dysfunction associated with serotonin reuptake inhibitors can be reversed by 5-HT$_2$ antagonists. The stimulatory effects on sexual behaviour that are sometimes seen with agents acting on other 5-HT receptors, such as with buspirone which acts on the 5-HT$_{1A}$ autoreceptor subtype, are probably due to inhibition of the release of serotonin (Baldwin and Thomas, 1996).

Acetylcholine appears to have only a limited role in regulating sexual activity. In male animal models, it reduces arousal but also reduces the threshold for ejaculation. Acetylcholine may have indirect effects, as optimal sexual function probably depends on a balance of adrenergic and cholinergic effects. Cholinergic agonists such as neostigmine and bethanechol can be helpful in reversing erectile dysfunction seen with certain antidepressant drugs (Segraves, 1993).

Gamma-aminobutyric acid (GABA) seems to have inhibitory effects on sexual behaviour, independent of its effects on motor activity. In animal models, benzodiazepine agonists such as diazepam (which exert their effects through actions on GABA) reduce male sexual activity, whereas benzodiazepine antagonists reverse the effects of agonists, but themselves have no effect on sexual behaviour (Wilson, 1993). In clinical practice, benzodiazepine use is associated with variable, but generally inhibitory, effects on sexual function and satisfaction. Many other neurotransmitters are involved in the regulation of sexual behaviour. These include oxytocin, arg-vasopressin, angiotensin II, gonadotrophin-releasing hormone, substance P, neuropeptide Y and cholecystokinin-8 (Wilson, 1993) (Table 13.1). In recent years, attention has focused on the role of endothelium-derived mediators such as nitric oxide and prostacyclin in the physiology of penile erection (Mellis and Argiolas, 1995; Ari et al, 1996).

Animal studies indicate that penile erection is mediated by oxytocinergic transmission from the paraventricular nucleus (PVN) of the hypothalamus. Injection of oxytocin into the hypothalamus of male rats produces erection, which can be prevented by the addition of nitric oxide synthase inhibitors (Mellis and Argiolas, 1995).

Adverse effects of antidepressant drugs on sexual function

Data derived from placebo-controlled treatment studies show that antidepressant drugs are often associated with the development of sexual dysfunction. These adverse effects arise from a range of pathophysiological mechanisms. For example, non-specific effects such as sedation can produce a decrease in sexual interest, whereas specific actions on certain neurotransmitters can lead to impairment of sexual function. Action within the autonomic nervous system may also lead to sexual difficulties. Furthermore, many psychotropic drugs have either direct or indirect effects on hormones that are involved in the regulation of sexual activity (Table 13.2).

Table 13.2 Adverse effects of antidepressant drugs on sexual function (Segraves, 1989).

Non-specific effects on central nervous system
Specific effects on neurotransmitters within central nervous system
Specific effects on neurotransmitters within autonomic nervous system
Direct effects on hormonal activity
Indirect effects on regulation of hormones

The true incidence of sexual difficulties with antidepressants is likely to be greater than that reported, for a number of reasons (Baldwin, 1995). Sexual problems are discussed in clinical settings only rarely. Many patients feel uncomfortable when discussing sexual problems, and although some report sexual difficulties when completing a questionnaire, others describe sexual dysfunction only after direct questioning by a doctor. However, recent studies suggest that many doctors do not feel comfortable when discussing sexual matters—for example, surgeons often fail to discuss potential sexual complications of urological procedures (Dunsmuir and Emberton, 1997), and psychiatrists frequently overlook the sexual history when admitting patients to hospital (Singh and Beck, 1997). Furthermore, the variation in description of clinical terms and absence of a generally accepted standardized schedule for eliciting sexual difficulties can lead to methodological problems when recording sexual problems.

As such, it seems likely that only the most troublesome sexual side effects of drugs are reported, there being a greater number of other problems that only come to light after direct questioning. For example, systematic enquiries in a sample of 60 patients, prescribed a number of different antidepressant drugs, including imipramine, fluoxetine, trazodone and desipramine, found that sexual dysfunction during treatment occurred in 43.3% of patients (Balon et al, 1993).

Tricyclic antidepressants

The sexual side effects of tricyclic antidepressants (TCAs) have not been investigated in detail. Until recently, most of the data were derived from single case reports or small case series. TCAs have been implicated in the development of most forms of sexual dysfunction, including decreased sexual interest, erectile failure, impaired ejaculation and impaired orgasm. Erectile difficulties and problems with ejaculation have been described in patients taking amitriptyline, imipramine, clomipramine, desipramine, lofepramine, nortriptyline and protryptiline. Anorgasmia has been reported with imipramine, clomipramine, desipramine, nortriptyline and doxepin (Ari et al, 1996). The relative incidence of these problems with differing drugs has not been determined reliably (Baldwin, 1995, 1996).

Sexual dysfunction may be especially common with the TCA clomipramine. In a placebo-controlled study of the treatment of patients with obsessive-compulsive disorder, 33% of those receiving clomipramine reported sexual problems. Furthermore, when completing a questionnaire, 66% of clomipramine-treated patients described sexual difficulties, this figure increasing to 95% after direct questioning by the research team. By contrast, none of the patients treated with placebo reported sexual dysfunction (Monteiro et al, 1987). Although reporting bias may account for some of the attention paid to the problem of sexual dysfunction with clomipramine, it is of some interest, as clomipramine possesses strong serotonin reuptake-inhibiting properties.

Monoamine oxidase inhibitors

As with tricyclic drugs, most reports of sexual dysfunction with monoamine oxidase inhibitors (MAOIs) are limited to single case reports or small case series. Like TCAs, MAOIs have been associated with the development of most forms of sexual dysfunction, including decreased sexual interest, erectile failure, impaired ejaculation and impaired orgasm (Baldwin, 1995).

Sexual difficulties may be more common with MAOIs than with TCAs. In a comparative study of phenelzine, imipramine and placebo, sexual dysfunction was reported by 80% of men and 57% of women taking phenelzine, compared with figures of 50% and 27% for imipramine, and 8% and 16% for patients taking placebo. Accurate evaluation of the presence of sexual dysfunction in the depressed women was especially dependent upon the use of specific enquiries (Harrison et al, 1986) (Table 13.3).

Although there are reports of increased sexual desire with isocarboxazid, its effects, and those of pargyline, on other aspects of sexual function are largely unknown (Baier and Philipp, 1994). By contrast, phenelzine has been linked to impairments of erection, ejaculation and orgasm. There are few published reports of erectile dysfunction or ejaculatory failure with tranylcpromine. Moclobemide, a reversible inhibitor of monoamine oxidase type A, may have fewer adverse effects on sexual function than conventional non-selective MAOIs (Philipp et al, 1993). In a study conducted in healthy volunteers, moclobemide did not appear to have any aphrodisiac properties (Kennedy et al, 1996).

Table 13.3 Relative incidence of sexual dysfunction with TCAs and MAOIs (Harrison et al, 1986).

	Imipramine	Phenelzine	Placebo
Sexual dysfunction: men (%)	50	80	8
Sexual dysfunction: women (%)	27	57	16

Selective serotonin reuptake inhibitors

As with TCAs and MAOIs, the selective serotonin reuptake inhibitors (SSRIs) have been implicated in the development of sexual dysfunction in a number of case reports and case series, as well as in the results of controlled clinical trials. During the course of development of the SSRIs, most studies suggested a relatively low incidence of sexual dysfunction. However, these findings had to be revised upwards as the drugs entered widespread use in clinical practice.

It is now clear that treatment with SSRIs can be associated with the development of most forms of sexual dysfunction, in particular delayed ejaculation in men and anorgasmia in women. The apparent increase in the incidence of sexual dysfunction is probably the result of more people being treated with SSRIs, and heightened awareness of the importance of sexual dysfunction, leading doctors to detect and report sexual side effects more frequently (Baldwin, 1996).

For example, in the case of fluoxetine, an early review of its tolerability and safety indicated that approximately 5% of patients developed 'treatment-emergent' sexual dysfunction (Stark and Hardison, 1985). Following the launch of fluoxetine, and its widespread clinical use, case reports and case series suggested that the incidence of sexual dysfunction was much higher than originally thought. Studies which have employed systematic questioning about the presence of sexual difficulties indicate that sexual dysfunction is present in 34–75% of patients treated with fluoxetine (Herman et al, 1988; Zajecka et al, 1991; Jacobsen, 1992; Balon et al, 1993; Patterson, 1993; Hsu and Shen, 1995; Shen and Hsu, 1995) (Table 13.4).

The problem of sexual dysfunction is not restricted to fluoxetine, but is also seen with other SSRIs. For example, in a placebo-controlled study of sertraline, the incidence of treatment-emergent male sexual dysfunction was found to be 8.5% at a dose of 50 mg/day, 7.5% at 100 mg/day, and 20.6 at 200 mg/day (Fabre et al, 1995). Evaluation of sexual dysfunction with paroxetine is somewhat difficult, as although the placebo-adjusted incidence of ejaculatory disturbance is 12.9%, a further 10% of

Table 13.4   Fluoxetine and sexual dysfunction.

Study	Year	N	Sexual dysfunction (%)
Stark and Hardison	1985	185	5.0
Herman et al	1990	60	8.3
Zajecka et al	1991	77	7.8
Jacobsen	1992	160	34.0
Balon et al	1993	14	42.9
Patterson	1993	60	75.0
Hsu and Shen	1995	32 (men)	43.0
Shen and Hsu	1995	48 (women)	30.0

patients experience 'other male genital disorders', which include erectile difficulties, delayed ejaculation and inhibited orgasm (Medical Economics Data, 1995).

The relative incidence of sexual dysfunction with the differing SSRIs is not yet known (Baldwin and Thomas, 1996). A recent review, drawing from a number of sources, suggests that sexual dysfunction may be rather more common with paroxetine than with fluoxetine, fluvoxamine or sertraline (Lane, 1997). This may be because of the high potency of paroxetine for serotonin reuptake inhibition, together with it having little or no effect on dopamine reuptake (Bolden-Watson and Richerson, 1993). Further head-to-head comparisons of SSRIs, in both the short-term and long-term treatment of depressed patients, are required before the relative potential of differing SSRIs to cause sexual problems can be determined reliably.

Similarly, the relative incidence of sexual dysfunction with SSRIs compared to other classes of antidepressant is also unknown. Although numerous comparator studies of SSRIs and other TCAs have been performed, few have examined the problem of sexual dysfunction in great detail. A recently completed study of imipramine and paroxetine found that sexual side effects were more common with the SSRI (Ontiveros et al, 1996). In this study, 38 outpatients suffering from DSM-III-R major depression received placebo for 1 week, prior to random allocation to either paroxetine 20 mg/day or imipramine 150–250 mg/day for 6 weeks. Patients were excluded from the study if they had other psychiatric diagnoses, or other relevant general medical conditions. The presence of sexual dysfunction was detected both before and after treatment. Paroxetine was associated with significantly more sexual dysfunction than imipramine, 16.6% of patients treated with imipramine having sexual side effects, compared to 35% of patients treated with paroxetine. Although the study was well designed, with systematic enquiries regarding sexual function, the findings need to be replicated in a larger investigation before any definitive conclusions can be drawn (Ontiveros et al, 1996). The exact mechanism of SSRI-induced sexual dysfunction is not known, although increased transmission in central serotonergic pathways, mediated by 5-HT receptors, produces a reduction in sexual activity in experimental animals (Wilson, 1993). Other mechanisms may be involved as well: for example, paroxetine has been found to significantly inhibit the activity of nitric oxide synthetase in depressed patients (Finkel et al, 1996).

Nefazodone

The antidepressant drug nefaxodone has a dual mechanism of action, having effects on two complementary sites in serotonergic neurons. It acts on the presynaptic neuron by inhibiting the reuptake of serotonin, though to a lesser degree than seen with the SSRIs, and is also an antagonist at 5-HT$_2$ receptors on postsynaptic neurons (Eison et al, 1990). This

Table 13.5   Relative incidence of sexual dysfunction with nefazodone (Robinson et al, 1996).

	Placebo	Imipramine	Fluoxetine	Nefazodone
All patients				
N	875	367	182	1310
Decreased libido (%)	0.5	1.6	2.2*	0.7
Psychosexual dysfunction (%)	0	1.1*	1.6*	0.1
Anorgasmia (%)	0.1	0.3	1.1	0.2
Men				
N	334	163	61	494
Impotence (%)	1.2	9.8*	1.6	1.4
Abnormal ejaculation (%)	0	3.1*	1.6	0.2

* $p < 0.5$ versus placebo.

dual mechanism of action may be responsible for the relatively low incidence of SSRI-like effects seen during clinical trials. For example, nausea and increased agitation appear less common with nefazodone than with SSRIs. Blockade of postsynaptic receptors may reduce the untoward effects of inhibiting the reuptake of 5-HT into the presynaptic neurons (Marcus, 1996).

The incidence of sexual dysfunction with nefazodone is low, in both men and women. The clinical trial database shows that there are no significant differences between nefazodone and placebo in the incidence of decreased libido, erectile dysfunction, abnormal ejaculation or anorgasmia, reported as a treatment-emergent side effect (Baldwin, 1996). In an overview of placebo-controlled studies involving nefazodone and placebo, both fluoxetine and imipramine were associated with a greater incidence of sexual dysfunction than was seen with placebo (Robinson et al, 1996) (Table 13.5).

These findings suggest that the incidence of sexual dysfunction with nefazodone is less than that with SSRIs. This inference is supported by the results of a comparative trial of the acute treatment of patients suffering from DSM-III-R major depression, which include a systematic evaluation of the effects of nefazodone and sertraline on sexual function, in addition to usual measures of efficacy and tolerability (Feiger et al, 1996). Nefazodone caused significantly less disturbance of sexual function than sertraline. In women, it was significantly superior to sertraline on measures of ease in achieving and satisfaction with orgasm. In men, treatment with nefazodone was associated with significantly less impairment of sexual enjoyment and satisfaction, and less difficulty with and delay of ejaculation. By contrast, treatment with sertraline was associated with significantly fewer reports of premature ejaculation, this observation being in line with other findings of delayed ejaculation with sertraline (Feiger et al, 1996).

The relative advantage of nefazodone over sertraline with regard to adverse effects on sexual function and satisfaction is supported by the results of a further study, again in patients suffering from DSM-III-R major depression (Ferguson et al, 1995). Patients who experienced sexual dysfunction with sertraline were withdrawn from the drug, and then followed up over a 7–10-day placebo washout interval. Those patients who no longer reported sexual dysfunction were then randomized to treatment with either sertraline or nefazodone for 8 weeks. At the end of the study, 71% of sertraline-treated patients experienced sexual dysfunction, compared to only 30% of patients treated with nefazodone (Ferguson et al, 1995).

Taken together, the findings of the placebo-controlled database and comparator studies with sertraline indicate that nefazodone has relatively few adverse effects on sexual function. The reason for this is unclear, but is possibly the blockade of postsynaptic 5-HT$_2$ receptors, as 5-HT$_2$ antagonism is found to enhance sexual behaviour in animal models, and to improve function in patients experiencing sexual side effects arising from treatment with serotonergic agonists (Baldwin, 1996).

Other antidepressants

Renewed interest in the importance of noradrenaline in the pathophysiology of depression has led to the development of a range of serotonin noradrenaline reuptake inhibitors (SNRIs) as potential antidepressants. Venlafaxine was the first of these to enter widespread clinical use. Treatment studies conducted prior to its launch showed that venlafaxine was associated with erectile failure in 12% and abnormal ejaculation in 6% of men, and with orgasmic problems in 2% of women. Sexual dysfunction did not appear to be a common problem in two recent studies (Cunningham et al, 1994; Schweizer et al, 1994), but these only described those side effects which were reported by more than 10% of patients, and the apparent lack of sexual side effects may be because most of the participating patients were women, whereas pre-launch investigations suggested that sexual dysfunction with venlafaxine was more common in men (Margolese and Assalian, 1996). A single case report has described the development of increased libido and frequent spontaneous erections early in the course of recovery from depression (Michael and Owen, 1997). The novel antidepressant drug milnacipran inhibits the reuptake of serotonin and noradrenaline both in vitro and in vivo, with no effects on dopamine reuptake (Briley et al, 1996). It may offer advantages over TCAs in terms of tolerability, and over SSRIs in terms of efficacy (Montgomery et al, 1996). During the course of development and in treatment studies conducted prior to its launch, milnacipran appeared to be associated with a low incidence of sexual dysfunction, the pattern in men suggesting a dose-dependent adverse effect (Table 13.6).

Table 13.6   Effects of milnacipran on male sexual function.

	Daily dose of milnacipran		
	<100 mg N = 123	100 mg N = 483	>100 mg N = 263
Impotence (%)	–	0.4	3.0
Reduction of libido (%)	–	0.8	0.8
Increase in libido (%)	0.8	–	0.4
Ejaculatory problems (%)	0.8	0.8	1.2
Testicular symptoms (%)	–	0.8	1.5
Penile problems (%)	–	–	0.4
Priapism (%)	–	0.2	–
Number of patients	1 (0.8%)	13 (2.7%)	17 (6.5%)

The antidepressant drug mirtazapine has a complex mechanism of action. It preferentially blocks the noradrenergic α_2–autoreceptors responsible for the release of both noradrenaline and serotonin. In addition, it blocks 5-HT$_2$ and 5-HT$_3$ receptors while having little affinity for the 5-HT$_{1a}$ receptor (de Boer, 1995). For these reasons, the incidence of sexual dysfunction with mirtazapine is expected to be low. Analysis of the clinical trial database supports this hypothesis, as sexual dysfunction with mirtazapine was no more common than with placebo, and apparently less common than with amitriptyline (Montgomery, 1995). However, more studies of sexual dysfunction during treatment with mirtazapine are required before further conclusions can be drawn.

The antidepressant drug bupropion is approved for use in the USA. Studies conducted prior to its launch found a low incidence of sexual dysfunction. For example, 3.1% of patients treated with bupropion reported reduced libido, compared to 1.6% of those receiving placebo, and erectile failure was described by 3.4% of men taking bupropion, and 3.1% of those receiving placebo (Margolese and Assalian, 1996). For these reasons, bupropion is sometimes used as an alternative treatment in patients who become troubled by sexual problems while taking other antidepressants. In an early study of substitution with bupropion, 86% of patients described a resolution of sexual dysfunction when switched to bupropion from other antidepressants, including TCAs, MAOIs and trazodone (Gardner and Johnston, 1985). A more recent investigation found that substitution with bupropion resolved sexual dysfunction in 94% of patients who developed this problem while previously treated with fluoxetine (Fabre et al, 1995).

Although lithium is widely used in the treatment of affective disorder, its effects on sexual function are unclear. Lithium alone has few effects on sexual health, but when combined with benzodiazepines, approximately half of patients experience sexual dysfunction (Aizenberg et al, 1996).

Beneficial effects of antidepressant drugs on sexual function

Although the adverse effects of antidepressant drugs on sexual function and satisfaction are being recognized more frequently, it should be remembered that treatment with antidepressants may improve sexual desire and satisfaction, in line with improvements in other depressive symptoms. The relative under-reporting of adverse sexual side effects may be accompanied by similar under-reporting of beneficial properties (Lane, 1997). For example, in an anonymous questionnaire survey of psychotropic drug-induced sexual side effects in women, 40% of women taking fluoxetine reported that it stimulated their sexual interest and performance (Post, 1996). Antidepressant drugs have been used to improve sexual desire and performance in non-depressed patients, on an open-label basis, and controlled studies have suggested that antidepressants may have a role in the overall management of patients suffering from premature ejaculation or paraphilic disorders.

Antidepressants in the treatment of premature ejaculation

Premature ejaculation is a common but under-reported disorder. In an analysis of 22 surveys of the general population, up to 35% of men had experienced premature ejaculation (Nathan, 1986). Although it is rather more common than erectile failure, fewer men present for treatment, usually consulting general practitioners rather than hospital specialists (Shahar et al, 1991). Some patients are helped by explanation and reassurance alone, and by the knowledge that premature ejaculation often resolves with increasing experience and confidence in sexual relationships. Others need to be helped by instruction in behavioural approaches, designed to gain greater control of sexual arousal and ejaculation, including the 'start–stop' technique and the 'squeeze technique' (Bancroft, 1989).

When premature ejaculation persists despite simple psychological and behavioural approaches, some patients benefit from treatment with antidepressant drugs. As might be expected from their association with the adverse effect of delayed ejaculation, clomipramine and the SSRIs have been evaluated in uncontrolled and controlled studies in men with persistent troublesome premature ejaculation. Clomipramine has been found to be beneficial in two double-blind placebo-controlled studies, doses of 25–50 mg being associated with longer ejaculatory delay, greater emotional satisfaction, and improvements in partner orgasmic attainment (Althof et al, 1995; Singh and Beck, 1997). Both paroxetine and sertraline have been found to be helpful in placebo-controlled studies (Waldinger et al, 1994; Mendels et al, 1995). These investigations used rather high doses of medication (paroxetine 40 mg/day; sertraline 200 mg/day), and the efficacy of lower daily doses or intermittent dosing is not yet established.

In addition to possessing beneficial effects in some patients with premature ejaculation, antidepressants may be of value in the management of patients suffering from other sexual disorders. Two open-label studies suggest that sertraline may have a role in the treatment of patients with paraphilia (a disorder of sexual preference). In the first, sertraline was associated with a significant reduction in unconventional sexual behaviour, while leaving more conventional sexual practice unchanged (Kafka, 1994). In the second, sertraline reduced 'abnormal' fantasies, sex drive and arousal, again without producing adverse effects on normal sexual relations (Bradford, 1995).

Unusual effects of antidepressant drugs on sexual function

Antidepressant drugs can occasionally produce rather unusual effects on sexual function. For example, tricyclic antidepressants have been associated with the development of painful ejaculation, which may occur in approximately 20% of men. The mechanism of this is unclear, but through blockade of peripheral sympathetic α-adrenergic receptors, TCAs can interfere with the coordinated contractions of smooth muscles involved in sperm transport and therefore cause painful ejaculation. Other unusual sexual side effects with antidepressants include penile anaesthesia with fluoxetine, and an unusual syndrome consisting of yawning, clitoral engorgement and multiple orgasm in the absence of sexual stimulation, which has been described in a few patients treated with clomipramine or SSRIs (Modell, 1994). Furthermore, a single case report has described the development of repeated spontaneous ejaculation in a man treated with nefazodone (Michael and Ramana, 1996).

Trazodone has been associated with both the development of priapism (prolonged painful erection) and an increase in sexual interest in both men and women. Priapism is an uncommon complication of treatment with trazodone (affecting between 1 in 1000 to 1 in 10 000 men), and is also seen with other psychotropic drugs, including SSRIs and antipsychotic agents (Thompson et al, 1990). Patients taking trazodone should be warned of the risk of priapism, and be advised to seek medical attention promptly should it occur. The initial treatment of priapism is medical, involving irrigation of the corpora cavernosa with either saline or metaraminol (an α-adrenoceptor agonist), which usually results in venous constriction and subsequent penile detumescence. However, if medical approaches are unsuccessful, surgical procedures may be necessary, which can sometimes result in permanent erectile dysfunction (Thompson et al, 1990).

Psychological approaches to sexual dysfunction in depression

Psychological factors play an extremely important role in the sexual response. Low mood and reduced self-esteem affect an individual's attractiveness and sense of being desired. Furthermore, depression can cause or contribute to relationship difficulties and thus affect a couple's sexual relationship. The management of sexual problems in depression is frequently complex and multifaceted, involving a combination of psychological and pharmacological approaches.

Depressed patients who are troubled by sexual dysfunction can be helped by some of the general psychological approaches to the management of people with sexual difficulties, which aim to reduce anxiety and foster feelings of security. By establishing better communication between partners, any sense of failure or resentment can often be reduced. Psychological approaches may be specifically targeted either at the particular sexual problem or at the overall relationship. The approaches which have been found to be successful include counselling and brief supportive psychotherapy, couple therapy, individual therapy and group therapy. Studies of the outcome of psychological interventions have revealed varying degrees of success. A survey of sex therapists suggests that up to 52% of men suffering from psychogenic erectile dysfunction can be helped by these approaches, particularly when the dysfunction is 'secondary', i.e. when at least one successful attempt at sexual intercourse has occurred (Kilmann et al, 1986). In addition to these individual, couple and group psychotherapeutic approaches, a number of specific behavioural techniques have been developed to improve particular aspects of sexual performance. These include intermittent penetration for men with erectile failure, and guided masturbation for delayed ejaculation or anorgasmia (Bancroft, 1989).

Pharmacological approaches to sexual dysfunction

The psychological and behavioural strategies used in the management of patients with sexual dysfunction can be complemented by a range of pharmacological approaches (Table 13.7). Clearly, treatment strategies should be tailored to the individual patient, taking into account the benefits and risks of each approach. The emergence of sexual dysfunction is thought to be an important cause of non-compliance in depressed patients treated with antidepressants. By contrast, effective management of sexual problems should be expected, at least in theory, to improve adherence to treatment, and therefore enhance long-term clinical outcome (Balon et al, 1993).

Table 13.7   Pharmacological management of sexual dysfunction (Segraves, 1993; Gitlin, 1994; Baldwin, 1995; Lane, 1997).

Continuation of current treatment
Delayed dosing
Reduction in dosage
Drug holidays
Withdrawal of medication
Adjunctive agents
Substitution with alternative treatment

Expectant management

Certain aspects of sexual dysfunction may remit simply with the passage of time. The rate of accommodation to the sexual side effects of antidepressant drugs is not known. Remission has been reported in some patients taking TCAs, MAOIs and SSRIs, but successful changes in sexual technique may give a misleading impression that an adverse effect has spontaneously resolved.

Delayed dosing

Some patients with drug-induced sexual dysfunction note improvements simply by postponing taking their medication until after sexual intercourse (Olivera, 1994). This approach allows them to continue with the same drug at the same dose, but is only helpful with antidepressant drugs that have a short half-life.

Reduction in dosage

Adverse effects on sexual function may be more common with higher doses of medication. Sexual dysfunction has been reported as being more common within higher doses of a range of antidepressant drugs, including imipramine, clomipramine, desipramine, maprotiline, protriptyline, fluoxetine and sertraline. However, many patients develop sexual problems, even while taking low doses of antidepressant drugs.

Withdrawal of medication

When distressing sexual dysfunction persists even after the passage of time and a reduction in dose (if possible), withdrawal of treatment may sometimes be appropriate. In most cases, this leads to the recovery of sexual function within a few days. With fluoxetine, resolution takes rather longer, probably because of the extended half-life of the drug and its principal active metabolite. Of course, withdrawal of medication runs the risk of precipitating a relapse of depression, and should only be considered when this risk is thought to be minimal.

Table 13.8   'Drug holidays' (Rothschild, 1995).

	Patients who reported 'much' or 'very much' improved sexual function in at least 2 of 4 weekends		
	Fluoxetine	Paroxetine	Sertraline
N	10	10	10
Mean daily dose	24 mg	26 mg	60 mg
Orgasm function	10%	50%	60%
Sexual satisfaction	0	50%	50%
Libido	0	50%	50%

'Drug holidays'

Recently, 'drug holidays' have been advocated in the management of patients with sexual dysfunction induced by SSRIs (Rothschild, 1995) (Table 13.8). Treatment is interrupted briefly, 1–2 days before anticipated sexual activity. Beneficial effects on sexual function have been seen in patients treated with paroxetine and sertraline, though not with fluoxetine (presumably because of its long half-life). Although encouraging, these findings are somewhat preliminary, as the published studies were of an 'open' design, and involved only small numbers of patients. Furthermore, it is likely that, if adopted more widely, many patients would find this approach aesthetically unacceptable.

Treatment substitution

A number of reports have described the beneficial effect of switching from one drug to another, in an attempt to reduce the incidence or severity of sexual dysfunction. There have been case reports of successful drug substitutions that include desipramine for imipramine and clomipramine, imipramine for amoxapine, nortriptyline for imipramine and doxepin, and bupropion for numerous antidepressants (Gardner and Johnston, 1985; Singh and Beck, 1997). Recent studies have suggested that nefazodone is a useful alternative in patients who develop sexual dysfunction with sertraline, and probably with other SSRIs (Ferguson et al, 1995). It is unclear whether greater benefit comes from substituting with a drug from the same class of antidepressant drug, or whether it is more helpful to choose a drug from a different class of compound.

Adjunctive treatments

Further pharmacological strategies in the management of drug-induced sexual dysfunction include the use of so-called adjunctive or adjuvant compounds (Table 13.9) (Baldwin, 1996).

Table 13.9   Adjunctive treatments (Segraves, 1989; Gitlin, 1994; Baldwin, 1995).

Class	Example
Serotonin antagonists	Cyproheptadine, mianserin
5-HT$_{1A}$ partial agonists	Buspirone
Adrenergic antagonists	Yohimbine, fluparoxan
Cholinergic agonists	Neostigmine, bethanechol
Dopamine agonists	Amantadine, dextroamphetamine, pemoline

Serotonin antagonists

Cyproheptadine, an antagonist at serotonin and histamine receptors, has been found useful in the management of anorgasmia associated with TCAs, MAOIs and SSRIs. Typically, 2–16 mg of cyproheptadine are taken 1–2 h prior to anticipated sexual activity. Unfortunately, use of cyproheptadine can sometimes result in the reversal of the therapeutic effects of antidepressants (Feder, 1991; Hollander et al, 1992). The antidepressant drug mianserin acts as an antagonist, both at 5-HT$_2$ and 5-HT$_3$ receptors and at α_2-adrenoceptors. As the 5-HT$_2$ antagonist properties of mianserin may be responsible for its efficacy in managing the akathisia occasionally seen with SSRIs (Poyurovsky et al, 1995), it should at least in theory be of some value in reversing SSRI-induced anorgasmia, although it has itself been linked to the development of sexual dysfunction (Kowalski et al, 1985).

5-HT$_{1A}$ partial agonists

Buspirone appears to have fewer adverse effects on sexual function than other anxiolytic drugs, and has been used in the management of sexual dysfunction in patients treated with SSRIs. Although the mechanism of action of these beneficial properties is unclear, it probably involves either inhibition of central serotonergic neurotransmission, arising from effects on presynaptic 5-HT$_{1A}$ autoreceptors (Norden, 1995), or α_2-antagonist properties of its major metabolite (Fuller and Perry, 1989).

Adrenergic antagonists

The adrenergic α_2-antagonists yohimbine and fluparoxan may have beneficial effects in relieving erectile dysfunction. The mechanism of action is not understood fully, but probably involves both a central effect in enhancing sexual interest, and a peripheral effect on α_2-receptors within the corpora cavernosa of the penis. Two approaches to treatment have been advocated—either a regular daily dose of 5.4 mg t.d.s., or a dose of 5.4–16.2 mg, taken 2–4 h before sex. The side effects of yohimbine are often unpleasant, including excessive perspiration, urinary frequency, anxiety, insomnia and fatigue (Segraves, 1993).

Cholinergic agonists

Both neostigmine and bethanechol have been reported to reverse the loss of sexual desire associated with amitriptyline, and anorgasmia linked to other TCAs. Treatment with bethanechol involves either a regular daily dose of 30–100 mg, or the use of 10–40 mg shortly before sexual intercourse. The side effects of bethanechol include diarrhoea, cramps and excessive perspiration (Segraves, 1989; 1993).

Dopamine agonists

Amantadine, dextroamphetamine and pemoline have been found to be helpful in reversing anorgasmia associated with the use of fluoxetine, sertraline and phenelzine. The mechanism of this effect is unclear, but probably involves either direct dopaminergic effects in increasing libido and facilitating ejaculation, or indirect actions, through reversing the inhibition of dopaminergic transmission that is seen with some serotonergic compounds (Segraves, 1993).

Unfortunately, there have been very few double-blind placebo-controlled trials of these drugs in depressed patients, most of the evidence of benefit coming from anecdotal case reports. In the absence of convincing evidence, doctors should be cautious when using unfamiliar treatments, particularly when they carry the risk of reversing the beneficial effects of antidepressant drugs.

Physical treatments of sexual dysfunction

The physical treatments of sexual dysfunction are directed mainly at men with erectile failure, usually secondary to an underlying chronic illness such as diabetes or multiple sclerosis. They are less appropriate when sexual dysfunction is psychologically based or secondary to the use of psychotropic medication, as these problems are most likely to respond to psychotherapeutic and pharmacological strategies. The physical treatments for men with organically determined sexual dysfunction differ in technique, efficacy and acceptability (Kirby, 1994) (Table 13.10). The importance of correct investigation and assessment cannot be overemphasized, and a multidisciplinary approach to the management of erectile dysfunction is

Table 13.10   Physical treatments for erectile dysfunction (Kirby, 1994).

Intracavernosal pharmacotherapy	Papaverine
	Alprostadil
Surgical treatments	Revascularization surgery
	Venous leak correction
Use of a vacuum device	
Penile prostheses	

ideal. Those patients with interpersonal or relationship difficulties are unlikely to find that these physical techniques for the management of erectile impotence do anything to improve their overall sexual function.

Conclusions

Adequate sexual expression is an essential component of human relationships, and may enhance quality of life and provide a sense of physical, psychological and social well-being. Unfortunately, depressive illness is associated with a range of impairments of sexual function and satisfaction, and the presence of these problems can worsen a quality of life already reduced by the effects of depression.

The existing established antidepressant drugs are far from ideal. Most antidepressants have adverse effects on sexual function, but the exact incidence of sexual dysfunction during treatment with antidepressants is not known. However, it is likely to be greater than presently thought, because of factors such as embarrassment, both in patients and health professionals, when discussing sexual problems. Disturbances of sexual interest and performance will only be detected in a reliable fashion when systematic enquiries are made during the course of the standard clinical interview. To facilitate the discussion of sexual function in depression, the UK self-help organization Depression Alliance has produced a simple questionnaire, for patients to complete prior to consultation with their doctor.

The growing awareness of the adverse effects of many antidepressants on sexual function should lead to some re-evaluation of earlier claims for the good tolerability of many of the newer drugs. There is a clear need for adequately designed controlled investigations of the effects of antidepressants on sexual function, so that the tolerability of different drugs can be assessed in a reliable fashion. But more than research is required. At present, doctors and nurses gain most of their professional knowledge of sexual function and health by a somewhat haphazard process. Little time and space is made available for teaching medical and nursing students about sexual matters, and this paucity of teaching continues into the postgraduate years. Teaching and training in human sexuality should become more fully incorporated into both undergraduate and postgraduate medical education.

References

Aizenberg D, Sigler M, Zemishlang Z et al (1996) Lithium and male sexual function in affective patients, *Clin Neuropharmacol* **19:**515–19.

Althof SE, Levine SB, Corty W et al (1995) A double-blind crossover trial of clomipramine for rapid ejaculation in 15 couples, *J Clin Psychiatry* **56:**402–7.

Ari G, Vardi Y, Hoffman A et al (1996) Possible role for endothelins in penile erection, *Eur J Pharmacol* **307:**69–74.

Baier D, Philipp M (1994) Effects of antidepressants on sexual function, *Fortschr Neurol Psychiatry* **62:**14–21.

Baldwin DS (1995) Psychotropic drugs and sexual dysfunction, *Int Rev Psychiatry* **7:**261–73.

Baldwin DS (1996) Depression and sexual function, *J Psychopharmacol* **10**(suppl 1):30–4.

Baldwin DS, Thomas SC (1996) *Depression and Sexual Function* (Martin Dunitz Ltd: London).

Balon R, Yeragani VK, Pohl R, Ramesh C (1993) Sexual dysfunction during antidepressant treatment, *J Clin Psychiatry* **54:**209–12.

Bancroft (1989) *Human Sexuality and its Problems*, 2nd edn (Churchill Livingstone: Edinburgh).

Bolden-Watson C, Richerson E (1993) Blockade by newly developed antidepressants of biogenic amine uptake into rat brain synaptosomes, *Life Sci* **52:**1023–9.

Bradford J (1995) An open pilot study of sertraline in the treatment of outpatients with pedophilia. Poster presented at the 148th annual meeting of the American Psychiatric Association, Miami, Florida, USA, 20–25 May.

Briley M, Prost JF, Moret C (1996) Preclinical pharmacology of milnacipran, *Int Clin Psychopharmacol* **11**(suppl 4): 9–14.

Cunningham LA, Borison RL, Carman JS et al (1994) A comparison of venlafaxine, trazodone and placebo in major depression, *J Clin Psychopharmacol* **14:**99–106.

de Boer T (1995) The effects of mirtazapine on central noradrenergic and serotonergic neurotransmission, *Int Clin Psychopharmacol* **10**(suppl 4): 19–23.

Dunsmuir WD, Emberton M (1997) Surgery, drugs and the male orgasm, *Br Med J* **314:**319–20.

Eison AS, Eison MS, Torrente JR et al (1990) Nefazodone: preclinical pharmacology of a new antidepressant, *Psychopharmacology (Berl)* **26:** 311–15.

Fabre LF, Abuzzahab FS, Amin M et al (1995) Sertraline safety and efficacy in major depression: a double-blind fixed-dose comparison with placebo, *Biol Psychiatry* **38:**592–602.

Fagan PJ, Schmidt CW Jr, Wise TN et al (1988) Sexual dysfunction and dual psychiatric diagnoses, *Comp Psychiatry* **29:**278–84.

Feder R (1991) Reversal of antidepressant activity of fluoxetine by cyproheptadine in three patients, *J Clin Psychiatry* **52:**163.

Feiger A, Kiev A, Shrivastava R et al (1996) Nefazodone versus sertraline in outpatients with major depression: focus on efficacy, tolerability, and effects on sexual function and satisfaction, *J Clin Psychiatry* **57**(suppl): 53–62.

Ferguson JM, Shrivastava R, Stahl SM et al (1995) Effects of double-blind treatment with nefazodone or sertraline on re-emergence of sexual dysfunction in patients with major depressive disorder. Presented at American College on Neuropsychopharmacology, San Juan, Puerto Rico, December.

Finkel MS, Laghrissi-Thode F, Pollock BG et al (1996) Paroxetine is a novel nitric oxide synthetase inhibitor, *Psychopharmacol Bull* **32:**653–8.

Fuller RW, Perry KW (1989) Effects of buspirone and its metabolite on brain monoamines and their metabolites in rats, *J Pharmacol Exp Ther* **248:** 50–56.

Gardner EA, Johnston JA (1985) Bupropion: an antidepressant without sexual pathophysiological action, *J Clin Psychopharmacol* **5:**24–9.

Gitlin MJ (1994) Psychotropic medications and their effects on sexual function: diagnosis, biology and treatment approaches, *J Clin Psychiatry* **5:** 406–13.

Harrison WM, Rabkin JG, Ehrhardt AA et al (1986) Effects of antidepressant medication on sexual function: a controlled study, *J Clin Psychopharmacol* **6:**144–9.

Herman JB, Brotman AW, Pollack E et al (1990) Fluoxetine-induced sexual dysfunction, *J Clin Psychiatry* **51:**25–7.

Hollander ER, Mullen LS, Carrasco JL et al (1992) Symptom relapse in bulimia nervosa and obsessive compulsive disorders after treatment with serotonin antagonists, *J Clin Psychiatry* **53:**207–9.

Hsu JH, Shen WW (1995) Male sexual side effects associated with antidepressants: a descriptive study of 32 patients, *Int J Psychiatry Med* **25:** 191–201.

Jacobsen FM (1992) Fluoxetine-induced sexual dysfunction and an open trial of yohimbine, *J Clin Psychiatry* **53:**119–22.

Kafka MP (1994) Sertraline therapy pharmacotherapy for paraphilias and paraphilia-related disorders: an open trial, *Ann Clin Psychiatry* **6:**139–45.

Kennedy JH, Ralevski E, Davis C, Neitzert C (1996) The effects of moclobemide on sexual desire and function in healthy volunteers, *Eur Neuropsychopharmacol* **6:**177–81.

Kilmann PR, Boland JP, Norton SP et al (1986) Perspectives of sex therapy outcome: a survey of AASECT providers, *J Sexual Marital Ther* **12:**116–38.

Kirby RS (1994) Impotence: diagnosis and management of male erectile dysfunction, *Br Med J* **308:**957–60.

Kivela S-L, Pahkala K (1988) Symptoms of depression in aged Finns, *Int J Social Psychiatry* **34:**274–84.

Kockott G, Pfeiffer W (1996) Sexual disorders in non-acute psychiatric outpatients, *Comp Psychiatry* **37:**56–61.

Kowalski A, Stanley RP, Dennerstein L et al (1985) The sexual side effects of antidepressant medication: a double-blind comparison of two antidepressants in a non-psychiatric population, *Br J Psychiatry* **147:**413–18.

Lane RM (1997) A critical review of selective serotonin re-uptake inhibitor-related sexual dysfunction: incidence, possible aetiology and implications for management, *J Psychopharmacol* **11:**72–82.

Marcus RN (1996) Safety and tolerability profile of nefazodone, *J Psychopharmacol* **10**(suppl):11–17.

Margolese HC, Assalian P (1996) Sexual side effcts of antidepresants: a review, *J Sexual Marital Ther* **22:** 209–17.

Matthew RJ, Weinman ML (1982) Sexual dysfunction in depression, *Arch Sexual Behav* **11:**323–8.

Medical Economics Data (1995) Paxil (paroxetine hydrochloride). In: *Physicians Desk Reference*, 49th edn (Medical Economics Data Production Company: Montvale, New Jersey) 2390–5.

Mellis MR, Argiolas A (1995) Nitric oxide donors induce penile erection and yawning when injected in the central nervous system of male rats, *Eur J Pharmacol* **294:**1–9.

Mendels J, Camera A, Sikes C (1995) Sertraline treatment for premature ejaculation, *Clin Psychopharmacol* **15:** 341–6.

Michael A, Owen A (1997) Venlafaxine-induced increased libido and spontaneous erections, *Br J Psychiatry* **170:**193.

Michael A, Ramana R (1996) Nefazodone-induced spontaneous ejaculation, *Br J Psychiatry* **169:**672–3.

Modell JG (1994) Repeated observations of yawning, clitoral engorgement and orgasm associated with fluoxetine treatment, *J Clin Psychopharmacol* **9:**63–5.

Monteiro WO, Norshirvani HF, Marks IM et al (1987) Anorgasmia from clomipramine in obsessive compulsive disorder: a controlled trial, *Br J Psychiatry* **151:**107–12.

Montgomery SA (1995) Safety of mirtazapine: a review, *Int Clin Psychopharmacol* **10**(suppl 4):37–45.

Montgomery JA, Prost JF, Solles A et al (1996) Efficacy and tolerability of minacipran: an overview, *Int Clin Psychopharmacol* **11**(suppl 4)47–51.

Nathan SG (1986) The epidemiology of DSM-III psychosexual dysfunctions, *J Sex Marital Ther* **12:**267–82.

Norden MJ (1995) Buspirone treatment of sexual dysfunction associated with selective serotonin re-uptake inhibitors, *Depression* **2:**109–12.

Olivera AA (1994) Sexual dysfunction due to clomipramine and sertraline: non-pharmacological resolution, *J Sex Educ Ther* **20:**119–22.

Ontiveros A, Valdes M, Costilla A (1996) Double-blind comparison of sexual dysfunction on imipramine and paroxetine. *Biol Psychiatry* **39:** 409.

Patterson WM (1993) Fluoxetine-induced sexual dysfunction, *J Clin Psychiatry* **54:**71.

Philipp M, Kohnen R, Benkert O (1993) A comparison study of moclobemide and doxepin in major depression with special reference to effects on sexual dysfunction, *Int Clin Psychopharmacol* **7:**123–32.

Post LL (1996) Sexual side effects of psychiatric medications in women, *Primary Psychiatry* **3:**47–51.

Poyurovsky M, Meerovich, Weizman A (1995) Beneficial effect of low-dose mianserin on fluvoxamine-induced

akathisia in an OCD patient, *Int Clin Psychopharmacol* **10:**11–114.

Robinson DS, Roberts DL, Smith JM et al (1996) The safety profile of nefazodone, *J Clin Psychiatry* **57**(suppl 2): 31–8.

Rothschild AJ (1995) Selective serotonin re-uptake inhibitor-induced sexual dysfunction: efficacy of a drug holiday, *Am J Psychiatry* **152:**514–16.

Schreiner-Engel P, Schiavi RC (1986) Lifetime psychopathology in individuals with low sexual desire, *J Nerv Ment Dis* **174:**646–51.

Schweizer E, Feighner J, Mandos LA et al (1994) Comparison of venlafaxine and imipramine in the acute treatment of major depression in out-patients, *J Clin Psychiatry* **55:**104–8.

Segraves RT (1989) Effect of psychotropic drugs on human erection and ejaculation, *Arch Gen Psychiatry* **46:**275–84.

Segraves RT (1993) Treatment-emergent sexual dysfunction in affective disorder: a review and management strategies, *J Clin Psychiatry* **11:**57–60.

Shahar E, Leder J, Herz MJ (1991) The use of a self-report questionnaire to assess the frequency of sexual dysfunction in family practice clinics, *Fam Practice* **8:**206–12.

Shen WW, Hsu JH (1995) Female sexual side effects associated with selective serotonin reuptake inhibitors: a descriptive clinical study of 33 patients. *Int J Psychiatry Med* **25:** 239–48.

Singh SP, Beck AJ (1997) 'No sex please, we're British.' Taking a sexual history from in-patients, *Psychiatr Bull* **21:**99–101.

Stark P, Hardison CD (1985) A review of multicenter controlled studies of fluoxetine versus imipramine and placebo in outpatients with major depressive disorder, *J Clin Psychiatry* **46:**53–8.

Swan M, Wilson MJ (1979) Sexual and marital problems in a psychiatric outpatient population, *Br J Psychiatry* **135:**310–14.

Thompson JW Jr, Ware MR, Blashfield RK (1990) Psychotropic medications and priapism: a comprehensive review, *J Clin Psychiatry* **51:**430–3.

Waldinger MD, Hengeveld MW, Zwinderman AH (1994) Paroxetine treatment of premature ejaculation: a double-blind, randomized, placebo controlled study, *Am J Psychiatry* **151:**1377–9.

Walker PW, Cole JO, Gardner EA et al (1993) Improvement in fluoxetine-associated sexual dysfunction in patients switched to bupropion, *J Clin Psychiatry* **54:**459–65.

Wilson CA (1993) Pharmacological targets for the control of male and female sexual behaviour. In: Riley A, Peet M, Wilson C, eds, *Sexual Pharmacology* (Oxford Medical Publications: Oxford) 1–58.

Zajecka J, Fawcett J, Schaff F et al (1991) The role of serotonin in sexual dysfunction: fluoxetine-associated orgasm dysfunction, *J Clin Psychiatry* **52:**66–8.

14

Non-pharmacological treatments for depression—focus on sleep deprivation and light therapy

Siegfried Kasper and Alexander Neumeister

Introduction

There are several pharmacological and non-pharmacological, though biologically based, treatment modalities for depression (Figure 14.1). Among the non-pharmacological treatments, electroconvulsive therapy (ECT) is used worldwide successfully with a refined methodology and specific treatment indications (American Psychiatric Association, 1990; Tauscher et al, 1997). Therapeutic sleep deprivation (SD), on the other hand, is mainly used in Germany and, with a few exceptions, primarily for research purposes, also in the USA. The therapeutic properties, as well as the proposed mechanisms underlying SD, have been recently summarized (Kasper and Möller, 1996). The effect of light therapy (LT) has been initiated and thoroughly studied by the group of Rosenthal (Rosenthal et al, 1984), and LT is now considered to be the standard treatment for seasonal affective disorder (SAD) and its subsyndromal form (Kasper et al, 1989a). In an effort to overcome the difficult procedure of ECT (e.g. anaesthesia) and to specifically stimulate brain areas which are thought

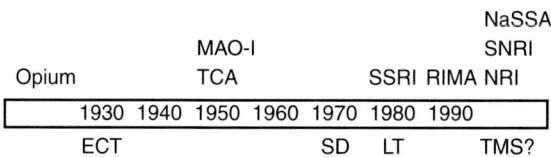

					NaSSA	
		MAO-I			SNRI	
Opium		TCA		SSRI	RIMA	NRI
1930	1940	1950	1960	1970	1980	1990
ECT			SD	LT		TMS?

Figure 14.1

Different pharmacological and non-pharmacological, though biologically based, therapies in depression. ECT, electroconvulsive treatment; SD, sleep deprivation; LT, light therapy TMS, transcranial magnetic stimulation; MAO-I, inhibitors of monoamine oxidase; TCA, tricyclic antidepressants; SSRI, selective serotonin reuptake inhibitors; NaSSA, noradrenaline serotonin specific antidepressant; SNRI, serotonin noradrenaline reuptake inhibitor; NRI, noradrenaline reuptake inhibitor; RIMA, reversible inhibitor of monoamine oxidase A.

to be responsible for regulating mood, we first set out to study the clinical usefulness of transcranial magnetic stimulation (TMS) (Höflich et al, 1993; Kolbinger et al, 1995). However, until now the different parameters necessary for clinical usefulness have not been settled (Puri and Lewis, 1996).

In this chapter the focus will be on the effects and possible psychophysiological explanations of SD and LT. Both treatment modalities have been extensively studied by our group, and we think that they are both clinically useful and serve as a model for state-dependent changes for biological research in depression.

Therapeutic sleep deprivation

Sleep deprivation as a treatment for depression

The beneficial effects of therapeutic SD in depression were initially described in 1966 by the German psychiatrist Schulte (1969) and then systematically studied by his associates Pflug and Tölle (1971). Up to now there have been over 1200 cases of therapeutic SD reported in the literature (Kuhs and Tölle, 1986; Wehr, 1990; Wu and Bunney, 1990). The different methods of SD are outlined in Table 14.1. For total sleep deprivation (TSD), patients are asked to stay awake for up to 40 h, starting from the morning before the night of SD until the evening after the deprivation night. For partial sleep deprivation (PSD) in the second half of the night, patients are asked to wake up at 1 AM or 2 AM and stay awake for the rest of the night and for all the following day. For PSD, patients may sleep for 4 h before they are awakened. In contrast to the beneficial effects of PSD of the second half of the night, controlled studies indicate that PSD in the first half of the night has little antidepressant efficacy (Sack et al, 1988).

Depression has also been treated by changing the timing of sleep using a phase advance paradigm (Sack et al, 1985; Berger et al, 1995). Phase advance of the sleep–wake cycle can be viewed as waking patients in the second half of the night, without depriving them of sleep (patients are asked to go to bed at 6 PM and get up at 1 AM). Sack et al (1985) have demonstrated that the antidepressant effect occurs after a few days and that there may not be a relapse if patients are shifted back to a normal sleep–wake cycle after 2 weeks. From a theoreti-

Table 14.1   Different forms of sleep deprivation therapies.

Total sleep deprivation (for the whole night)
Partial sleep deprivation (second half of the night)
Phase advance therapy
Selective REM sleep deprivation

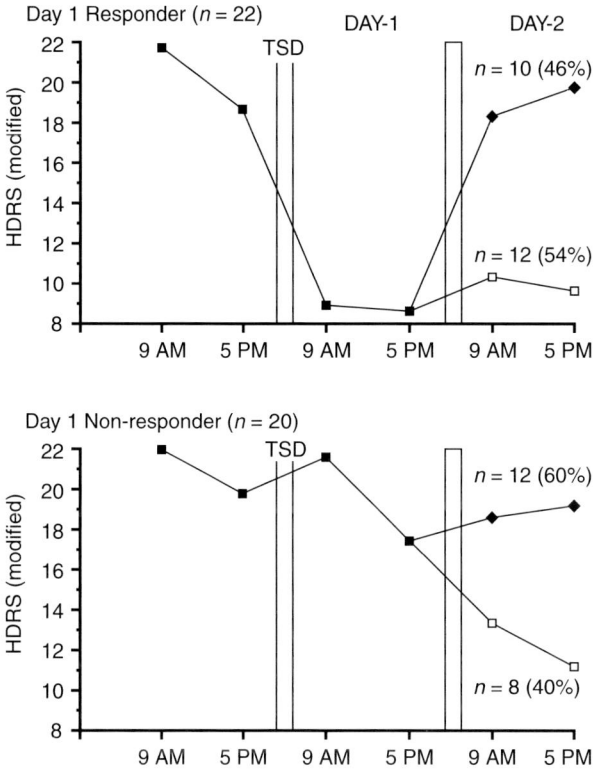

Figure 14.2

Psychopathological changes after total sleep deprivation (TSD) in 42 patients with major depression. Twenty-two patients (53%) have been classified as day 1 responders and 20 patients (47%) as day 1 non-responders. It is apparent that on the second day after TSD there are still patients who respond to TSD, regardless of whether they responded on the first day after TSD or not. Vertical rectangular boxes indicate the night of TSD (left) and the night when patients slept again (recovery night) (right). HDRS (modified): Hamilton Rating Scale for Depression without items 4, 5, 6, 16, 18. Data from Kasper et al (1990c).

cal perspective, it is interesting that a selective reduction of REM sleep has also been reported to have antidepressant properties (Vogel et al, 1980).

On the first day after SD (day 1 response) there is an improvement of depression in about 50–60% of major depressed patients (Kuhs and Tölle, 1986; Wehr, 1990). However, this rapid and dramatic antidepressive response is often reversed by recovery sleep, i.e. when patients sleep again in the night after the SD night (see Figure 14.2). The psychopathological course during TSD is exemplified by data obtained in 42 major depressed inpatients which have been described by our group elsewhere (Kasper et al, 1990c). In this sample of patients, 22 patients (52%) have been classified as day 1 responders, and from this group

Table 14.2   Response to SD and antidepressive medication.

Medication status	Total sleep deprivation		Partial sleep deprivation	
	N	% Response	N	% Response
Drug-free ≥2 weeks	99	56.6	53	56.7
Drug free <2 weeks	456	62.1	36	50.0
On drug	318	51.0	94	61.7
Total	873	56.6	183	56.1

Summary of studies published in detail in Wehr (1990)

approximately half of the patients relapsed on the second day. Researchers and clinicians should be aware that a subgroup of day 1 responders (28% of the total group) also remained well on the second day after SD. Furthermore, an improvement on day 2 (day 2 responders) has been observed in the group of patients who did not respond on the first day (19% of the total group).

Table 14.2 summarizes the day 1 response to TSD and PSD in relation to the concomitant use of antidepressive medication. The results indicate that for the acute antidepressant effect of SD, the type of medication that patients receive does not influence response. For practical reasons we recommend against giving sedating antidepressants during the SD night in order to facilitate the patients staying awake. However, the type of medication plays a role in preventing the relapse after the recovery night, since a number of studies indicate that antidepressants with a serotonergic mechanism of action, like clomipramine (Loosen et al, 1976) or fluvoxamine (Kasper et al, 1990a), but also lithium (Baxter et al, 1986) or LT (Neumeister et al, 1996) are capable of preventing the relapse, at least partly. Interestingly, for both lithium and LT, a serotonergic mechanism of action has been discussed (Kasper et al, 1996).

The following clinical variables have been associated with a favourable outcome of SD in depressed patients (Kuhs and Tölle, 1986): diurnal variation, severity of depression, and psychotic features. The response to SD has also been studied in different diagnostic groups, and good responses have been documented whenever a depressive symptomatology was prevalent, regardless of diagnosis. For example, there are a few studies that indicate that SD is effective for treatment of depressive symptomatology in schizophrenia (Fähndrich, 1982; Wehr, 1990) or Parkinson's disease (Bertolucci et al, 1987). There is one study that documents this therapeutic effect for premenstrual syndrome (Parry and Wehr, 1987). No improvement after SD was found for obsessive-compulsive disorder (OCD) or panic disorder, and, in fact, SD may aggravate panic disorder (Roy Burne et al, 1986).

Worsening of depression after recovery sleep

Systematic studies have shown that patients whose depressions improve after SD often relapse after recovery sleep. Wiegand et al (1987) suggest that the occurrence of episodes of REM sleep may be an important factor in this depressogenic effect. Results of Berger et al (1991) which have been obtained in 58 SD responders indicate that, after a night of SD, afternoon naps were better tolerated than morning naps. In contrast to the findings of Wiegand et al (1987), the occurrence of REM sleep in the Berger et al (1991) study did not turn out to be correlated with relapses into depression. The authors discuss their findings in connection with a two-process model of sleep regulation (Borbély, 1982) and a choliner-gic–aminergic interaction model of REM sleep regulation. Since trypto-phan depletion was not capable of inducing a relapse into depression in SD responders, it seems unlikely that short-term availability of serotonin is necessary for the maintenance of the antidepressant response (Neumeister et al, 1997b). Changes in receptor function could be responsible for the immediate psychopathological changes induced by SD.

Sleep deprivation and mania/hypomania

Like other antidepressant treatment modalities, SD appears to be capable of inducing mania or hypomania. In reviewing the literature, it is apparent that most SD studies report on the antidepressant effects of SD, but neglect to address the hypomanic/manic side effects of SD. Among the 11 reports in the literature in which mania or hypomania was apparent after SD, there is just one investigation (Wehr et al, 1982) in which mania ratings or criteria for mania/hypomania were included prospectively (Table 14.3). Based on these reports, there is some evidence that

Table 14.3   Studies reporting mania/hypomania after sleep deprivation.

Authors	Number	Mania	Hypomania
Pflug (1972)	12	1 (8%)	ND
Banji and Roy (1975)	2	0	1
Svendson (1976)	17	0	ND
Post et al (1976)	9	0	1 (11%)
Wirz-Justice et al (1975)	7	0	2 (29%)
Cole and Müller (1976)	3	1 (33%)	ND
Yamaguchi et al (1978)	7	1 (14%)	ND
Vovin et al (1982)	7	1 (14%)	ND
Wehr et al (1982)	12	4 (33%)	5 (42%)
Dessauer et al (1985)	4	1 (25%)	1 (25%)
Kasper et al (1992b)	93	0	14 (15%)
Total	173	9 (5%)	24 (14%)

ND, not determined.

switches into mania occur after SD, but switches into hypomania are more common. In a group of rapid-cycling bipolar patients studied by Wehr et al (1982), mania/hypomania was a frequent side effect of this procedure. For this group of patients, the authors report that in over two-thirds of the cases mania/hypomania was induced by SD, and lasted between 1 and 50 days (mean 7 days). The authors also note that mania/hypomania could usually be reproduced in the same patient if SD was repeated. There is a lack of prospective data concerning the occurrence of mania/hypomania after PSD, selective REM SD and phase advance of sleep. The experiences of the NIMH group indicate that bipolar patients may become manic or hypomanic after a phase advance of the sleep period (Wehr, 1990). The data of Kasper et al (1992b) obtained in a sample of predominantly unipolar depressed patients (78 unipolar, 15 bipolar) indicate that in 14% of the patients hypomania symptoms may occur. From a long-term therapeutic perspective, the induction of mania/hypomania after SD in a patient previously viewed as having unipolar depression may also help the clinician to better understand the diagnosis of the patient. SD may therefore be able to unmask a bipolar component and guide the clinician to use prophylactic lithium, carbamazepine or valproic acid in the patient in addition to antidepressants.

Mechanism of action of therapeutic sleep deprivation

Various attempts have been made to understand the antidepressant properties of SD (Table 14.4) but there is still a lack of knowledge on the underlying mechanism of action. From a theoretical perspective, SD appeals to researchers because the effects on depression are immediate and not confounded by drug effects. SD can therefore be viewed as a

Table 14.4   Proposed mechanism of action of SD.

Placebo effect (intensive care)
Psychological effect ('self-punishment')

Non-specific stress

Increased hypothalamic–pituitary activity
Changes in monoaminergic activity

Resynchronization of biological rhythms
Prevention of sleep during 'critical phase'
Phase advance hypothesis

Sleep-released depressogenic substance

Antidepressive substance released during wakefulness

Prevention of 'depressogenic' REM

Prevention of 'relative hyperthermia'

useful model for studying state-dependent changes, and its effects may yield important information about the pathophysiology of depression.

Among the theories that have been advanced to explain the antidepressant mechanism of SD, it is generally believed that psychological mechanisms can be ruled out (Buddeberg and Dittrich, 1981), including the assumption that intensive care leads to the beneficial effects of SD, or a more psychodynamic perspective that the deprivation of sleep is a most welcome punishment for depressive patients who have feelings of guilt and desire to be punished due to their strong super-ego. Some approaches focus on chronobiological considerations (Wehr and Wirz-Justice, 1981; Borbély and Wirz-Justice, 1982). Although there is no evidence that biological rhythms are resynchronized by SD (Gerner et al, 1979), it does seem to be of importance that patients are awake during a critical phase of the night (Wehr and Wirz-Justice, 1981), e.g. the second half of the night. Wu and Bunney (1990) have presented a theory that depressogenic substances are released during sleep, a process that is avoided with SD. However, we do not have biochemical or direct experimental evidence to support this theory. Vogel et al (1980) hypothesized that suppression of REM sleep was the therapeutic mechanism of antidepressant drugs and SD. This theory is supported by the findings of Wiegand et al (1987), who reported that, following SD, the presence of REM sleep in short naps tended to be associated with relapses, a result that could not, however, be replicated by the same group in a recent study that included a larger number of patients (Berger et al, 1991). In their hypothesis about the therapeutic mechanism of sleep deprivation, Borbély and Wirz-Justice (1982) focus on a process related to slow-wave sleep. Different investigators have attempted to relate changes in hormonal and neurotransmitter patterns to the antidepressant effect of SD (Yamaguchi et al, 1978; Gerner et al, 1979; Kasper et al, 1988a,b; Baumgartner et al, 1990). For example, an increase in hypothalamic–pituitary–thyroid activity has been reported to be associated with clinical response (Baumgartner et al, 1990; Wehr, 1990).

A new theory which includes the regulation of body temperature in depression and its interaction with SD has been proposed by Wehr (1990). There is a physiological drop in body temperature during the night in healthy controls as well as in depressed patients. Compared with healthy controls and recovered depressed patients, acutely depressed patients have elevated nocturnal body temperature. During SD, body temperature is higher than during sleep, but the temperature controller responds as though the body were cooler because its set point is higher (Satinoff and Hendersen, 1977; Bligh, 1979). SD therefore prevents the relative hyperthermia that is associated with sleep onset. Thus, SD can be viewed as a type of relative heat deprivation. The results of a study in which patients were sleep deprived on two occasions, once in an ambient temperature of 18°C, and once in an ambient temperature of 33°C, indicate that a better response of SD can be achieved in the cold environment (Kasper et al, 1989c). These results suggest that many of the observations on the effects of sleep–wake manipulations in affective illness might be understood within the framework of thermoregulatory physiology. These results also raise the possibility that heating and cooling manoeuvres might be used to treat or prevent episodes of affective illness. These approaches were, at least partially, known to psychiatrists at the turn of the century (Ross et al, 1988) (e.g. wet sheet packs and cold baths) and can now be studied with new technologies and a better understanding of the underlying physiology of manic–depressive illness.

Light therapy

LT has become increasingly popular in various countries around the world in the last decade. For instance, according to a survey carried out in Germany in 1992, 13% ($n = 56$) of all German psychiatric hospitals ($n = 422$) used LT for different treatment indications and another 8% indicated their interest in doing so (Kasper et al, 1994a). Among university facilities, LT is even more popular, with a percentage of 57%. Although the most frequently used treatment indication for LT is SAD or its subsyndromal form (S-SAD), it is apparent that other forms of depression, e.g. non-seasonal forms, either acute or chronic, are also a target for this new treatment modality (see Table 14.5). A number of studies support the use of LT for SAD (review: Terman et al, 1989); however there are just a few studies on non-seasonal depression or the other treatment indications (review: Kasper et al, 1994b).

Table 14.5   Use of LT for different treatment indications in Germany (Kasper et al, 1994a).

Diagnosis	Usage	
	Percentage[a]/Number of hospitals	
SAD	86	48
Subsyndromal SAD	43	24
Depression, acute	49	27
Depression, chronic	57	32
Neurosis	18	10
Schizophrenia, negative symptoms	11	6
Premenstrual syndrome	7	4
Circadian rhythm disturbance	7	4
Other	9	5
All	56 hospitals	

[a] Relates to the number of hospitals which use LT in Germany (56 of 422).

Seasonal affective disorder

SAD is a variant of recurrent major depressive disorder or bipolar disorder and is characterized by the regular occurrence of depressive episodes at characteristic times of the year. In most cases the episodes being in autumn and winter and remit in the following spring and summer (Rosenthal et al, 1984; Kasper et al, 1989b). SAD patients typically fulfil for their longitudinal course the diagnostic criteria of the seasonal pattern specifier of the *Diagnostic and Statistical Manual of Mental Disorders*, 4th edn (DSM-IV) (American Psychiatric Association, 1994). Furthermore, the clinical syndrome is characterized, although not exclusively, by the presence of atypical symptoms, such as hypersomnia, hyperphagia, and carbohydrate craving with consecutive weight gain and fatigue. Although several studies have been carried out to gain insights into the pathophysiology of SAD, there remain numerous unanswered questions. There is some evidence that the neurotransmitter serotonin (5-HT) is involved in the pathogenesis of SAD and possibly also in the mechanism of action of LT (Kasper et al, 1996).

Light therapy in SAD patients

Since the first anecdotal observations and the first systematic study (Rosenthal et al, 1984), knowledge about LT for treatment of SAD and its subsyndromal form has increased rapidly (Blehar and Rosenthal, 1989). Numerous groups have documented robust antidepressant responses to bright artificial light in depressed patients with SAD (Terman et al, 1989). Whereas most observations obtained in uncontrolled settings would support the treatment of SAD patients for the whole 'dark season', there are hints in the literature that LT administered at the beginning of the winter season, when subjects are still free of symptoms, could be successful in preventing the development of SAD symptomatology during the rest of the season (Meesters et al, 1991; Partonen and Lönnqvist, 1996b). Anecdotally, the NIMH group has found that those relatively rare SAD patients afflicted with severe endogenous depression respond worst to LT. The antidepressant effect usually appears after 3 days, and when the lights are withdrawn, relapse into depression frequently takes at least a few days (Figure 14.3).

Light therapy in non-seasonal depression

Kantor (1983) suggested that LT might be a potential new treatment for a subgroup of depressed patients and not just limited to those with seasonal mood cycles. However, since then it has become apparent that the efficacy of LT is less impressive in non-seasonal depression than in SAD patients (see Table 14.6). One of the major drawbacks is that there are just

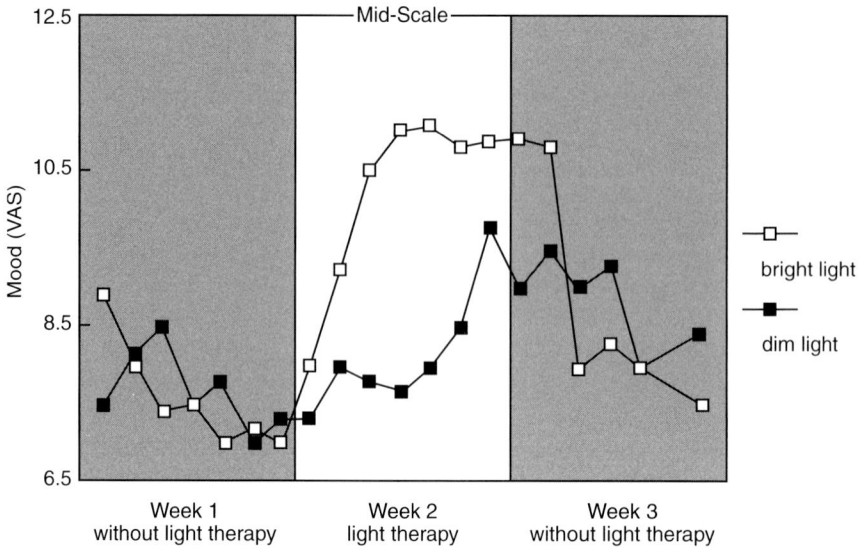

Figure 14.3

Characteristic course under LT with either bright (2500 lux) or dim (<300 lux) light in patients with SAD. VAS, visual analog scale.

a few studies in this area, most of them including only a small number of patients. With the exception of one study (Schuchardt and Kasper, 1997), all of them have been carried out over a short period of time (mostly 1 week). The results of these studies are therefore not directly comparable to those of pharmacological studies for non-seasonal depression.

Kripke et al (1983) studied the effects of LT in non-seasonal depression most extensively and reported encouraging results. In the first published report (Kripke et al, 1983), a positive antidepressant effect was achieved with 1 h of LT for 1 day. However, the patients received LT in early morning hours, so SD might have confounded these results. In the report of 1992, Kripke et al (1992) described the effects of LT with bright light in 25 drug-free hospitalized patients and compared its efficacy with 26 depressed patients who received a dim red light placebo control treatment (76% of the patients were treated with 3 h/day for 1 week in the evening hours, and 24% of patients with 1 h in the morning and 1 h in the evening). A global composite depression score showed a statistically significant ($p = 0.02$) difference, favouring bright white light treatment. Whereas the bright light group exhibited an 18% drop of the total score of the Hamilton Rating Scale for Depression (HDRS, 17-item version), there was just a 6% drop of these values in the dim light group. There was no difference in the therapeutic effect according to the time (evening or morning and evening) when treatment was applied. In addition, it was apparent that patients treated in summer responded as well as those treated in winter.

Table 14.6   Controlled studies for LT in non-seasonal depression.

Authors	Number	Duration of LT		Result
		Days	Hours per day	
Kripke et al (1983)	12	1	1	BL > DL
Kripke et al (1987)	14	5	1–2	BL (>) DL
Kripke et al (1989)[a]	12	5	2	BL = DL
Kripke et al (1989)[a]	26	7	3	BL > DL
Volz et al (1990)[b]	30	7	2	BL = DL
Stewart et al (1990)	8	14	4	BL no efficacy
Kasper et al (1990b)	7	7	2	BL = DL
Mackert et al (1991)	42	7	2	BL = DL
Kripke et al (1992)	51	7	3	BL > DL
Schuchardt and Kasper (1997)	30	28	2	BL + Med > DL + Med

LT, light therapy; BL, bright light (≥2500 lux); DL, dim light (<300 lux); Med, antidepressant medication.
[a] Patients of these reports are also included in Kripke et al (1992).
[b] Patients of this report are also included in Mackert et al (1991).

The report of Mackert et al (1991) summarizes the findings of 2 h of LT daily (morning) conducted over 1 week in 42 drug-free hospitalized non-seasonally depressed patients. There was a 22% decrease (from 19.5 ± 4.1 to 15.3 ± 5.0) of the HDRS total score (21-item version) in the bright light group and a 9% decrease (from 19.1 ± 4.2 to 17.3 ± 6.2) in the dim light group. This difference was not statistically significant but there was a significant reduction over time in both groups.

Schuchardt and Kasper (1997) studied 30 non-seasonal major depressed outpatients who were refractory to previous antidepressant treatment modalities. Over the period of 4 weeks, patients received either fluoxetine (20 mg) plus bright light (3000 lux) or fluoxetine (20 mg) plus dim light (<300 lux). After 1 week of treatment, there was a 10% decrease of HDRS total scores in both groups. Whereas there was a significant further decline in the bright light group, there was just a modest reduction in the dim light group. At the end of the 4-week trial, the bright light group exhibited a 53% decrease of HDRS total scores whereas there was just a 26% decrease in the dim light group. This is the first study in which the effects of LT have been evaluated over a period of 4 weeks in non-seasonal depressed patients, and it allows comparison of the results with those of psychopharmacological studies reported in the literature. The results of this study indicate that LT with bright light might be a valuable addition to pharmacotherapy in patients resistant to antidepressants alone. Since this study was conducted in a private practice setting, it also allows us to conclude that this form of treatment can be performed outside of research facilities. However, the mechanism of reimbursement by health insurance providers is still unclear and needs to be settled before a wide range of acceptance can be expected.

Light therapy as an addition to pharmacotherapy or sleep deprivation in non-SAD depression

Based on the published reports in the literature, it is apparent that there is only a modest response to LT in non-seasonal depression if LT is used as the only treatment modality. The question therefore arises of whether LT can be used as an adjunct to pharmacotherapy (Prasko, 1988; Prasko et al, 1988; Schuchardt and Kasper, 1997). The controlled study of Schuchardt and Kasper (1997) and the open study of Prasko et al (1987) indicate that there is an additive effect of LT and pharmacotherapy, as is the case for SD, one of the other non-pharmacological treatment modalities. However, there is a difference between these reports. Whereas the group of Prasko et al (1987) found that LT hastens the onset of action of antidepressants after 1 week, this effect was found in the studies of Schuchardt and Kasper (1997) and Levitt et al (1991) only after 2 weeks. It is our personal experience that the effects of LT have a slower onset of action in non-SAD patients compared with SAD patients, and a final judgement of whether LT is effective should not be made before 4 weeks. Neumeister et al (1996) showed recently that light therapy (4 h) administered in the morning and evening after PSD and continued for 1 week is capable of preventing the otherwise naturally occurring relapse after SD in non-SAD patients.

Further treatment indications for light therapy

Further treatment indications, besides non-seasonal depression, are summarized in Table 14.7. Among these treatment indications, the treatment of jet-lag is probably the best studied area. The psychophysiological problems after crossing time-zones can probably be explained by the observation that the human organism does not have a problem in prolonging the period of the circadian rhythm to a certain extent (as is the case, for instance, when travelling from Europe to North America). However, an advance of the circadian phase, as is the case with a flight from North America to Europe, can cause serious adjustment problems, since it shortens the circadian period considerably. In order to adjust for the desynchronization of internal and external rhythms, it is important that the light exposure does not fall within a part of the phase–response curve which would further shorten the phase (Daan and Lewy, 1984; Minors et al, 1991).

Shiftwork, which influences the circadian rhythm of physiological parameters, is, in vulnerable individuals, often accompanied by sleeping difficulties, daytime tiredness, low work efficiency, digestion problems and irritability. Researchers working in the field of shiftwork (e.g. Eastman, 1991) recommend, therefore, that specifically vulnerable individuals should shift their sleeping schedule before the new shift starts, e.g. by

Table 14.7 Treatment indications for bright light therapy as reported in the literature.

Non-seasonal depression
  Kripke et al (1983, 1987, 1989, 1992), Mackert et al (1991), Kasper et al (1990a), Schuchardt and Kasper (1997), Yerevanian et al (1986), Peter et al (1986), Fleischhauer et al (1988), Heim (1988), Prasko et al (1987, 1988), Prasko (1988), Levitt et al (1991)

Subsyndromal SAD
  Kasper et al (1989a)

Recurrent brief SAD
  Kasper et al (1992a)

Jet-lag syndrome
  Daan and Lewy (1984), Wever (1985), Czeisler and Allan (1987), Czeisler et al (1989), Sasaki et al (1989)

Shiftwork
  Eastman (1986, 1989, 1991), Powers et al (1989), Czeisler et al (1990); Campbell and Dawson (1992)

Delayed-sleep-phase syndrome
  Joseph-Vanderpool et al (1989), Rosenthal et al (1990)

Premenstrual syndrome
  Parry et al (1987, 1989)

Depression, 'negative symptoms' within schizophrenia
  Heim (1990), Kasper et al (1990a)

OCD seasonal
  Höflich et al (1992)

Alcohol withdrawal syndrome
  Dietzel et al (1986)

Bulimia
  Lam et al (personal communication)

Postpartum blues
  Unpublished observation

2 h every day. This regimen can be supported by bright light exposure during the working hours of the new time schedule. However, in the hours after a night shift the eyes should be protected from bright light, e.g. by wearing sunglasses (Eastman, 1994). It has been shown that this regimen works in research conditions (Eastman, 1991). However, in everyday life it may not be practical.

Patients with a delayed-sleep-phase syndrome usually go to bed between 2 and 6 o'clock in the morning and experience trouble when they are forced to start working in the morning, which is an unphysiological time for these individuals (Weitzman et al, 1981). First results indicate that LT in the morning hours, after waking up, might be of therapeutic value (Rosenthal et al, 1990).

There are two reports on the effects of LT in patients with schizophrenia and concomitant depressive or so-called 'negative' symptomatology (Heim, 1990; Kasper et al, 1990a). In the report of Heim (1990), 20 medicated schizophrenic patients were studied and there was a good response after 5 days (2 h daily) of LT. We studied three schizophrenic patients (two with neuroleptics, one without medication) who were currently depressed and/or exhibited negative symptoms. The diagnosis of schizophrenia was established during a previous phase when patients exhibited positive symptoms. None of the patients suffered from positive symptoms at the time when we initiated LT. In these patients it was apparent that the depressive and/or 'negative' symptomatology was independent of schizophrenic symptoms and that it was recurrent in autumn/winter. One patient previously suffering from a schizophrenic episode was without medication and was treated with LT (2 h daily, 1 week). In this patient it is apparent that there was a reduction of negative symptoms (apathic syndrome) without exacerbation of positive symptoms. The other two patients, who were on stable neuroleptic medication, also exhibited a favourable outcome with LT. These observations warrant further controlled studies.

Another, as yet not thoroughly studied, treatment indication for LT is premenstrual syndrome. Parry et al (1989) found good therapeutic efficacy for this syndrome when patients were exposed to LT in the evening hours. Dietzel et al (1986) reported that the addition of LT to conventional psychotropic drugs helps to reduce the amount of the necessary medication in alcohol withdrawal syndrome.

The role of serotonin in the pathophysiology of SAD and light therapy

Besides the annual reoccurrence of depressive episodes in SAD, it has emerged that SAD patients have a characteristic psychopathological profile, with a predominance of atypical symptoms. Many of the neurovegetative functions, which seem to be disturbed in SAD, have been shown to have an important relationship with the 5-HT system. Serotonergic mechanisms seem to be involved in the regulation of appetite and weight (Rosenthal et al, 1987). It has been discussed in the literature whether the frequently reported high carbohydrate intake of SAD patients during autumn/winter represents a behavioural–biochemical feedback loop for raising the available 5-HT content (Fernstrom, 1977). More evidence that 5-HT might be involved in the pathophysiology of SAD is derived from the finding that seasonal fluctuations occur in the 5-HT system of healthy subjects as well as of depressed patients (Carlsson et al, 1980; Egrise et al, 1986; Klompenhouwer et al, 1990). These findings suggest that the serotonergic system is responsive to seasonal changes and that this physiological variation may turn into a pathological variant.

The behavioural responses to the administration of the serotonergic agent *m*-chlorophenylpiperazine (m-CPP) before and after LT imply that SAD patients may have an underlying dysregulation within the 5-HT system which is influenced by LT (Jacobsen et al, 1989; 1994). Before the beginning of LT, the depressed SAD patients reported feelings of euphoria after the intravenous application of m-CPP, whereas healthy controls did not. After exposure to bright light, which induced a remission of the depressive syndrome, the patients' subjective responses no longer differed from those of the normal controls. This finding can be interpreted as showing that LT may result in changes in serotonergic function which are associated with a remission of the depressive syndrome. Hormonal challenge tests with serotonergic agents resulted in blunted responses in SAD patients (Jacobsen et al, 1989; Coiro et al, 1993). These data are consistent with a decrease of central serotonergic activity in SAD patients which is influenced by LT.

The assumption that a dysfunction of the brain serotonergic function might be one aetiological factor in the pathophysiology of SAD is indirectly supported by the preferential efficacy of serotonergic compounds in the psychopharmacological treatment of SAD patients (Kasper et al, 1996). The only study to exhibit a SSRI/placebo difference is the one of Blashko et al (1997), using 50–150 mg (mean 111 mg daily) sertraline. Fluoxetine (Ruhrmann et al, 1993) and citalopram (Wirz-Justice et al, 1992) are also probably effective in SAD. However, a significant difference to placebo has not been demonstrated, as yet, for these compounds. It has been shown that these compounds not only reduce the depression ratings of the patients but also decrease the subjects' calorie and nutrient intakes, which are typically enhanced during the depressive episodes. Therefore, serotonergic drugs, especially selective serotonin reuptake inhibitors (SSRIs), which might have a greater 5-HT neurotransmitter specificity as compared to other drugs, e.g. tricyclics, seem to be especially efficient in the treatment of SAD patients, since their depression is frequently associated with weight gain. The antidepressants used until now for SAD are summarized in Table 14.8.

Exacerbation of depressive symptoms in LT-induced remission from depression after short-term tryptophan depletion

Because all the evidence for a 5-HT dysregulation in SAD which might be normalized by the use of LT is indirect, the effects of lowering brain 5-HT function were studied in a more direct manner (Lam et al, 1995; Neumeister et al, 1997a). Tryptophan depletion, as described by Young et al (1985), provides a tool for investigating 5-HT mechanisms in the pathophysiology of affective disorder and its treatment (Delgado et al, 1990, 1994; Miller et al, 1992). Using a double-blind placebo-controlled balanced crossover design, we therefore assessed whether short-term

Table 14.8   Antidepressant medication in patients with SAD.

Author	No. of patients	Antidepressants
Open studies		
O'Rourke et al (1989)	N = 7	d-Fenfluramine
Jacobsen et al (1989)	N = 3	Fluoxetine, Trazodone
McGrath et al (1990)	N = 9	L-Tryptophan
Dilsaver et al (1990)	N = 47	Bupropion, desipramine, tranylcypromine
Dilsaver and Jaeckle (1990)	N = 14	Tranylcypromine
Teicher and Glod (1990)	N = 6	Alprazolam
Wirz-Justice et al (1992)	N = 1	Citalopram
Lingjaerde and Haggag (1992)	N = 5	Moclobemide
Heßelmann et al (1997)	N = 8	Mirtazapine
Controlled studies		
Ruhrmann et al (1993)	N = 40	Fluoxetine versus bright light
Martinez et al (1994)	N = 20	Hypericine ± bright light
Partonen and Lönnqvist (1996a)	N = 32	Fluoxetine versus moclobemide
Placebo-controlled studies		
Lingjaerde et al (1993)	N = 34	Moclobemide versus placebo
Lam et al (1995)	N = 78	Fluoxetine versus placebo
Blashko et al (1997)	N = 187	Sertraline versus placebo
Schlager (1994)	N = 23	Propranolol versus placebo
Oren et al (1994)	N = 25	Levodopa + carbidopa versus placebo

depletion of the essential amino acid tryptophan, the precursor of 5-HT, leads to a depressive relapse in drug-free SAD patients who had previously responded to LT. Before entering the study period, the patients were remitted for at least 2 weeks. Twelve patients were given a 24-h, 160 mg/day, low-tryptophan diet, followed the next morning by a 15-amino acid drink (tryptophan depletion); in the control testing, the patients received a 16-amino acid drink containing 2.3 g tryptophan.

The patients experienced a depressive relapse after the tryptophan-free amino acid drink, which was apparent 7 h after ingestion of the drink and was more pronounced on the following day. Control testing did not produce any significant behavioural effects. These findings seem to be indicative that short-term availability of 5-HT is a necessary condition for the antidepressant efficacy of LT. Additionally, our results support the hypothesis that serotonergic dysfunction may be involved in the pathophysiology of SAD and that 5-HT may be intimately involved in the mechanism of action of bright light therapy. However, tryptophan depletion did not worsen depressive symptomatology in depressed SAD patients, which indicates that mechanisms other than serotonergic ones might also be involved in the pathophysiology of SAD (Neumeister et al, 1997c). Since a depressive symptomatology could also be triggered by tryptophan depletion in asymptomatic SAD patients in summer (e.g. free of symptoms for at least 4–5 months), this could be indicative of a trait phenomenon (Neumeister et al, 1997d).

Several lines of evidence suggest that a dysfunction of brain 5-HT function is involved in the pathophysiology of SAD and also in the mechanism of action of LT. However, it is obvious that a simple model of the pathobiology of SAD and the underlying mechanism of action of LT is inadequate and that other neurotransmitter systems (e.g. the noradrenergic system) are also likely to be involved. The current results from the literature and our own findings support the hypothesis that disturbances in the brain 5-HT function contribute to the pathophysiology of SAD as a state and also a trait marker, and that the short-term availability of 5-HT is an important factor for the maintenance of the antidepressant effects of LT.

Conclusion

Non-pharmacological treatments for depression, like ECT, SD, LT and possibly also TMS, are powerful. Additionally, SD and LT can also be used as a model for state-dependent changes, since psychopathological alterations during these treatment procedures are not confounded by drug effects. These treatments therefore enable the direct interpretation of psychopathological changes according to a proposed mechanism of action. Since both SD and LT, but especially SD, are characterized by a fast antidepressant onset, their mechanism of action can help pharmacological developmental plans to characterize a profile which share with SD a rapid antidepressant onset. Furthermore, SD and LT can be used as the only treatment, but also in combination with antidepressant medication, exerting additive therapeutic properties. Therefore, besides their interesting possibilities for basic research, a large therapeutic potential exists for both treatment modalities, which warrants their recognition by researchers and therapists in everyday practice.

References

American Psychiatric Association (1990) *The Practice of Electroconvulsive Therapy: Recommendations for Treatment, Training and Privileging. A Task Force Report* (American Psychiatric Association: Washington DC).

American Psychiatric Association (1994) *Diagnostic and Statistical Manual of Mental Disorders*, 4th edn (American Psychiatric Association: Washington DC).

Banji S, Roy GA (1975) The treatment of psychotic depression by sleep deprivation. A replication study, *Br J Psychiatry* **127:**222–6.

Baumgartner A, Riemann D, Berger M (1990) Neuroendocrinological investigations during sleep deprivation in depression. II. Longitudinal measurement of thyrotropin, TH, cortisol, prolactin, GH, and LH during sleep and sleep deprivation, *Biol Psychiatry* **28:**569–87.

Baxter LR, Liston EH, Schwartz JM et al (1986) Prolongation of the antidepressant response to partial sleep deprivation by lithium, *Psychiatry Res* **19:**17–23.

Berger M, Riemann D, Wiegand M (1991) Pathogenetic considerations on the antidepressive effect of sleep deprivation and the depressiogenic effects of naps. In: *Proceedings of the 5th World Congress of Biological Psychiatry*, Florence, 9–14 June.

Berger M, Vollmann J, Hohagen F, König A, Lohner H, Riemann D (1995) Treating depression with sleep deprivation and consecutive sleep phase advance therapy, *Acta Neuropsychiat* **7**(2):50–1.

Bertolucci PHF, Andrade LAF, Lima JGC, Carlini EA (1987) Total sleep deprivation and parkinson disease, *Arq Neuropsyquiatr* **45:**224–30.

Blashko CA, Moscovitch A, Eagles JM, Darcourt G, Thompson C, Kasper S (1997) A placebo-controlled study of sertraline in the treatment of outpatients with seasonal affective disorder, *Arch Gen Psychiatry* (submitted).

Blehar MC, Rosenthal NE (1989) Seasonal affective disorders and phototherapy. Report of a National Institute of Mental Health-sponsored workshop, *Arch Gen Psychiatry* **46:** 469–74.

Bligh J (1979) The central neurology of mammalian thermoregulation, *Neuroscience* **4:**1213–36.

Borbély AA (1982) A two process model of sleep regulation, *Hum Neurobiol* **1:**195–204.

Borbély AA, Wirz-Justice A (1982) Sleep, sleep deprivation, and depression, *Hum Neurobiol* **1:**205–10.

Buddeberg CA, Dittrich A (1981) Psychologische Aspekte des Schlafentzugs, *Arch Psychiatr Nervenkr* **225:**249–61.

Campbell SS, Dawson WA (1992) Bright light effects on human sleep and alertness during simulated night shift work. In: Holick MF, Kligman AM, eds, *Biologic Effects of Light* (de Gruyter: Berlin, New York) 188–95.

Carlsson A, Svennerholm L, Winblad B (1980) Seasonal and circadian monoamine variations in human brains examined post mortem, *Acta Psychiatr Scand* **61**(suppl 280):75–85.

Coiro V, Volpi R, Marchesi C et al (1993) Abnormal serotonergic control of prolactin and cortisol secretion in patients with seasonal affective disorder, *Psychoneuroendocrinology* **18:** 551–6.

Cole MG, Müller HF (1976) Sleep deprivation in treatment of elderly depressed patients, *J Am Geriat Soc* **24:**308–13.

Czeisler CA, Allan JS (1987) Acute circadian phase reversal in man via bright light exposure: application to jet lag, *Sleep Res* **18:**605.

Czeisler CA, Kronauer RE, Allan JS et al (1989) Bright light induction of strong (Type 0) resetting of the human circadian pacemaker, *Science* **244:**1328–33.

Czeisler CA, Johnson MP, Dufy JF, Brown EN, Ronda JM, Kronauer RE (1990) Exposure to bright light and darkness to treat physiologic maladaptation to night work, *N Engl J Med* **322:**1253–9.

Daan S, Lewy AJ (1984) Scheduled exposure to daylight: a potential strategy to reduce 'jet lag' following transmeridian flight, *Psychopharmacol Bull* **20:**566–8.

Delgado PL, Charney DS, Price LH, Aghajanian GK, Landis H, Heninger GR (1990) Serotonin function and the mechanism of antidepressant action. Reversal of antidepressant-induced remission by rapid depletion of plasma tryptophan, *Arch Gen Psychiatry* **47:**411–18.

Delgado PL, Price LH, Miller HL et al (1994) Serotonin and the neurobiology of depression. Effects of tryptophan depletion in drug-free depressed patients, *Arch Gen Psychiatry* **51:** 865–74.

Dessauer M, Goetze U, Tölle R (1985) Periodic sleep deprivation in drug-refractory depression, *Neuropsychobiology* **13:**111–16.

Dietzel A, Saletu B, Lesch OM, Sieghart W, Schjerve M (1986) Light treatment in depressive illness: polysomnographic, psychometric, and neuroendocrinological findings, *Eur Neurol* **25**(suppl 2):93–103.

Dilsaver SC, Jaeckle RS (1990) Winter depression responds to an open trial of tranylcypromine, *J Clin Psychiatry* **51:**326–9.

Dilsaver SC, Del Medico VJ, Quadri A, Jaeckle RS (1990) Pharmacological responsiveness of winter depression, *Psychopharmacol Bull* **26:**303–9.

Eastman CJ (1986) Bright light improves the entrainment of the circadian rhythm of body temperature to a 26-hr sleep–wake schedule in humans, *Sleep Res* **15:**271.

Eastman CJ (1989) Circadian rhythms during gradually advancing and delaying bright light and sleep schedules, *Sleep Res* **18:**418.

Eastman CJ (1991) Squashing vs. nudging circadian rhythms with artificial bright light: solutions for shift work? *Perspect Biol Med* **34:**181–95.

Egrise D, Rubinstein M, Schoutens A, Cantraine F, Mendlewicz J (1986) Seasonal variation of platelet serotonin uptake and 3H-imipramine binding in normal and depressed subjects, *Biol Psychiatry* **21:**283–92.

Fähndrich E (1982) Schlafentzugstherapie depressiver Syndrome bei schizophrener Grunderkrankung, *Nervenarzt* **53:**279–85.

Fernstrom JD (1977) Effects of the diet on brain neurotransmitters, *Metabolism* **26:**207–23.

Fleischhauer J, Glauser G, Hofstetter P (1988) The influence of light therapy in depressive patients, *Pharmacopsychiatry* **21:**414–15.

Gerner RO, Post RM, Gillin JC, Bunney WE (1979) Biological and behavioral effects of one night's sleep deprivation in depressed patients and normals, *J Psychiatr Res* **15:**21–40.

Heim M (1988) Effectiveness of bright light therapy in cyclothymic axis syndromes. A cross-over study in comparison with partial sleep deprivation, *Psychiatr Neurol Med Psychol* **40:** 269–77.

Heim M (1990) Bright-Light-Therapie bei schizophrenen Erkrankungen, *Psychiatr Neurol Med Psychol* **42:**146–50.

Heßelmann B, Habeler A, Praschak-Rieder N, Willeit M, Kasper S (1997) Mirtazapine in seasonal affective disorder (SAD)—a preliminary report, *Eur Neuropsychopharmacol* (in press).

Höflich G, Kasper S, Möller H-J (1992) Erfolgreiche Behandlung eines saisonalen Zwangs-syndroms mit Lichttherapie, *Nervenarzt* **63:**701–4.

Höflich G, Kasper S, Hufnagel A, Ruhrmann S, Möller HJ (1993) Application of transcranial magnetic stimulation for treatment of drug-resistant major depression—a report of two cases, *Hum Psychopharmacol* **8:** 361–5.

Jacobsen FM, Murphy DL, Rosenthal NE (1989) The role of serotonin in seasonal affective disorder and the antidepressant response to phototherapy. In: Rosenthal NE, Blehar MC, eds, *Seasonal Affective Disorder and Phototherapy* (Guilford Press: New York) 333–41.

Jacobsen FM, Mueller EA, Rosenthal NE, Rogers S, Hill JL, Murphy DL (1994) Behavioral responses to intravenous meta-chlorophenylpiperazine in patients with seasonal affective disorder and control subjects before and after phototherapy, *Psychiatry Res* **52:**181–97.

Joseph-Vanderpool JR, Rosenthal NE, Levendosky AA et al (1989) Phase-shifting effects of bright morning light as treatment for delayed sleep phase syndrome, *Sleep Res* **18:**422.

Kantor JS (1983) Light as a treatment for nonseasonal depression, *Am J Psychiatry* **140:**1262.

Kasper S, Möller HJ (1996) *Therapeutischer Schlafentzug. Klinik und Wirkmechanismen* (Springer Verlag: Wien, New York).

Kasper S, Vieira A, Wehr TA et al (1988a) Serotonergically induced hormonal responses and the antidepressant effect of total sleep deprivation in patients with major depression, *Psychopharmacol Bull* **50:**450–3.

Kasper S, Sack DA, Wehr TA, Kick H, Voll G, Vieira A (1988b) Nocturnal TSH and prolactin secretion during sleep deprivation and prediction of antidepressant response in patients with major depression, *Biol Psychiatry* **24:**631–41.

Kasper S, Rogers S, Yancey A, Schulz PM, Skwerer RG, Rosenthal NE (1989a) Phototherapy in individuals with and without subsyndromal seasonal affective disorder, *Arch Gen Psychiatry* **46:**837–44.

Kasper S, Wehr TA, Bartko JJ, Gaist PA, Rosenthal NE (1989b) Epidemiological findings of seasonal changes in mood and behavior. A telephone survey of the Montgomery County, Maryland, *Arch Gen Psychiatry* **46:**823–33.

Kasper S, Sack DA, Wehr TA (1989c) Therapcutischer Schlafentzug und Energiehaushalt. In: Pflug B, Lemmer B, eds, *Chronobiologie und Chronopharmakologie, Antidepressiva—Schlafentzug—Licht* (Gustav Fischer Verlag) 53–79.

Kasper S, Peters S, Maienberg P, Wicharz G, Pastoors L, Zinner J (1990a) Erfahrungen mit einer Spezialambulanz für saisonal abhängige Depressionen (SAD) und Phototherapie, *Zentralbl Neurol Psychiatr* **255:**218–19.

Kasper S, Rogers SLB, Madden PA, Joseph-Vanderpool JR, Rosenthal NE (1990b) The effects of phototherapy in the general population, *J Affect Disord* **18:**211–19.

Kasper S, Voll G, Vieira A, Kick H (1990c) Response to total sleep deprivation before and during treatment with fluvoxamine or maprotiline in patients with major depression—results of a double blind study, *Pharmacopsychiatry* **23:**135–42.

Kasper S, Ruhrmann S, Haase T, Möller HJ (1992a) Recurrent brief depression and its relationship to seasonal affective disorders, *Eur Arch Psychiatry Clin Neurosci* **242:**20–6.

Kasper S, Danos P, Ruhrmann S, Wittkopf B (1992b) Hypomania after therapeutic sleep deprivation in major depression, *Biol Psychiatry* **31:**100A.

Kasper S, Ruhrmann S, Neumann S, Möller HJ (1994a) Use of light therapy in German psychiatric hospitals, *Eur Psychiatry* **9:**288–92.

Kasper S, Ruhrmann S, Schuchardt HM (1994b) The effects of light therapy in treatment indications other than seasonal affective disorder (SAD). In: Holick MF, Jung EG, eds, *Biologic Effects of Light 1993* (Walter de Gruyter & Co.: Berlin, New York) 206–18.

Kasper S, Neumeister A, Rieder-Praschak N, Hesselmann B, Ruhrmann S (1996) Serotonergic mechanisms in the pathophysiology and treatment of seasonal affective disorder. In: Holick MF, Jung EG, eds, *Biological Effects of Light 1995* (Walter de Gruyter & Co.: Berlin, New York) 325–31.

Klompenhouwer JL, Fekkes D, Moleman HP, Pepplinkhuizen L, Mudler PGH (1990) Seasonal variations in binding of 3H-paroxetine to blood platelets in healthy volunteers: indications for a gender difference, *Biol Psychiatry* **28:**509–17.

Kolbinger HM, Höflich G, Hufnagel A, Möller H-J, Kasper S (1995) Transcranial magnetic stimulation (TMS) in the treatment of major depression—a pilot study, *Hum Psychopharmacol* **10:** 305–10.

Kripke DF, Risch SC, Janowsky D (1983) Bright white light alleviates depression, *Psychiatry Res* **10:** 105–12.

Kripke DF, Gillin JC, Mullaney DJ, Risch SC, Janowsky DS (1987) Treatment of major depressive disorders by bright white light for 5 days. In: Halaris A, ed., *Chronobiology and Psychiatric Disorders* (Elsevier: Amsterdam).

Kripke DF, Mullaney DJ, Savides TJ, Gillin JC (1989) Phototherapy for nonseasonal major depressive disorders. In: Rosenthal NE, Blehar MC, eds, *Seasonal Affective Disorders and Phototherapy* (Guilford: New York) 342–56.

Kripke DF, Mullaney DJ, Klauber MR, Risch SC, Gillin JC (1992) Controlled trial of bright light for nonseasonal major depressive disorders, *Biol Psychiatry* **31:**119–34.

Kuhs H, Tölle R (1986) Schlafentzug (Wachtherapie) als Antidepressivum, *Fortschr Neurol Psychiat* **54:**341–55.

Lam RW, Gorman CP, Michalon M et al (1995) Multi-centre, placebo-controlled study of fluoxetine in seasonal affective disorder, *Am J Psychiatry* **152:**1765–70.

Levitt AJ, Joffe RTJ, Kennedy SH (1991) Bright light augmentation in antidepressant nonresponders, *J Clin Psychiatry* **52:**336–7.

Lingjaerde O, Haggag A (1992) Moclobemide in winter depression: some preliminary results from an open trial, *Nord J Psychiatry* **46**(3):201–3.

Lingjaerde O, Reichborn-Kjennerud T, Haggag A, Gärtner I, Narud K, Berg EM (1993) Treatment of winter depression in Norway. II. A comparison of the selective monoamine oxidase A inhibitor moclobemide and placebo, *Acta Psychiatr Scand* **88:**372–80.

Loosen PT, Merke N, Amelung N (1976) Combined sleep deprivation and clomipramine in primary depression, *Lancet* **i:**156–7.

Mackert A, Volz HP, Stieglitz RD, Müller-Oerlinghausen B (1991) Phototherapy in nonseasonal depression, *Biol Psychiatry* **30:**257–68.

Martinez B, Kasper S, Ruhrmann S, Möller HJ (1994) Hypericum in the treatment of seasonal affective disorders, *J Geriatr Psychiatry Neurol* **7:**S29–33.

McGrath RE, Buckwald B, Resnick EV (1990) The effect of L-tryptophan on seasonal affective disorder, *J Clin Psychiatry* **51:**162–3.

Meesters Y, Lambers PA, Jansen JHC, Bouhuys AL, Beersma DGM, van den Hoofdakker RH (1991) Can winter depression be prevented by light treatment? *J Affect Disord* **23:**75–9.

Miller HL, Delgado PL, Salomon RM, Licinio J, Barr LC, Charney DS (1992) Acute tryptophan depletion: a method of studying antidepressant action, *J Clin Psychiatry* **53**(suppl 10):28–35.

Minors DA, Waterhouse JM, Wirz-Justice A (1991) A human phase-response curve to light, *Neurosci Lett* **133:**36–40.

Neumeister A, Gössler R, Lucht M, Kapitany T, Barnas C, Kasper S (1996) Bright light therapy stabilizes the antidepressant effect of partial sleep deprivation, *Biol Psychiatry* **39:**16–21.

Neumeister A, Rieder-Praschak N, Heßelmann B, Rao ML, Glück J, Kasper S (1997a) Effects of tryptophan depletion on drug-free patients with seasonal affective disorder during a stable response to bright light therapy, *Arch Gen Psychiatry* **54:**133–8.

Neumeister A, Praschak-Rieder N, Heßelmann B et al (1997b) Effects of acute tryptophan depletion in drug-free depressed patients who responded to total sleep deprivation, *Arch Gen Psychiatry* (in press).

Neumeister A, Praschak-Rieder N, Heßelmann B et al (1997c) Rapid tryptophan depletion in drug-free depressed patients with seasonal affective disorder, *Am J Psychiatry* **154:**1153–5.

Neumeister A, Praschak-Rieder N,

Heßelmann B et al (1997d) Effects of tryptophan depletion in fully remitted patients with seasonal affective disorder during summer, *Psychol Med* (in press).

Neumeister A, Praschak-Rieder N, Heßelmann B et al (1997e) The tryptophan depletion paradigm—methods and clinical relevance, *Nervenarzt* **68:**556–62.

O'Rourke D, Wurtman JJ, Wurtman RJ, Chebli R, Gleason R (1989) Treatment of seasonal affective disorder with d-fenfluramine, *J Clin Psychiatry* **50:** 343–7.

Oren DA, Mould DE, Schwartz PJ, Wehr TA, Rosenthal NE (1994) A controlled trial of levodopa plus carbidopa in the treatment of winter seasonal affective disorder: a test of the dopamine hypothesis, *J Clin Psychopharmacol* **14:**196–200.

Parry BL, Wehr TA (1987) Therapeutic effect of sleep deprivation in patients with premenstrual syndrome, *Am J Psychiatry* **144:**808–10.

Parry BL, Rosenthal NE, Tamarkin L, Wehr TA (1987) Treatment of a patient with seasonal premenstrual syndrome, *Am J Psychiatry* **144:**762–6.

Parry BL, Berga SL, Mostofi N, Sependa PA, Kripke DF, Gillin JC (1989) Morning versus evening bright light treatment of late luteal phase dysphoric disorder, *Am J Psychiatry* **146:**1215–17.

Partonen T, Lönnqvist J (1996a) Moclobemide and fluoxetine in treatment of seasonal affective disorder, *J Affect Disord* **41:**93–9.

Partonen T, Lönnqvist J (1996b) Prevention of winter seasonal affective disorder by bright-light treatment, *Psychol Med* **26:**1075–80.

Peter K, Räbinger U, Kowalik A (1986) Erste Ergebnisse mit Bright-Light (Phototherapie) bei affektiven Psychosen, *Psychiatr Neurol Med Psychol* **38:**384–90.

Pflug B (1972) Sleep deprivation as an ambulant therapy for endogenous depression, *Nervenarzt* **12:**614–22.

Pflug B, Tölle R (1971) Therapie endogener Depressionen durch Schlafentzug—Praktische und theoretische Konsequenzen, *Nervenarzt* **42:**117–24.

Post RM, Kopin J, Goodwin FK (1976) Effects of sleep deprivation on mood and central amine metabolism in depressed patients, *Arch Gen Psychiatry* **33:**627–32.

Powers LL, Terman M, Link MJ (1989) Bright light treatment of night shift workers, *Soc Light Treatment Biol Rhythms Abst* **1:**34.

Prasko J (1988) The acceleration of antidepressants' effects by using phototherapy in endogenous depression, *Psychopharmacol Bull* **96**(suppl):398.

Prasko J, Goldmann P, Zindr R, Zindr V (1987) Hastening the onset of action of tricyclic antidepressants by using white light, *Cs Psychiatr* **83:**376–84.

Prasko J, Goldmann P, Praskova H, Zindr V (1988) Hastened onset of the effect of antidepressive drugs when using three types of timing of intensive white light, *Cs Psychiatr* **84:**373–83.

Puri BK, Lewis SW (1996) Transcranial magnetic stimulation in psychiatric research, *Br J Psychiatry* **169:**675–7.

Rosenthal NE, Sack DA, Gillin JC et al (1984) Seasonal affective disorder; a description of the syndrome and preliminary findings with light therapy, *Arch Gen Psychiatry* **41:**72–80.

Rosenthal NE, Genhart M, Jacobsen FM, Skwerer RG, Wehr TA (1987) Disturbances of appetite and weight regulation in seasonal affective disorder, *Ann NY Acad Sci* **499:**216–30.

Rosenthal NE, Joseph-Vanderpool JR, Levandowsky AA et al (1990) Phase-shifting effects of bright morning light as treatment for delayed sleep phase syndrome, *Sleep* **13:**354–61.

Ross DR, Lewin R, Gold K et al (1988) The psychiatric uses of cold wet sheet packs, *Am J Psychiatry* **145:**242–5.

Roy Burne PP, Uhde TW, Post RM (1986) Effects of one night's sleep deprivation on mood and behavior in patients with panic disorder, *Arch Gen Psychiatry* **43:**895–9.

Ruhrmann S, Kasper S, Hawellek B et al (1993) Fluoxetine as a treatment alternative to light therapy in seasonal affective disorder (SAD), *Pharmacopsychiatry* **26:**193.

Sack DA, Nurnberger J, Rosenthal NE, Ashburn E, Wehr TA (1985) The potentiation of antidepressant medications by phase-advance of the sleep–wake cycle, *Am J Psychiatry* **142:**606–8.

Sack DA, Duncan W, Rosenthal NE, Mendelson WE, Wehr TA (1988) The timing and duration of sleep in partial sleep deprivation therapy of depression, *Acta Psychiatr Scand* **77:**219–24.

Sasaki M, Kurosaki Y, Onda M et al (1989) Effects of bright light on circadian rhythmicity and sleep after transmeridian flight, *Sleep Res* **18:**442.

Satinoff E, Hendersen R (1977) Thermoregulatory behavior. In: Honig WK, Staddon JER, eds, *Handbook of Operant Behavior* (Springer) 153–73.

Schlager DS (1994) Early-morning administration of short-acting β-blockers for treatment of winter depression, *Am J Psychiatry* **151:**1383–5.

Schuchardt HM, Kasper S (1997) Lichttherapie in der psychiatrischen Praxis. In: Peters UH, ed., *150 Jahre DGPN (Deutsche Gesellschaft für Psychiatrie und Nervenheilkunde), Proceedings of Jubiläumskongreß*, Köln (in press).

Schulte W (1969) Über die Bedeutung des klinischen Details: Protrahiertes Herausgeraten aus melancholischen Phasen. In: Hippius H, Selbach H, eds, *Das Depressive Syndrom* (Karger: Basel) 415–20.

Stewart JW, Quitkin FW, Terman M, Terman JS (1990) Is seasonal affective disorder a variant of atypical depressive disorder? *Psychiatry Res* **33:**121–8.

Svendson K (1976) Sleep deprivation therapy in depression, *Acta Psychiatr Scand* **54:**184–92.

Tauscher J, Neumeister A, Fischer P, Frey R, Kasper S (1997) Die Elektrokonvulsionstherapie in der klinischen Praxis, *Nervenarzt* **68:**410–16.

Teicher MH, Glod CA (1990) Seasonal affective disorder: rapid resolution by low-dose alprazolam, *Psychopharmacol Bull* **26:**197–202.

Terman M, Terman JS, Quitkin FM, McGrath PJ, Steward JW, Rafferty B (1989) Light therapy for seasonal affective disorder. A review of efficacy, *Neuropsychopharmacology* **2:**1–22.

Vogel GW, Vogel C, Mcabee RS, Thurmond AJ (1980) Improvement of depression by REM sleep deprivation: new findings and a theory, *Arch Gen Psychiatry* **37:**247–53.

Volz HP, Mackert A, Stieglitz RD, Müller-Örlinghausen M (1990) Effect of bright white light therapy on non-seasonal depressive disorder: preliminary results, *J Affect Disord* **19:**15–21.

Vovin RY, Aksenova IO, Sverdlov LS (1982) Sleep deprivation in the treatment of chronic depressive states, *Neurosci Behav Physiol* **12:**92–6.

Wehr TA (1990) Effects of wakefulness and sleep on depression and mania. In: Montplaisier J, Godbout R, eds, *Sleep and Biological Rhythms, Basic Mechanisms and Applications to Psychiatry* (Oxford University Press: New York, Oxford) 42–86.

Wehr TA, Wirz-Justice A (1981) Internal coincidence model for sleep deprivation and depression. In: Koella WP, ed., *Sleep 1980* (Karger: Basel) 26–33.

Wehr TA, Goodwin FK, Wirz-Justice A, Breitmaier J, Craig C (1982) 48-hour sleep–wake cycles in manic-depressive illness, *Arch Gen Psychiatry* **39:**559–65.

Weitzman ED, Czeisler CA, Coleman RM, Spielman AJ, Zimmerman JC, Dement W (1981) Delayed sleep phase syndrome: a chronobiological disorder with sleep onset insomnia, *Arch Gen Psychiatry* **38:**737–46.

Wever RA (1985) Use of light to treat jet lag: differential effects of normal and bright artificial light on human circadian rhythms, *Ann NY Acad Sci* **453:**282–304.

Wiegand M, Berger M, Zulley J, Lauer C, Von Zerssen D (1987) The influence of daytime naps on the therapeutic effect of sleep deprivation, *Biol Psychiatry* **22:**386–9.

Wirz-Justice A, Pühringer W, Hole G (1975) Sleep deprivation in depression: effects on the diurnal rhythm of plasma free tryptophan and relation to clinical response. Presented at the Second International Sleep Research Congress, Edinburgh, 1975.

Wirz-Justice A, van der Velde P, Nil R (1992) Comparison of light treatment with citalopram in winter depression: a longitudinal single case study, *Int Clin Psychopharmacol* **7:**109–16.

Wu JC, Bunney WE Jr (1990) The biological basis of an antidepressant response to sleep deprivation and relapse: review and hypothesis, *Am J Psychiatry* **147:**14–21.

Yamaguchi N, Maeda K, Kuromaru S (1978) The effects of sleep deprivation on the circadian rhythm of plasma cortisol levels in depressive patients, *Folia Psychiatr Neurol Jpn* **32:**479–87.

Yerevanian BJ, Anderson JL, Grota LJ, Bray M (1986) Effects of bright incandescent light on seasonal and nonseasonal major depressive disorder, *Psychiatry Res* **18:**355–64.

Young SN, Smith SE, Pihl RO, Ervin FR (1985) Tryptophan depletion causes a rapid lowering of mood in normal males, *Psychopharmacology* **87:** 173–77.

15

Adjunct treatments for rapid onset of action and greater efficacy in major depression

Pierre Blier, Richard Bergeron and Claude de Montigny

Introduction

There are several pharmacologic strategies which can be used for treatment-resistant major depression. They produce an antidepressant response in a significant percentage of patients and thus provide a greater therapeutic effect than a single drug used alone. These include the addition of lithium, T3, the serotonin (5-HT)$_{1A}$ agonist buspirone and the β-adrenoceptor/5-HT$_{1A}$ antagonist pindolol to an antidepressant-drug regimen in resistant patients (Joffe and Schuller, 1993; Artigas et al, 1994; de Montigny, 1994; Aroson et al, 1996; Figure 15.1). A rapid titration of the 5-HT/norepinephrine (NE) reuptake blocker venlafaxine to 300 mg/day or more has also been shown to produce a robust and a more rapid antidepressant effect in a significant proportion of patients (Guelfi et al, 1995). Perhaps related to the mechanism of action of venlafaxine, the effectiveness of the combined use of a selective 5-HT reuptake inhibitor (SSRI) and an NA reuptake blocker has also been reported to induce a therapeutic response in treatment-resistant patients (Weilburg et al, 1989; Nelson et al, 1991; Zajecka et al, 1995). Finally, electroconvulsive shock treatment (ECT) still remains a most valuable option for the treatment of drug-resistant depression. While there is a general consensus that at least some of the above-mentioned strategies have a greater efficacy, there is much more controversy with regard to the fact that some treatments may exert a rapid response. Indeed, whatever the antidepressant drug used, there is in general a 2-week delay before a clear therapeutic effect is obtained. The introduction of antidepressant drugs which can be given at a therapeutic dose from the beginning of the treatment, and which reach a steady-state level within a few days, has not shortened the delayed onset of action of antidepressant drugs. Consequently, the antidepressant response must be explained by adaptive changes that gradually develop secondary to the acute biochemical effects of the antidepressant drugs.

Before providing a brief description of the putative mechanisms by

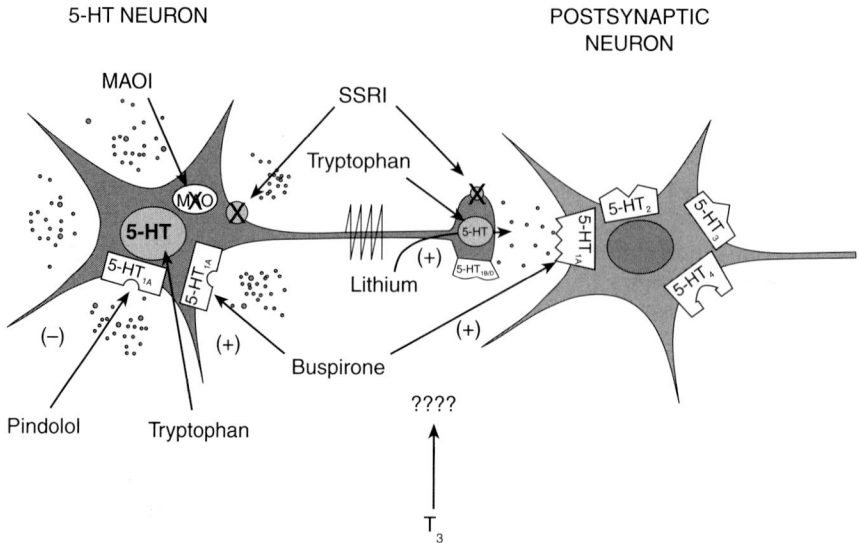

Figure 15.1

Presynaptic and postsynaptic factors regulating the effectiveness of serotonin (5-HT) neurotransmission and sites of action of selected antidepressant drugs/augmentation strategies. Only the subtypes of 5-HT receptors for which an electrophysiologic response has been identified in unitary recordings are depicted. 5-HT$_{1A}$ receptors on the cell body of 5-HT-containing neurons mediate an inhibitory effect on firing activity by the opening of potassium channels. 5-HT$_{1B/D}$ receptors on the terminals exert an inhibitory action on 5-HT release. The two small circles on the 5-HT neuron represent the high-affinity reuptake carrier. The different symbols used to depict the pre- and postsynaptic 5-HT$_{1A}$ receptors are to indicate that they have different pharmacologic properties. The question marks above T3 signify that the mechanism of action of this potentiating agent is not known. (+) represents an activation or an increase, (−) an inhibition and X a blockade.

which antidepressant drugs exert a therapeutic response in major depression, one has to consider whether it is possible to obtain a rapid antidepressant response. This is a crucial issue, as it would be impossible to obtain such an early onset of action, e.g. by bypassing the neurobiological events which would lead to the return of euthymic mood, if this response were endowed with an inertia of the order of weeks.

The following lines of clinical evidence can be mentioned in support of the notion that a rapid antidepressant effect can be obtained. First, a one-night sleep deprivation produces a marked antidepressant effect the following day in at least 50% of patients (Benca et al, 1992). Second, ECT often produces a marked antidepressant effect in the first week of treatment (Rich et al, 1984; Post et al, 1987; Rodger et al, 1994; Segman et al, 1995). Third, in patients markedly improved by an antidepressant drug, acute tryptophan depletion produces a relapse within 5 h, in most cases with the symptomatology being identical to that presented before the antidepressant regimen was initiated. Subsequently, when the normal diet is restored, the antidepressant response returns within 24–48 h (Delgado et al, 1990). These three series of clinical observations indicate that not only can a depressive state be reversed rapidly but that, within 24 h, an individual may have few or no depressive symptoms, present a major depressive syndrome and regain a euthymic mood.

Mechanisms of action of antidepressant treatments

Extensive electrophysiologic investigations carried out in our laboratory have documented that several types of antidepressant treatments enhance 5-HT neurotransmission in the rat hippocampus (see Blier and de Montigny, 1994). This net effect, which is common to the major types of antidepressant treatments, is, however, mediated via different mechanisms (Figure 15.1; Table 15.1). All tricyclic antidepressant (TCA) drugs, independently of their capacity to inhibit the reuptake of 5-HT and/or NE, progressively enhance the responsiveness of postsynaptic $5-HT_{1A}$ receptors in the hippocampus with a time course that is congruent with the delayed onset of action of these drugs in major depression (de Montigny and Aghajanian, 1978). It has also been demonstrated by our group and other laboratories that this enhanced responsiveness to 5-HT also occurs in other, but not all, brain regions and that the sensitivity of 5-HT receptor subtypes other than that of the $5-HT_{1A}$ receptors is also altered. For instance, in the facial motor nucleus, the effect of 5-HT is mediated by

Table 15.1   Effects of long-term administration of antidepressant treatments on 5-HT neurotransmission[a].

	Somatodendritic autoreceptor responsiveness[b]	Terminal autoreceptor responsiveness[c]	Postsynaptic responsiveness[b]	Net effect[d]
Tricyclic antidepressants	0	0	↑	↑
Electroconvulsive shocks	0	0	↑	↑
Monoamide oxidase inhibitors	↓	0	0/↓	↑
Selective 5-HT reuptake inhibitors	↓	↓	0	↑
$5-HT_{1A}$ agonists	↓	0	↑	↑[e]

[a] Rats were treated for at least 14 days.
[b] Assessed by microiontophoresis or systemic injection of 5-HT receptor agonists.
[c] Assessed by comparing the effects of agonists or antagonists in control and treated rats.
[d] Determined from the firing activity of the presynaptic neurons and the effect of stimulating 5-HT fibers.
[e] Effect obtained by an enhanced tonic activation of postsynaptic $5-HT_{1A}$ receptors resulting from a normal amount of 5-HT (normalized 5-HT neuronal firing) and the presence of the exogenous $5-HT_{1A}$ agonist. ↑, increased; ↓, decreased; 0, no change.

(A)   (B)

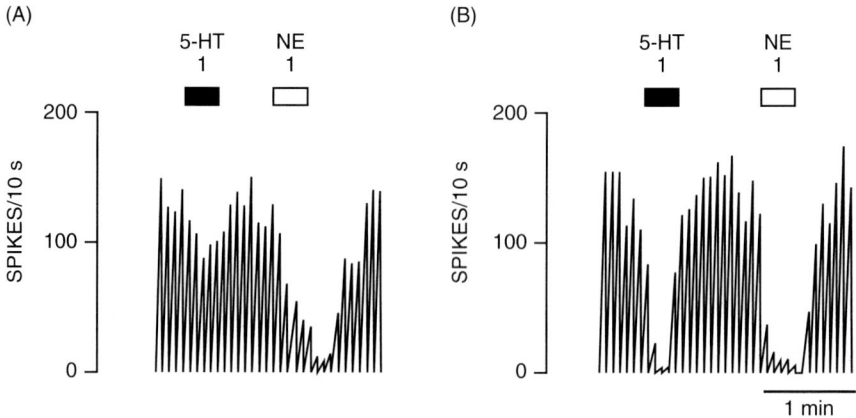

Figure 15.2

Integrated firing rate histograms of two CA$_3$ dorsal hippocampus pyramidal neurons showing their response to microiontophoretic applications of 5-HT and NE in a control rat (A) and in a rat treated with six electroconvulsive shocks over a 2-week period (B). The shocks were delivered under halothane anesthesia and the recordings were carried out under chloral hydrate anesthesia. The bars above the traces indicate the duration of the application (50 s) for which the ejection current is given in nanoamps. The time base applies to both traces. Note that only the responsiveness to 5-HT is increased.

5-HT$_2$ receptors and that of NE by α_2-adrenoceptors, yet both types are sensitized following repeated TCA administration (Menkes et al, 1980). Repeated, but not single, electroconvulsive shocks also induce this sensitization of 5-HT$_{1A}$ receptors in the dorsal hippocampus (de Montigny, 1984; Chaput et al, 1991; Figure 15.2). This is consistent with the clinical effectiveness of repeated ECT sessions.

Monoamine oxidase inhibitors (MAOIs), SSRIs and 5-HT$_{1A}$ agonists all induce an initial attenuation of the firing activity of 5-HT neurons upon treatment initiation because they increase the degree of activation of the somatodendritic 5-HT$_{1A}$ autoreceptors which control the firing rate of 5-HT neurons (Blier and de Montigny, 1983, 1985a, 1987). This is followed by a gradual recovery to normal firing activity of 5-HT neurons when the treatment is continued for 2–3 weeks, due to a desensitization of the 5-HT$_{1A}$ autoreceptors (Figure 15.3). At this point in time, MAOIs enhance 5-HT transmission by increasing the amount of 5-HT released per action potential as a result of a greater concentration of 5-HT in the terminals (Blier et al, 1986). SSRIs produce the same effect, not by augmenting the releasable pool of 5-HT like MAOIs do, but rather by desensitizing the terminal 5-HT$_{1B/1D}$ autoreceptor, which exerts a negative influence on the amount of 5-HT that is released per impulse (Chaput et al, 1986; Blier and Bouchard, 1994). 5-HT$_{1A}$ agonists produce an enhanced tonic activation of postsynaptic 5-HT$_{1A}$ receptors, as a result of a normalized firing activity of 5-HT neurons (and of 5-HT release as well) in the presence of

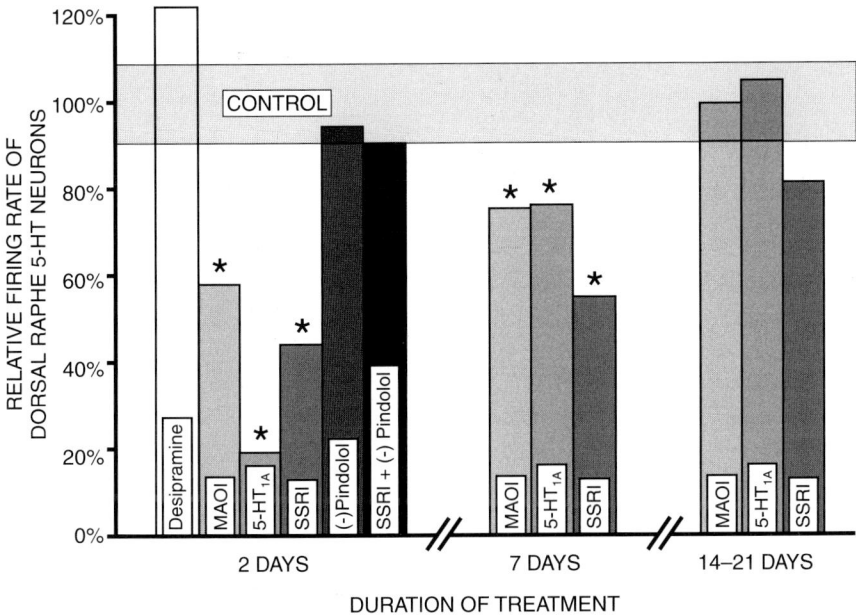

Figure 15.3

Effects of various types of drug treatment on the firing activity of dorsal raphe 5-HT neurons recorded in anesthetized rats. The values are expressed relative to controls carried out in the same experimental series for the various treatment groups. The mean firing rate in controls varied from 0.9 to 1.2 action potentials per second, with a standard error of the mean of about 10%. All drugs were administered using osmotic minipumps implanted subcutaneously, with the exception of the type A MAOI clorgyline, which produced a sustained inhibition of the enzyme with a once-daily administration, and the SSRI citalopram, which was given intraperitoneally once a day and the experiments carried out 10–12 h after the last dose. $p < 0.05$ using a Student's t-test.

the exogenous 5-HT$_{1A}$ agonist acting on normosensitive postsynaptic 5-HT$_{1A}$ receptors (Blier and de Montigny, 1987).

Considering that some treatment strategies have a greater efficacy and that it is possible to rapidly induce an antidepressant response, the issue of whether these two aspects of the treatment of depression are related from a mechanistic point of view will be examined. The strategy of adding and/or combining lithium and pindolol with antidepressant drugs will be examined as there are now controlled trials which have addressed and confirmed these aspects of the antidepressant response to these two agents.

Lithium

It is now well established that the addition of lithium to the therapeutic regimen of depressed patients treated with but not responding to their antidepressant drug, rapidly induces a response in a significant number of cases (de Montigny, 1994). The rate of response is about 50% after about 2 weeks of lithium addition (see Joffe and Schuller, 1993; Baumann et al, 1996). In most cases, the type of response obtained is of the all or none type and is therefore readily detectable. The effectiveness of this strategy in comparison to a reference treatment for resistant depression has been examined (Dinan and Barry, 1989). In TCA-resistant patients, lithium addition and ECT addition were shown to produce the same degree of improvement after 14 and 21 days, respectively. In that particular study, the beneficial effect of lithium was already maximal after 7 days of lithium administration, whereas the therapeutic effect of ECT given twice weekly was present only at day 14.

The capacity of lithium to accelerate the antidepressant response has been examined, i.e. combining lithium with an antidepressant from the beginning of the therapeutic trial. Thus far, four controlled studies have been published (Table 15.2). They were all carried out using TCA drugs. None of them showed a significant difference between the lithium and the placebo group in the first 2–3 weeks of treatment with respect to the rapidity of action. This clearly indicates that combining lithium with an antidepressant drug is not a strategy that provides an early onset of action in untreated patients, in contrast to the rapid improvement observed in resistant patients, as described above. In contrast, in two of these studies, there was a significantly greater effect in the lithium group than in the placebo group at the end of the trial. In the study by Ling-jaerde et al (1974), 80% of the patients responded to clomipramine plus lithium versus 53% in the clomipramine plus placebo group, whereas in the trial by Ebert et al (1995), the mean scores on the Hamilton Rating Scale were 13 and 6 in the TCA alone and the TCA plus lithium groups, respectively, at the end of the 5-week study period. The lack of a greater efficacy of lithium combination in two of the four controlled trials thus far conducted does not constitute evidence that this strategy is not more

Table 15.2   Published data on the possibility that lithium potentiates (acceleration/augmentation) tricyclic antidepressant drugs.

Placebo-controlled studies	N[a]	Rapid onset[b] (2–3 weeks)	Greater efficacy[b] (4–5 weeks)
Lingaerde et al (1974)	45	–	+
Nick et al (1976)	30	–	NA
Ebert et al (1996)	40	–	+
Shahal et al (1996)	20	–	–

[a] Total number of patients.

[b] As assessed either by a greater percentage of patients achieving a 50% degree of improvement or statistically different (lower) score on the Hamilton scale for depression in the lithium than in the placebo group.

NA, not applicable.

effective. Rather, these negative results underscore the fact that this type of trial design is not optimal for detecting greater efficacy. Considering that about 60% of depressed patients will respond to an antidepressant drug alone, and that lithium should produce such a response in about half of the resistant patients, one needs to have a relatively large number of patients in a study to be able to demonstrate a statistically significant difference between the 60% rate of response with the antidepressant drug alone and the expected 80% rate of response with the lithium combination (see Baumann et al, 1996).

The prompt response to lithium addition in treatment-resistant patients is thought to result from its capacity to enhance 5-HT release in several, but not all, brain regions (Blier and de Montigny, 1985b, 1992). Although lithium has been shown to interfere with some second messenger systems in concentrations effective in the treatment of mania/hypomania (approximately 1 mmol/l or more), the beneficial effect of lithium in treatment-resistant depression can be obtained at a low range of plasma levels (0.4–0.7 mmol/l) (de Montigny et al, 1993). In parallel with these clinical observations, we have shown that a short-term treatment (2–3 days) markedly enhances the electrically evoked release of 5-HT in anesthetized rats with blood levels as low as 0.4 mmol/l (Blier and de Montigny, 1985b). The mechanism by which lithium enhances 5-HT release has not yet been elucidated. However, it appears to be different from those of other types of antidepressant drugs. It is thus not surprising that lithium addition has been reported to be effective with all antidepressant treatments. From a theoretical point of view, the lithium combination would not be expected to produce a more rapid onset of antidepressant action. In the case of TCA drugs, the therapeutic effect of lithium resulting from enhanced 5-HT release should not be expected until the post-synaptic 5-HT receptors are sensitized (Blier and de Montigny, 1994). The therapeutic effect of this strategy would thus result from a marked potentiation of 5-HT neurotransmission resulting from pre- and post-synaptic factors. In support of this possibility, the lack of an immediate antidepressant effect of SSRIs can be mentioned despite their capacity to enhance extracellular 5-HT concentration upon acute administration. However, after long-term SSRI administration, the levels of 5-HT in various brain structures are enhanced to a much greater degree than upon their acute administration (Bel and Artigas, 1992; Rutter et al, 1994; Kreiss and Lucki, 1995; Invernizzi et al, 1996). This difference is most likely attributable to an attenuated negative feedback mediated by the cell body and terminal 5-HT autoreceptors, which normally exert a suppressant effect on the function of 5-HT neurons (Blier and de Montigny, 1994).

Cell body 5-HT$_{1A}$ autoreceptor antagonism

A novel strategy has recently been devised to accelerate the antidepressant response (de Montigny et al, 1993). It consists of combining an SSRI with the 5-HT$_{1A}$/β-adrenoceptor antagonist pindolol (Artigas et al, 1994; Blier and Bergeron, 1995; Figure 15.4). This approach is based on the capacity of pindolol to block the 5-HT$_{1A}$ autoreceptor on the cell body of 5-HT neurons in order to prevent the initial decrease of the firing activity of these neurons at the beginning of the SSRI treatment, as described in the preceding section (Figure 15.3). It is important to emphasize that pindolol does not block certain postsynaptic 5-HT$_{1A}$ receptors (Romero et al, 1996). Otherwise, the simultaneous blockade of both pre- and postsynaptic 5-HT$_{1A}$ receptors would prevent a net increase in 5-HT neurotransmission via postsynaptic 5-HT$_{1A}$ receptors, which are present at

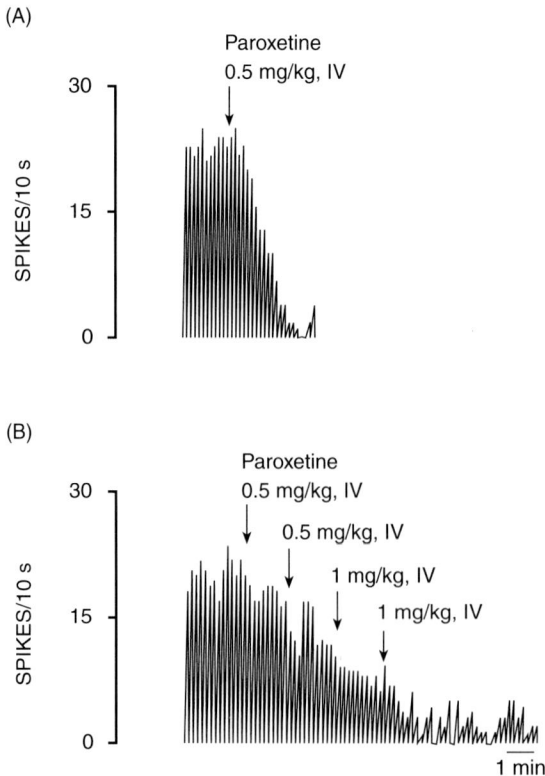

Figure 15.4

Effect of the administration of the selective 5-HT reuptake inhibitor paroxetine on the spontaneous firing activity of dorsal raphe 5-HT neurons recorded in chloral hydrate-anesthetized rats, (A) in a control, and (B) in a rat which received the 5-HT$_{1A}$ antagonist (−)pindolol subcutaneously (15 mg/kg per day for 2 days) using an osmotic minipump. The time base applies to both traces.

particularly high density in the limbic system and are thought to play an important role in the antidepressant response. Obviously, such a mechanism relies on the distinct pharmacologic nature of 5-HT_{1A} receptors. Although a single amino acid sequence encoding the 5-HT_{1A} receptor has thus far been identified, several lines of evidence have been gathered which clearly show that 5-HT_{1A} receptors are heterogenous. First, most exogenous 5-HT_{1A} agonists are full agonists at presynaptic sites but partial agonists in the hippocampus. Second, upon long-term administration of 5-HT_{1A} agonists, 5-HT_{1A} autoreceptors become desensitized, whereas 5-HT_{1A} receptors in the hippocampus remain normosensitive (Blier and de Montigny, 1994). Third, the 5-HT_{1A} antagonist spiperone readily blocks the 5-HT_{1A} autoreceptor in the dorsal raphe but not the 5-HT_{1A} receptors in the dorsal hippocampus, whereas the buspirone derivative BMY 7378 blocks the post- but not the presynaptic 5-HT_{1A} receptors in the same two brain structures (Chaput and de Montigny, 1988; Blier et al, 1993). Finally, the potent and selective 5-HT_{1A} antagonist WAY 100,635 blocks 5-HT_{1A} receptors on the cell body of 5-HT neurons in the dorsal raphe and of pyramidal neurons in the hippocampus but not those located in the orbitofrontal cortex (Fletcher et al, 1996; El Mansari and Blier, 1997; Haddjeri et al, 1997). Taken together, these four lines of evidence indicate that there would be at least three pharmacologically distinct subtypes of 5-HT_{1A} receptors.

Since 5-HT release in most postsynaptic regions is highly dependent on electrical impulse flow in 5-HT axons, the prevention of the initial decrease of 5-HT neuronal firing activity by pindolol should physiologically mimic the desensitization of the 5-HT_{1A} autoreceptor, which has been documented to occur after a 2-week SSRI treatment. There are now four open-labeled studies which have examined the capacity of pindolol to accelerate the therapeutic effect of antidepressant drugs (Table 15.3). In the very first trial by Artigas et al (1994), five of seven patients had a greater than 50% improvement within 1 week of initiating paroxetine (20 mg/day) and pindolol (2.5 mg t.i.d.). In a subsequent trial, seven of nine patients also presented a greater than 50% improvement with the same therapeutic regimen (Blier and Bergeron, 1995; Figure 15.4). Viñar et al (1996) documented an acceleration of the antidepressant response to the same SSRI when individuals presenting a second episode were concomitantly treated with pindolol. The onset of action was shorter in 15 of 22 patients. Bakish et al (1996) have observed a rapid improvement in patients receiving a higher dose of the 5-HT reuptake blocker nefazodone together with pindolol in comparison with historical controls treated with nefazodone in one of their previous trials.

There are three placebo-controlled trials which have addressed this putative accelerating effect of pindolol. Two studies confirm it and one was negative. In the trial carried out in Barcelona, there were 55 patients in the fluoxetine (20 mg/day) plus placebo group and 56 in the fluoxetine

Table 15.3   Published data on the possibility that pindolol potentiates (acceleration/augmentation) antidepressant drugs.

	N [a]	Rapid onset[b]	Greater efficacy[b]
Open-labeled studies			
Artigas et al (1994)	15	+	+
Blier and Bergeron (1995)	28	+	+
Vinar et al (1996)	27	+	NA
Blier and Bergeron (1996)	11	−	+
Moreno et al (1996)	10	−	−
Bakish et al (1997)	20	+	+
Blier et al (1997)	30	+	+
Placebo-controlled studies			
Maes et al (1996)	33	−	+
Perez et al (1997)	111	+	+
Tome et al (1997)	80	+	−
Berman et al (1997)	43	−	−

[a] Total number of patients.
[b] As assessed either by a greater percentage of patients achieving a 50% degree of improvement or statistically different (lower) score on the Hamilton scale for depression in the pindolol than in the placebo group.
NA, not applicable.

plus pindolol group (2.5 mg t.i.d.). The mean time to a sustained response (a 50% or more improvement) was 29 days in the placebo group and 19 days in the pindolol group (Perez et al, 1997). In the trial using paroxetine (20 mg/day), the time to onset of action using the 50% improvement criterion was 10 days in the SSRI plus pindolol group (2.5 mg t.i.d.) and 24 days in the SSRI plus placebo group (Tome et al, 1997). In the third study, there was no difference observed with the use of pindolol (2.5 mg t.i.d. or 5 mg b.i.d.) together with fluoxetine (20 mg/day) (Berman et al, 1997). There are two factors which may account for the negative results obtained in the latter study. First, the mean weight of the patients was 84 kg whereas, in most other studies, patients on average were about 15 kg lighter. Since the optimal dose of pindolol is not known, it is conceivable that these patients did not receive a dose sufficient to block the 5-HT$_{1A}$ autoreceptor. The authors claim that, on the contrary, an adequate dose was administered, as they observed a significant decrease in pulse and blood pressure in the patients receiving pindolol. In contrast, we have never observed such a consistent change of these cardiovascular parameters (Blier and Bergeron, 1995, 1996; Blier et al, 1997). Consequently, obese patients may be more sensitive to the β-adrenergic properties of pindolol than are individuals of normal weight. The fact that several of these patients were overweight also suggests that perhaps more than 4 of the 23 patients in their fluoxetine plus pindolol group were presenting, in fact, an atypical depression. It is as yet unknown whether the pindolol combination is effective in this subtype of depression characterized mainly by hyperphagia and hypersomnia. Considering that TCA drugs are of little use while MAOIs are very effective in this subtype of depression (Liebowitz et al, 1988) and that these agents act at least in part via the 5-HT system by different mechanisms, it is conceivable that pindolol may not be useful in this situation. A second confounding factor is that half of the patients in that third study had a history of substance abuse or dependence. Such patients are generally more difficult to treat and it is not mentioned in the latter article whether a drug screen test was carried out before allowing entrance into the trial. Nevertheless, it is interesting to note that 3 of 20 patients demonstrated a clinical deterioration upon double-blind pindolol discontinuation at the end of this 6-week trial, thus providing evidence that pindolol had exerted a beneficial effect at least in some patients.

Taken together, these results indicate that pindolol is effective in some patients to accelerate the antidepressant response. However, the main question is whether there are any factors which predict a favorable response. It is noteworthy with respect to this issue that in the trial carried out with paroxetine (Tome et al, 1997), the patients who were referred mainly from primary care settings had an extremely rapid response when given pindolol (mean time to 50% improvement: 8 days on pindolol versus 42 days on placebo addition). In fact, this group of patients entirely accounted for the decrease in the onset of action of paroxetine, as the other group of patients, referred mostly from psychiatrists, failed to show any acceleration of the antidepressant response of the SSRI. Similarly, in the negative double-blind trial (Berman et al, 1997), there were less patients without a history of prior treatment in the pindolol group than in the placebo group. Clearly, further research is needed to clarify this issue.

In order to provide further evidence that pindolol accelerates the antidepressant effect of SSRIs via the preferential antagonism of the cell body 5-HT_{1A} autoreceptor, the capacity of pindolol to potentiate the antidepressant effect of the 5-HT_{1A} agonist buspirone was examined (Blier et al, 1997). Buspirone, in a dose range higher than that used for the treatment of generalized anxiety disorder, has been shown to be an antidepressant drug in a large placebo-controlled trial, exerting a more robust effect in patients meeting the criteria for melancholia (Robinson et al, 1990). Since buspirone activates both pre- and postsynaptic 5-HT_{1A} receptors, and the desensitization of the autoreceptor results in an enhancement of 5-HT neurotransmission, it was postulated that its combination with pindolol would lead to a preferential activation of postsynaptic 5-HT_{1A} receptors. This effect was postulated to exert a rapid antidepressant effect (de Montigny and Blier, 1991). After 1 week of this treatment regimen (buspirone 20 mg/day plus pindolol 2.5 mg t.i.d.), 8 of 10 patients with major depression presented a 50% or more degree of improvement. These results provide further evidence that the 5-HT_{1A}

antagonist pindolol does not block all the 5-HT_{1A} receptors that the 5-HT_{1A} agonist buspirone is activating, as otherwise this drug combination would have been inactive. In the same trial, 10 patients were also treated with pindolol and TCA drugs which do not block the reuptake of 5-HT. The rationale for this combination was that pindolol should not accelerate the antidepressant effect of these drugs because they do not initially decrease the firing rate of 5-HT neurons (Figure 15.3). The use of the selective NE reuptake blocker desipramine with pindolol leads patients to discontinue their medication in the first 7 days due to an exacerbation of their anxiety, irritability or insomnia. The combination with trimipramine, a TCA which does not block the reuptake of either 5-HT or NE, produced a gradual but modest antidepressant effect after 4 weeks of treatment. The lack of a potentiation of the antidepressant response of trimipramine using pindolol also supports the notion that the β-adrenergic properties of pindolol do not contribute to the beneficial effect of this adjunct in the treatment of depression.

Pindolol addition is not only an accelerating strategy but it has also been reported in open-labeled trials to produce an antidepressant effect in patients not responding to an SSRI or an MAOI (Artigas et al, 1994; Blier and Bergeron, 1995; Figure 15.6). This greater efficacy was detected in one of two double-blind trials carried out in non-resistant patients. The response rate in the SSRI plus placebo group was 59%, whereas in the SSRI plus pindolol group it was 75% with remission rates (a Hamilton score of 8 or less) of 45% and 60%, respectively, at the end of the 6-week trial (Perez et al, 1997). The latter results constitute evidence of a greater efficacy of the pindolol augmentation strategy. In another controlled trial using mainly resistant patients, the response rates were 73% in the trazodone (a weak 5-HT reuptake blocker with sedative properties) plus pindolol group, 75% in the fluoxetine plus trazodone group, and 20% in the trazodone plus placebo group (Maes et al, 1996). One may speculate that depressed patients who are rapidly and markedly improved by the addition of the 5-HT_{1A} antagonist pindolol may have failed to respond to their antidepressant drug regimen because their 5-HT_{1A} autoreceptors did not desensitize, thus precluding a recovery of the firing activity of 5-HT neurons. It will be interesting to test this hypothesis when a probe for the 5-HT_{1A} autoreceptor in humans becomes available.

Conclusion

In summary, there are now controlled studies indicating that pindolol addition leads to both a rapid onset of action and a greater efficacy in major depression. However, not all strategies having a greater effectiveness also provide a more rapid onset of action, as is the case of lithium addition to antidepressant drugs. Consequently, greater efficacy does

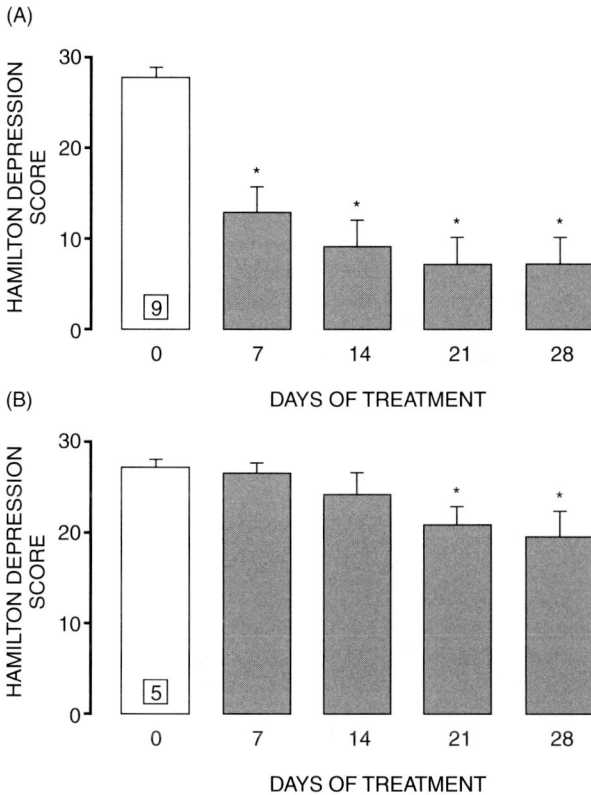

(A)

(B)

Figure 15.5

Hamilton depression scores on the 21-item scale depicting the intensity of depressive symptomatology in depressed unipolar patients. Paroxetine was given at a 20 mg/day dose throughout the 28 days (A), whereas the TCA trimipramine was administered at 75 mg at bedtime for the first week and at 150 mg at bedtime for the subsequent 3 weeks (B). Pindolol was given in both groups at a dose of 2.5 mg three times daily throughout the trials. The degree of improvement obtained in the trimipramine plus pindolol group is generally that obtained with an antidepressant drug used alone.* $p < 0.05$ when compared to the corresponding baseline values (day 0).

not invariably imply rapid onset of action, and the mechanism of action of the treatment strategies can help predict outcome. The data reviewed in the present chapter also indicate that appropriate trial design and patient populations are two crucial factors when these two characteristics of treatment response are being examined. A better understanding of the mechanism of action of the different pharmacologic strategies to treat depression may help us to obtain an optimal response in depressed patients with the drugs presently available, and will help us to develop drugs with a rapid antidepressant effect in a greater proportion of patients.

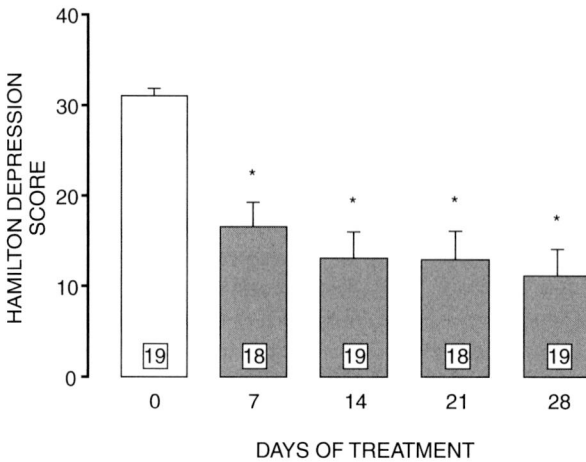

Figure 15.6

Intensity of the depressive syndrome, using the 21-item Hamilton depression scale, in drug-resistant patients who received pindolol 2.5 mg three times daily without altering their antidepressant drug regimen. Eight patients were on paroxetine (20–40 mg/day), five were on sertraline (50–100 mg/day), three were on fluoxetine (20–40 mg/day), and two were on moclobemide (900 mg/day). The unequal numbers at the bottom of the columns are because one patient could not be assessed at day 7 and 21. None of the five patients on sertraline responded to pindolol addition. * $p < 0.01$ when compared with the corresponding day 0 value using a one-way analysis of variance.

References

Aroson R, Offman HJ, Joffe RT, Naylor D (1996) Triiodothyronine augmentation in the treatment of refractory depression. A meta-analysis, *Arch Gen Psychiatry* **53:**842–8.

Artigas F, Perez V, Alvarez E (1994) Pindolol induces a rapid improvement of depressed patients with serotonin reuptake inhibitors, *Arch Gen Psychiatry* **51:**248–51.

Bakish D, Hooper CL, Thornton M, Wiens A, Miller C, Thibaudeau C (1997) Fast onset: an open labelled study of the treatment of major depressive disorder with nefazodone and pindolol combination treatment, *Int Clin Psychopharmacol* **12:**91–8.

Baumann P, Nil R, Souche A et al (1996) A double-blind, placebo-controlled study of citalopram with and without lithium in the treatment of ther-

apy-resistant depressive patients: a clinical, pharmacokinetic, and pharmacogenetic investigation, *J Clin Psychopharmacol* **16:**307–14.

Bel N, Artigas F (1992) Fluvoxamine preferentially increases extracellular 5-hydroxytryptamine in the raphe nuclei: an in vivo microdialysis study, *Eur J Pharmacol* **229:**101–3.

Benca RM, Obermeyer WH, Thisted RA, Gillin JC (1992) Sleep and psychiatric disorders: a meta-analysis, *Arch Gen Psychiatry* **49:**651–68.

Berman RM, Darnell AM, Miller HL, Anand A, Charney DS (1997) Effect of pindolol in hastening response to fluoxetine in the treatment of major depression: a double-blind, placebo-controlled trial, *Am J Psychiatry* **154:**37–43.

Blier P, Bergeron R (1995) Effectiveness of pindolol with selected antidepressant drugs in the treatment of major depression, *J Clin Psychopharmacol* **15:**217–22.

Blier P, Bergeron R (1996) Sequential administration of augmentation strategies in treatment-resistant obsessive-compulsive disorder: preliminary findings, *Int Clin Psychopharmacol* **11:**37–44.

Blier P, de Montigny C (1983) Electrophysiological studies on the effect of repeated zimelidine administration on serotonergic neurotransmission in the rat, *J Neurosci* **3:**1270–8.

Blier P, de Montigny C (1985a) Serotonergic but not noradrenergic neurons in rat CNS adapt to long-term treatment with monoamine oxidase inhibitors, *Neuroscience* **16:**949–55.

Blier P, de Montigny C (1985b) Short-term lithium administration enhances serotonergic neurotransmission: electrophysiological evidence in the rat CNS, *Eur J Pharmacol* **113:**69–77.

Blier P, de Montigny C (1987) Modifications of 5-HT neuron properties by sustained administration of the 5-HT$_{1A}$ agonist gepirone: electrophysiological studies in the rat brain, *Synapse* **1:**470–80.

Blier P, de Montigny C (1992) Lack of efficacy of lithium augmentation in obsessive-compulsive disorder: the perspective of different regional effects of lithium on serotonin release in the central nervous system, *J Clin Psychopharmacol* **12:**65–6.

Blier P, de Montigny C (1994) Current advances and trends in the treatment of depression, *Trends Pharmacol Sci* **15:**220–6.

Blier P, de Montigny C, Azzaro AJ (1986) Modification of serotonergic and noradrenergic neurotransmission by repeated administration of monoamine oxidase inhibitors: electrophysiological studies in the rat CNS, *J Pharmacol Exp Ther* **227:**987–94.

Blier P, Lista A, de Montigny C (1993) Differential properties of pre- and postsynaptic 5-hydroxytryptamine$_{1A}$ receptors in the dorsal raphe and hippocampus: I—Effect of spiperone, *J Pharmacol Exp Ther* **265:**7–15.

Blier P, Bergeron R, de Montigny C (1997) Selective activation of postsynaptic 5-HT$_{1A}$ receptors produces a rapid antidepressant response, *Neuropsychopharmacology* **16:**333–8.

Chaput Y, de Montigny C, Blier P (1986) Effects of a selective 5-HT reuptake blocker, citalopram, on the sensitivity of 5-HT autoreceptors: electrophysiological studies in the rat, *Naunyn Schmiedebergs Arch Pharmacol* **333:**342–8.

Chaput Y, de Montigny C and Blier P (1991) Presynaptic and postsynaptic modifications of the serotonin system by long-term antidepressant treatments: electrophysiological studies in the rat brain, *Neuropsychopharmacology* **5:**219–29.

de Montigny C (1984) Electroconvulsive shock treatments enhance responsiveness of forebrain neurons to serotonin, *J Pharmacol Exp Ther* **228:**230–4.

de Montigny C (1994) Lithium addition in treatment-resistant depression, *Int Clin Psychopharmacol* **9**(suppl 2): 31–5.

de Montigny C, Aghajanian GK (1978) Tricyclic antidepressants: long-term treatment increases responsivity of rat forebrain neurons to serotonin, *Science* **202:**1303–6.

de Montigny C, Blier P (1991) Development of selective agonists of postsynaptic 5-HT$_{1A}$ receptors: a future direction in the pharmacotherapy of affective disorders? In: Meltzer HY, Nerozzi D, eds, *Current Practices and Future Developments in the Pharmacotherapy of Mental Disorders* (Elsevier: Amsterdam) 99–104.

de Montigny C, Chaput Y, Blier P (1993) Classical and novel targets for antidepressant drugs, *Int Acad Biomed Drug Res* **5:**8–17.

Delgado PL, Charney DS, Price LH, Aghajanian GK, Landis H, Heninger GR (1990) Serotonin function and the mechanism of antidepressant action. Reversal of antidepressant induced remission by rapid depletion of plasma tryptophan, *Arch Gen Psychiatry* **47:**411–18.

Dinan TG, Barry S (1989) A comparison of electroconvulsive therapy with a combined lithium and tricyclic combination among depressed tricyclic nonresponders, *Acta Psychiatr Scand* **80:**97–100.

Ebert D, Jaspert A, Murata H, Kaschka WP (1995) Initial lithium augmentation improves the antidepressant effects of standard TCA treatment in non-resistant depressed patients, *Psychopharmacology* **118:**223–5.

El Mansari M, Blier P (1997) *In vivo* electrophysiological characterization of 5-HT receptors in the guinea pig head of caudate nucleus and orbitofrontal cortex, *Neuropharmacology* (in press).

Fletcher A, Forster EA, Bill DJ et al (1996) Electrophysiological, biochemical, neurohormonal and behavioural studies with WAY-100635, a potent, selective and silent 5-HT 1A, *Behav Brain Res* **73:**337–53.

Guelfi JD, White C, Hackett D, Guichoux JY, Magni G (1995) Effectiveness of venlafaxine in patients hospitalized for major depression and melancholia, *J Clin Psychiatry* **56:**450–8.

Haddjeri N, de Montigny C, Blier P (1997) Modulation of the firing activity of norepinephrine neurons in the locus coeruleus by the serotonin system, *Br J Pharmacol* **120:**865–75.

Invernizzi R, Bramante M, Samanin R (1996) Role of 5-HT$_{1A}$ receptors in the effects of acute and chronic fluoxetine on extracellular serotonin in the frontal cortex, *Pharmacol Biochem Behav* **54:**143–7.

Joffe RT, Schuller DR (1993) An open study of buspirone augmentation of serotonin reuptake inhibitors in refractory depression, *J Clin Psychiatry* **54:**269–71.

Kreiss DH, Lucki I (1995) Effects of acute and repeated administration of antidepressant drugs on extracellular levels of 5-hydroxytryptamine measured in vivo, *J Pharmacol Exp Ther* **274:**866–76.

Liebowitz MR, Quitkin FM, Steward JW et al (1988) Antidepressant specificity in atypical depression, *Arch Gen Psychiatry* **45:**129–37.

Lingjaerde O, Edbend AH, Gormsen CA et al (1974) The effect of lithium carbonate in combination with tricyclic antidepressants in endogenous depression, *Acta Psychiatr Scand* **50:**233–42.

Maes M, Vandoolaeghe E, Desnyder R (1996) Efficacy of treatment with trazodone in combination with pindolol or fluoxetine in major depression, *J Affect Disord* **41:**201–10.

Menkes DB, Aghajanian GK, McCall RB (1980) Chronic antidepressant treatment enhances alpha-adrenergic and serotonergic responses in the facial nucleus, *Life Sci* **27:**45–55.

Moreno FA, Delgado PL, Bachark, Gelenberg AJ (1996) Pindolol augmentation in treatment-resistant depressed patients, *Psychopharmacol Bull* **32:**492.

Nelson JC, Mazure CM, Bowers MB, Jaltow PI (1991) A preliminary, open study of the combination of fluoxetine and desipramine for rapid treatment of major depression, *Arch Gen Psychiatry* **48:**303–7.

Nick J, Wante JP, Des Lauriers A, Moinet A, Monfort J (1976) L'Association clomipramine-lithium: essay contrôle *Encephale* **2:**5–26.

Perez V, Gilaberte I, Faries D, Alvarez E, Artigas F (1997) Randomised, double-blind, placebo-controlled trial of pindolol in combination with fluoxetine antidepressant treatment, *Lancet* (in press).

Post RM, Uhde TW, Rubinow DR, Huggins T (1987) Differential time course of antidepressant effects after sleep deprivation, ECT, and carbamazepine: clinical and theoretical implications, *Psychiatr Res* **22:**11–19.

Rich CL, Spiker DG, Jewell SW, Neil JF, Black NA (1984) The efficiency of ECT: I. Response in depressive episodes, *Psychiatr Res* **11:**167–76.

Robinson DS, Rickels K, Feighner J et al (1990) Clinical effects of the 5-HT$_{1A}$ partial agonists in depression: a composite analysis of buspirone in the treatment of depression, *J Clin Psychopharmacol* **10:**67S–76S.

Rodger CR, Scott AI, Whalley LJ (1994) Is there a delay in the onset of the antidepressant effect of electroconvulsive therapy? *Br J Psychiatry* **164:**106–9.

Romero L, Bel N, Artigas F, de Montigny C, Blier P (1996) Effect of pindolol at pre- and postsynaptic 5-HT$_{1A}$ receptors: in vivo microdialysis and electrophysiological studies in the rat brain, *Neuropsychopharmacology* **15:**349–60.

Rutter JJ, Gundlah C, Auerbach SB (1994) Increase in extracellular serotonin produced by uptake inhibitors is enhanced after chronic treatment with fluoxetine, *Neurosci Lett* **171:**183–6.

Segman RH, Shapira B, Gorfine M, Lerer B (1995) Onset and time course of antidepressant action: psychopharmacological implications of a controlled trial of electroconvulsive therapy, *Psychopharmacology* **119:** 440–8.

Shahal B, Piel E, Mecz C, Kremer I, Klein E (1996) Lack of advantage for imipramine combined with lithium versus imipramine alone in the treatment of major depression. *Biol Psychiat* **40:**1181–3.

Tome MB, Isaac MT, Harte R, Holland C (1997) Paroxetine and pindolol: a randomized trial of serotonergic autoreceptor blockade in the reduction of antidepressant latency, *Int Clin Psychopharmacol* **12:**81–90.

Vinar O, Vinarova E, Horacek J (1996) Pindolol accelerates the therapeutic action of selective serotonin reuptake inhibitors (SSRI) in depression, *Homeostasis* **37:**93–5.

Weilburg JB, Rosenbaum JF, Biederman J, Sachs GS, Pollack MH, Kelly K (1989) Fluoxetine added to non-MAOI antidepressants converts nonresponders to responders: a preliminary report, *J Clin Psychiatry* **50:**447–9.

Zajecka JM, Jeffriess H, Fawcett J (1995) The efficacy of fluoxetine combined with a heterocyclic antidepressant in treatment-resistant depression: a retrospective analysis, *J Clin Psychiatry* **56:**338–43.

16

Synergistic effects of serotonergic and noradrenergic antidepressants in combination

J Craig Nelson

During the past decade, several new antidepressants have been introduced. The clinician now has an array of different antidepressants available to treat depression. Yet all available antidepressants have a delayed onset of action. Quitkin reported that 'true drug effects' may take 5–6 weeks to develop or to be distinguishable from those of placebo (Quitkin et al, 1984). The design of that study included gradual dosing over the first 18 days, and this may account for part of the delay; nevertheless, there is general agreement that all antidepressants show some delay in their effects. Furthermore, 25–35% of depressed patients fail to respond to the first antidepressant agent (Nelson, 1997a). For these reasons, the development of antidepressants which have more rapid effects and which are more effective would be highly desirable.

Recently, the selective serotonin reuptake inhibitors (SSRIs) have become popular for the treatment of depression (Nelson et al, 1995). These drugs appear to cause fewer subjective side effects, and fewer serious side effects which result in termination of treatment. They are safe in overdose, and appear to be relatively free of cardiac complications. They are more convenient to use than the tricyclic antidepressants. SSRIs are usually given once a day and often require minimal dose adjustment.

Nevertheless, there have been concerns that these agents, which are relatively selective for the serotonin system, may have a narrower spectrum of action than the tricyclic antidepressants. In two previous studies (Danish University Antidepressant Group, 1986, 1990) comparing clomipramine with either citalopram or paroxetine, the Danish University group demonstrated greater efficacy for the tricyclic in the treatment of severely depressed inpatients. The differences were significant and meaningful.

It is possible that drugs with a broader spectrum of action might be more effective. Specifically, drugs that have both noradrenergic and serotonergic effects might treat a broader range of patients and, perhaps, would be more rapidly acting. The latter was suggested by a preclinical study of Baron et al (1988) which found that the combination of desipramine and fluoxetine downregulated β-adrenergic receptors more rapidly than either agent alone. This downregulation occurred quickly, within 4 days of treatment. An alternative hypothesis, although not contradictory to the former, suggests that adequate serotonergic function is necessary for noradrenergic downregulation. This has sometimes been referred to as the permissive hypothesis (Brunello et al, 1982).

Finally, it appears that both norepinephrine and serotonin (5-HT) are involved in mediating antidepressant response. A series of studies using tryptophan depletion or α-methyl-p-tyrosine (AMPT) have demonstrated that both neurotransmitters are involved in the regulation of antidepressant action. In the first study (Delgado et al, 1990), depressed patients, who had been successfully treated, were rapidly depleted of tryptophan using an amino acid diet. Relapse occurred within hours of the administration of this diet. On inspection of the data, Delgado et al found that patients who had been treated with serotonergic antidepressants were more likely to relapse, while those treated with noradrenergic agents were relatively unaffected. Administration of this amino acid drink to untreated, depressed patients had little effect (Delgado et al, 1994). The authors concluded that the findings of this challenge paradigm suggested that serotonin is involved in mediating antidepressant action, but that the study did not directly address the role of serotonin in the neurophysiology of depression.

Subsequently, studies using AMPT to block synthesis of catecholamines produced relapse in depressed patients who had been successfully treated with noradrenergic antidepressants, while those treated with serotonergic agents were relatively unaffected (Miller et al, 1996). Taken together, these findings suggest that both norepinephrine and serotonin are involved in mediating antidepressant response. From this, it is hypothesized that drugs combining both effects might have a broader spectrum of action.

Open clinical trials

Weilberg et al (1989) at Massachusetts General Hospital in Boston demonstrated the possible advantages of this combination in a series of 30 depressed outpatients, who had been refractory to prior treatment. Most of these patients had been treated for an extended period, an average of 11 months, without response. Most patients were receiving tricyclic antidepressants, the agents commonly used at that time. Fluoxetine was added to their ongoing antidepressant treatment. Twenty-six of the 30 patients responded.

Seth et al (1992) described a series of eight patients, most of whom were elderly, who had been quite refractory to prior treatments, including electroconvulsive therapy (ECT). Each of the patients responded to the combination of a noradrenergic tricyclic, usually nortriptyline, with an SSRI.

Boyer and Feighner (1995) described an open trial, using the combination of fluoxetine and bupropion in 23 patients. The noradrenergic effects of bupropion and its metabolites were intended to complement the serotonergic effects of fluoxetine. The 23 patients described had been refractory to treatment with either fluoxetine or bupropion alone. The second drug was then added to the first. Both sequences occurred. Eight of 23 (35%) of the patients had a moderate or marked response. Six of 23 (26%) had minimal response. The remaining nine patients (39%) had an adverse reaction which required termination of treatment. The adverse reactions were described as typical of either drug individually. No seizures were observed. Nevertheless, this rate of adverse reactions is one of the highest reported for any augmentation strategy (Nelson, 1997b).

Studies with desipramine and fluoxetine

On the basis of an earlier preclinical report suggesting rapid effects with the combination of desipramine and fluoxetine (Baron et al, 1988), we conducted a preliminary, open study with this combination (Nelson et al, 1991). Fourteen patients received desipramine (DMI) and fluoxetine. They were compared with 52 patients, previously treated in the same setting, with DMI alone. All patients had non-psychotic, unipolar, major depression. Desipramine was administered in a standardized fashion to the patients in the combined treatment group, as well as to those receiving DMI alone. A 24-h blood level was obtained after a standardized test dose. This level was determined and then used to calculate the dose necessary to achieve an adequate plasma level of desipramine (Nelson et al, 1982). This method has been previously described (Nelson et al, 1987). In patients receiving the combination, the dose was further adjusted, anticipating the enzyme-inhibiting effects of fluoxetine (Preskorn et al, 1990). Desipramine was then administered for a 4-week period. In the combined treatment group, fluoxetine was administered for the first 2 weeks, and then discontinued. This was done for two reasons. First, we were interested in differences in response during the first 2 weeks. Second, patients receiving fluoxetine for 2 weeks will continue to have significant plasma levels of fluoxetine for at least another 2 weeks following its withdrawal. All patients were treated in the same setting, and depression was rated using the 17-item Hamilton Depression Scale.

The demographic characteristics of the two groups were comparable, in terms of age, gender, initial Hamilton score, prior episodes and episode duration. Other characteristics were examined, some of which, e.g. prior drug failure and personality disorder, have previously been shown to predict poor response to DMI (Nelson et al, 1994). Again, the combined treatment group appeared comparable to the group receiving DMI alone with respect to these variables.

The group receiving combined treatment responded more quickly to the combination. Hamilton scores dropped more quickly, they were significantly different after 1 week of treatment, and they remained significantly different throughout the 4 weeks of the trial (Figure 16.1). Percentage improvement on the Hamilton scale was also significantly different in the two groups, with patients receiving combined treatment showing, essentially, twice the level of improvement as those receiving DMI alone during the first 2 weeks of treatment. At 1 week, the combined treatment group had improved 42% on the Ham-D versus 20% in the patients on DMI alone. At 2 weeks, the rates of improvement were 60% and 30%, respectively. Both differences were significant (Mann Whitney U test, $p < 0.01$).

Mean Hamilton scores, however, are of limited value for assessing speed of response. Mean Hamilton scores reflect two different dimensions—speed of response and frequency of response. If speed of onset is the issue, then inclusion of Ham-D scores of non-responders obscures the results. For this reason, another analysis was performed, limiting the sample to those patients who were rated as either much improved or very much improved on a CGI rating at the conclusion of the trial. In these responders, mean Hamilton scores were assessed again, and now more clearly reflected speed of response. Again, significant differences were noted as early as 1 week (Figure 16.2). The magnitude of the difference appeared to increase at the second week.

Another method of assessing response is to determine the time to achieve a response criterion. Figure 16.3 shows the cumulative number

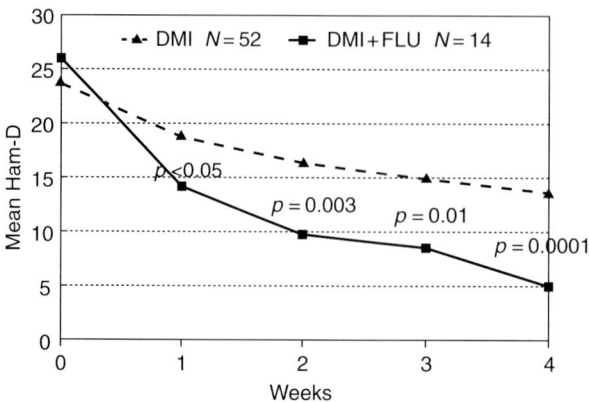

Figure 16.1

Weekly Hamilton Depression Rating (Ham-D) scores in 14 patients on desipramine and fluoxetine and 52 patients receiving desipramine alone.

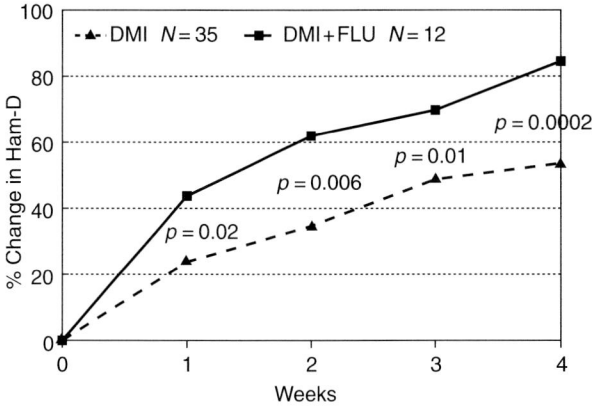

Figure 16.2

Weekly percentage improvement in Ham-D scores in responders who were rated as much or very much improved on the CGI scale at the end of treatment.

of responders for each week during the trial. In this case, we used a stringent criterion for remission. The criterion required 75% improvement in the Hamilton Scale and a final score of less than 7. In this analysis, differences were not apparent in the first week. However, from the second week on, there is a substantially higher percentage of the sample remitting each week with the combination. Relatively few patients receiving DMI alone actually remitted during the 4 weeks of the trial.

An important question relative to efficacy is to what extent the drug interaction might explain the greater effectiveness of the combination. It is well established that fluoxetine inhibits the cytochrome P450 2D6

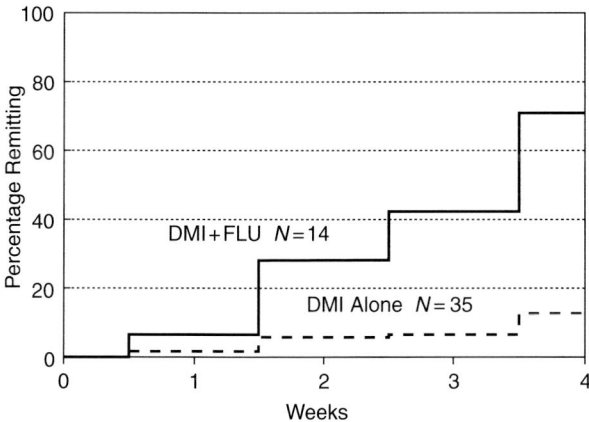

Figure 16.3

Cumulative percentage remitting over 4 weeks of treatment with the combination of fluoxetine and desipramine or desipramine alone. Remission = 75% improvement on the Ham-D and a final Ham-D <7.

isoenzyme which metabolizes desipramine (Preskorn et al, 1990), resulting in higher DMI blood levels. However, we anticipated this interaction
and reduced the DMI dose in the combined treatment group. In fact, total
blood levels of DMI and the active metabolite hydroxydesipramine were
nearly identical at week 1 in the combined treatment and DMI-alone
groups, and were not significantly different at weeks 3 and 4. At week 2,
there was a trend for higher levels to be achieved in the combined treatment group ($p = 0.09$). However, in fact, the patient with the highest
blood level did less well. It appeared unlikely that differences in blood
levels explained the greater effectiveness of the combination.

We now have information about the interaction of fluoxetine and DMI in
27 patients treated with the combination. Comparing the actual plasma
concentration obtained with the initial predicted level, we found a three-
fold increase in DMI levels in patients who were initially rapid metabolizers of DMI (as indicated by their 24-h level). In patients who were slow
metabolizers of DMI, fluoxetine has less effect, raising DMI levels only
about 50%. Another way to conceptualize this interaction is that fluoxetine converts rapid metabolizers of DMI to slow metabolizers. If a patient
is already a slow metabolizer, that patient will be less affected. During
combined treatment, the actual doses of DMI ranged from 50 to 225 mg,
but most patients received doses of 75–125 mg per day.

Overall, this combination was safe. There were no unusual side effects.
The side effects that did occur appeared to be typical of each agent, e.g.
nausea or orthostatic hypotension. Because of the drug interaction
between the compounds and the potential for toxicity during combined
treatment, blood level monitoring is advised.

Implications of the findings

The data from the preliminary study described above, as well as the other
open studies described, suggest that the combination of a noradrenergic
agent and a serotonergic agent may enhance efficacy and may be more
rapidly effective. The mechanism of this enhanced efficacy is less clear. The
findings would be consistent with the hypothesis of rapid downregulation of
β-adrenergic receptors, but another study found that the combination of
yohimbine and DMI, which rapidly downregulates β-receptors, was not clinically effective (Charney et al, 1986). Furthermore, Sulser has suggested that
the initial studies reporting a permissive action of the serotonin system,
enabling downregulation of noradrenergic receptors, were misinterpreted
(see Chapter 5). Perhaps the simplest and most compelling hypothesis is
that if serotonin and norepinephrine both mediate antidepressant response,
then a combination of the two might enhance treatment. This hypothesis has
been the basis of recent drug development. For example, both venlafaxine
and mirtazepine appear to have effects on both serotonergic and noradren-

ergic systems, and at least one study has suggested greater efficacy of one of these dual-action agents than fluoxetine in severely depressed, melancholic inpatients (Clerc et al, 1994).

Although the logical hypothesis that combination of a noradrenergic and a serotonergic effect might have a broader spectrum of action seems plausible, it is less clear why this combination would necessarily be more rapidly acting. If the preliminary findings described here for the combination of fluoxetine and DMI are replicated in controlled studies, the basis for the more rapid effects would need to be further explored.

It is difficult to separate rapid onset of action from greater general efficacy. They may reflect the same pharmacologic action. It is noted, however, that there have been two augmentation studies adding T_3 (Prange et al, 1969) or lithium (Price et al, 1995) at the beginning of treatment, in which greater improvement was noted with augmentation after 1–2 weeks of treatment, but not after 4 weeks. In these two studies, the combination was more rapid but not more effective in the long run. These findings suggest that it might be possible to enhance speed of onset without affecting final outcome.

Conclusions

The findings of the current preliminary study, as well as the previous open studies which have combined serotonergic agents with noradrenergic antidepressants, suggest enhanced efficacy and, perhaps, greater speed of response for the combination. This has important implications for future drug development. It also has implications for augmentation strategies in patients started on selective agents who fail to respond. In these patients, a second agent can be added to complement the first. Finally, the data presented do not tell us much about the side effects encountered. In the study of fluoxetine and bupropion described above (Boyer and Feighner, 1995), the discontinuation rate because of side effects was relatively high, although this has not been described in the other studies. It is logical to assume that the addition of two agents, which have effects on two different systems, will increase side effects, i.e. the side effects associated with serotonin will be added to the side effects associated with norepinephrine. There are some differences in terms of the drugs employed. If a tricyclic antidepressant is employed, orthostatic hypotension will be more frequent and cardiac conduction problems may occur. The newer agents, which employ combined mechanisms, do not appear to have cardiac effects and do not appear to be associated with orthostatic hypotension. Finally, the concept of additive side effects may be simplistic and there may be conditions in which the addition of a second agent may actually reduce side effects. For example, it has been suggested that bupropion helps to reduce or reverse sexual dysfunction associated with an SSRI (Labbate and Pollack, 1994). Although there are no controlled data to support this finding, it is an interesting possibility that combined-action drugs might reduce some side effects.

● Acknowledgment

This work was supported in part by MH 47894 from the NIMH.

References

Baron BM, Ogden AM, Siegel BW, Stegman J, Ursillo RC, Dudley MW (1988) Rapid down regulation of β-adrenoceptors by co-administration of desipramine and fluoxetine, *Eur J Pharmacol* **154:**125–34.

Boyer WF, Feighner JP (1995) The combined use of fluoxetine and bupropion. Presented at the Annual Meeting of the APA, 27 May.

Brunello N, Baraccia ML, Chuang D-M, Costa E (1982) Down-regulation of B-adrenergic receptors following repeated injections of desmethylimipramine: permissive role of serotonergic axons, *Neuropharmacology* **21:** 1145–9.

Charney DS, Price LH, Heninger GR (1986) Desipramine–yohimbine combination treatment of refractory depression, *Arch Gen Psychiatry* **43:**1155–61.

Clerc GE, Ruimy P, Verdeau-Pailles J (1994) A double-blind comparison of venlafaxine and fluoxetine in patients hospitalized for major depression and melancholia, *Int Clin Psychopharmacol* **9:**138–43.

Danish University Antidepressant Group (1986) Citalopram: clinical effect profile in comparison with clomipramine. A controlled multicenter study, *Psychopharmacology* **90:**131–8.

Danish University Antidepressant Group (1990) Paroxetine: a selective serotonin reuptake inhibitor showing better tolerance, but weaker antidepressant effect than clomipramine in a controlled multicenter study, *J Affect Disord* **18:**289–99.

Delgado PL, Charney DS, Price LH et al (1990) Serotonin function and the mechanism of antidepressant action. Reversal of antidepressant-induced remission by rapid depletion of plasma tryptophan, *Arch Gen Psychiatry* **47:**411–18.

Delgado PL, Price LH, Miller HL et al (1994) Serotonin and the neurobiology of depression, *Arch Gen Psychiatry* **51:**865–74.

Labbate LA, Pollack MH (1994) Treatment of fluoxetine-induced sexual dysfunction with bupropion: a case report, *Ann Clin Psychiatry* **6:**13–15.

Miller HL, Delgado P, Salomon R et al (1996) Clinical and biochemical effects of catecholamine depletion on antidepressant-induced remission of depression, *Arch Gen Psychiatry* **53:** 117–28.

Nelson JC (1997a) Treatment of refractory depression, *Depression* (in press).

Nelson JC (1997b) Augmentation strategies for treatment of unipolar major depression. In: Rush AJ, ed., *Modern Problems of Pharmacopsychiatry*, Vol. 25 Treatment Algorithms (S Karger: Basel) in press.

Nelson JC, Jatlow P, Quinlan DM, Bowers MB Jr (1982) Desipramine plasma concentrations and antidepressant response, *Arch Gen Psychiatry* **39:**1419–22.

Nelson JC, Jatlow PI, Mazure C (1987) Rapid desipramine dose adjustment using 24-hour levels, *J Clin Psychopharmacol* **7:**72–7.

Nelson JC, Mazure CM, Bowers MB et al (1991) A preliminary, open study of the combination of fluoxetine and desipramine for rapid treatment of major depression, *Arch Gen Psychiatry* **48:**303–7.

Nelson JC, Mazure CM, Jatlow PI (1994) Characteristics of desipramine refractory depression, *J Clin Psychiatry* **55:**12–19.

Nelson JC, Casper S, Docherty JP, Henschen GM, Nierenberg AA, Ward NG (1995) Algorithm for the treatment of unipolar depression (for the International Algorithm Project), *Psychopharmacol Bull* **31:**475–82.

Prange AJ, Wilson IC, Rabon AM et al (1969) Enhancement of imipramine antidepressant activity by thyroid hormone, *Am J Psychiatry* **126:**457–69.

Preskorn SH, Beber JH, Faul JC, Hirschfeld RMA (1990) Serious adverse effects of combining fluoxetine and tricyclic antidepressants, *Am J Psychiatry* **147:**532.

Price LH, Cappiello AC, McDougle CJ, Malison RT, Charney DS, Heninger GR (1995) Lithium plus desipramine versus desipramine alone in the treatment of major depression: a controlled study. Annual Meeting of the APA, 23 May, 1995.

Quitkin FM, Rabkin JG, Ross D, McGrath P (1984) Duration of antidepressant drug treatment, *Arch Gen Psychiatry* **41:**238–45.

Seth R, Jennings AL, Bindman J et al (1992) Combination treatment with noradrenaline and serotonin reuptake inhibitors in resistant depression, *Br J Psychiatry* **161:**562–5.

Weilburg JB, Rosenbaum JF, Biederman J et al (1989) Fluoxetine added to non-MAOI antidepressants converts nonresponders to responders: a preliminary report, *J Clin Psychiatry* **50:**447–9.

17
Suicide prevention: the role of antidepressants

Luc Mequies, Martine Jasson, Claudine Soubrie and Alain J Puech

While suicide is one of the most severe and frequent complications of depressive states, proof of antidepressant efficacy in preventing suicide and attempted suicide is lacking.

This chapter reviews available data from clinical trials and pharmacoepidemiology.

Direct effects of antidepressants on suicidal behavior

It is obvious that clinical trials attempting to assess the effectiveness and tolerance of a specific antidepressant lack the power to determine if it has a positive (or negative) effect on the suicidal behavior of depressed patients, given the incidence of suicidal behavior, the small number of patients included and the usually short treatment period of these trials.

A clinical trial of sufficient power (i.e. one with a placebo control group) is unimaginable for technical (several thousand patients treated for 6 months to 1 year) as well as ethical reasons. In theory, only a meta-analysis that brings together several weak studies can shed some light on this question.

However, a clinical trial by Rouillon et al (1989) obtained unexpected results. The objective of this trial was to assess the effectiveness of two different doses of maprotiline against a placebo in preventing relapses of depressive episodes. Patients who responded after 2 months of open treatment with maprotiline were then randomly assigned to one of three groups and treated for 12 months. The statistical power of this trial was calculated in order to differentiate the two doses of maprotiline. For this reason, the number of patients included was unusually high (placebo = 374, maprotiline = 777).

The results showed that relapse rates for the maprotiline group were significantly lower than for the placebo control group, and better results were obtained with the higher of the two doses of maprotiline. On the contrary, and unexpectedly so, suicidal behavior was more common in the maprotiline groups. This difference was statistically significant (for suicide attempts): maprotiline, 5 suicides and 9 attempts; placebo, 1 suicide and 0 attempts.

As is the case in the majority of clinical trials, patients not responding to treatment were not followed up once they dropped out of the study. The length of time for which the placebo group was observed was therefore shorter than for the maprotiline groups, due to the unequal rates of failure to respond to the different treatment doses.

After this trial was published, various authors speculated on the possibility that a treatment could alleviate depressive symptoms while leaving suicidal behavior unchanged or, worse still, aggravating it.

Conversely, the various published meta-analyses conducted favor

Table 17.1   Fluoxetine meta-analysis (Tollefson et al, 1993).

	Suicidal acts (%)	Risk difference (95% CI)	p
Placebo n = 637	0.8	−0.2	NS
Fluoxetine n = 1.434	0.3	(−1.1, 0.6)	
TCA n = 1.560	0.5	0.4	NS
Fluoxetine n = 1.623	1	(−0.2, 1.0)	

NS, not significant; TCA, tricyclic antidepressant; CI, confidence interval.

Table 17.2   Paroxetine meta-analysis (Montgomery et al, 1995).

	Placebo n = 554 72 PEY	Paroxetine n = 2963 1008 PEY	Active controls n = 1151 218 PEY
Suicides n (%)	2 (0.36)	5 (0.17)	3 (0.26)
n/PEY	0.028	0.005	0.014
Attempted suicides n (%)	6 (1.1)	40 (1.3)	12 (1.0)
n/PEY	0.083	0.04	0.055

PEY, patient exposure years.

Table 17.3   Milnacipran meta-analysis (unpublished data).

	Placebo n = 394 59 PEY	Milnacipran n = 4006 975 PEY	TCA n = 940 177 PEY	SSRI n = 344 47 PEY
Suicides (n)	4	14	3	1
n/PEY	0.066	0.014	0.017	0.02
Suicide attempts (n)	10	49	13	10
n/PEY	0.16	0.049	0.07	0.2

TCA, tricyclic antidepressant; SSRI, selective serotonin reuptake inhibitor; PEY, patient exposure years.

treatment with active products even if, as we shall see, the differences observed are not statistically significant (see Tables 17.1, 17.2 and 17.3).

The results of a meta-analysis of the effects of fluoxetine on suicide (Tollefson et al, 1993) show that fluoxetine is a more effective treatment than a placebo but it is less effective than tricyclics. This difference is not statistically significant in spite of the large number of patients studied.

It is worth noting that the incidence of suicidal behavior in the fluoxetine group varies (0.3 versus 1) with the product it is compared with, suggesting that, regardless of the inclusion criteria retained, patients participating in studies for which there is no placebo control group are more severely depressed.

The paroxetine meta-analysis published by Montgomery et al (1995) (Table 17.2) analyzes the results in a different way: patients receiving paroxetine were placed in one of two groups, depending on whether they had just completed a placebo control group trial or a leading treatment control group trial. The frequency of events was adjusted for the length of treatment. The results are thus expressed in PEY (patient exposure years). This meta-analysis found a 2–4-fold decrease in the number of suicides and attempted suicides, but these results are not significant in spite of the large number of subjects included.

As can be seen, the incidence of suicide in the placebo control group is small (0.028%). This is lower than the rate found by Jick et al (1995) for treated depressed patients not included in the study. There is, then, an inclusion bias in placebo control group trials that are carried out on low-risk subjects.

The milnacipran meta-analyses (Table 17.3) give the same types of result. The placebo control group has a suicide risk of 0.06% and an attempted suicide risk of 0.16%. Milnacipran reduces these figures by three or four times, as do the tricyclics, but these differences are not statistically significant.

These three meta-analyses show that the patients included in these placebo control group trials were selected because they presented a low suicide risk, and rightly so. Under these circumstances, even when a large number of patients is studied, the reduction in suicide risk is not significant. It is likely that, if four or five of these analyses were grouped together, this reduction in suicide risk would become significant. These results can be considered reassuring. Contrary to what happened in the maprotilin study, an increase in the risk of suicide was never reported; in fact, it was reduced by a factor of two to four.

Effects of antidepressants on suicidal ideation

The most common assessment criterion used in antidepressant trials is the global score on a depression scale (Hamilton or MADRS) or the percentage of subjects improved by more than 50% based on these scales.

If the effects of antidepressants on suicide are to be studied, the question of the extent to which antidepressants work in a homogeneous manner on all symptoms and how effective they are on suicidal ideation in particular should be raised. Their demonstrated effectiveness on the 'suicidal ideation' item of the depression scales is relevant only if there are compelling reasons to think that it is more predictive of suicide attempts than any other item in the scale or the global score. Lately, there has been much debate on this subject. Some authors have implied that antidepressants (or certain antidepressants) can aggravate suicidal ideation or increase suicide attempts at the beginning of treatment.

In 1990, Fawcett et al (1990) published a significant article on factors predicting suicide based on a study of 954 depressed patients with a 10-year follow-up. Thirty-two suicides occurred, approximately 3% of the group. This study showed that suicidal ideation is not a short-term predictor of suicide, while loss of interest or pleasure, anxiety and insomnia are. Suicidal ideation, on the contrary, is a long-term predictor of suicide but to a lesser degree than hopelessness.

Another study with the same objectives (Goldstein et al, 1991) (Table 17.4) treated 1906 depressed subjects for 2–3 years. Forty-six suicides (2.4%) occurred. Among the risk factors assessed by these authors, the significative ones were sex, the number of prior attempts and, above all, the presence or absence of suicidal ideation at the time of inclusion in the study (odds ratio significant to 1.8).

A case-control study was also conducted on the milnacipran trials database. The cases are suicides or attempted suicides. The controls are subjects matched by sex, age, antidepressant, length of treatment and clinical trial.

When the odds ratios for the different items of the MADRS at inclusion (D_0) as well as just prior to an attempted suicide (D_n) are examined (Table 17.5), the greatest ratio (and also the most significant) is that

Table 17.4   Factors influencing suicide in 1906 depressed patients (Goldstein et al, 1991).

	Odds ratio (95% CI)
Sex M/F	1.9 (1.0, 3.4)
Suicidal ideation on index admission	1.8 (1.0, 3.4)
Number of prior suicide attempts	
None (reference)	1
1	1.4 (1.1, 1.7)
2	1.9 (1.2, 3.0)
3	2.7 (1.4, 5.3)
⩾4	3.7 (1.5, 9.2)

CI, confidence interval.

Table 17.5   Milnacipran database.

	Cases n = 74	Controls[a] n = 182	Odds ratio	95% CI	p
MADRS, Day 0	m (sd)	m (sd)			
Total score	34.3 (6.2)	32.3 (6.8)	1.05	1.00–1.09	0.05
Apparent sadness	4.2 (1.1)	3.9 (1.1)	1.4	1.0–1.8	0.04
Reported sadness	4.1 (0.9)	3.9 (1.0)	1.2	0.9–1.7	0.25
Inner tension	3.3 (1.1)	3.4 (1.0)	0.9	0.7–1.2	0.65
Inability to feel	3.6 (1.1)	3.3 (1.0)	1.2	0.9–1.6	0.13
Suicidal thought	2.6 (1.4)	2.1 (1.3)	1.4	1.1–1.9	0.005
MADRS, Day n					
Total score	21.6 (13.1)	18.1 (11.8)	1.05	1.02–1.08	0.002
Apparent sadness	2.5 (1.7)	2.0 (1.6)	1.5	1.1–1.8	0.002
Reported sadness	2.3 (1.6)	2.1 (1.5)	1.2	1.0–1.6	0.08
Inner tension	2.3 (1.4)	2.2 (1.4)	1.2	0.9–1.5	0.20
Inability to feel	2.2 (1.4)	1.8 (1.4)	1.4	1.1–1.7	0.01
Suicidal thought	1.7 (1.5)	1.0 (1.1)	1.9	1.4–2.6	0.0001

[a]Paired on: sex, age, antidepressant, follow-up and trial; m, mean; sd, standard deviation.

obtained for suicidal ideation. These three studies show that it is reasonable to believe that suicidal ideation is a more significant predictor of suicide attempts than any other item and that it is therefore relevant to observe the effect of antidepressants on suicidal ideation.

Several meta-analyses have been published to evaluate the effect of antidepressants on the 'suicidal ideation' item.

A fluoxetine meta-analysis was published by Beasley et al (1991). This meta-analysis looked at 17 trials, or the equivalent of 1765 depressed patients treated with fluoxetine, 731 with tricyclics and 569 in the placebo groups. Patients were categorized according to whether suicidal ideation emerged, increased or decreased (Table 17.6). For this population, which at the beginning of the trials had low suicidal ideation scores (item 3, Hamilton = 1, 2), the percentage of emergence or aggravation was of the same magnitude and not significant for any of the three groups. However, suicidal ideation, on the contrary, decreased significantly for groups receiving active products compared to the placebo control group.

Table 17.6   Meta-analysis of fluoxetine.

	Emergence %	Worsening %	Improvement %
Placebo	2.6	17.9	54.8
Fluoxetine	1.2	15.3	72.2
TCA	3.6	16.3	69.8

Baseline HDRS total ≃ 26, Item 3 ≃ 1.2.
Emergence = 0 or 1 → 3 or 4.
Worsening = any increase, any time.
Improvement = any decrease from baseline to the last observation.

Another meta-analysis (Tollefson et al, 1993) was carried out on all flu-oxetine trials for conditions other than depression (e.g. bulimia, obesity, obsessive-compulsive disorder). As subjects did not present suicidal ideation at the beginning of the study, it is difficult to assess treatment effects on ideation. However, this group is especially interesting if the emergence of suicidal ideation, however weak it may be, is to be studied. This meta-analysis shows that the emergence of suicidal ideation was not more frequent in the fluoxetine group as compared to the placebo control group.

A meta-analysis was conducted (Montgomery et al, 1995) that included 2852 patients treated with paroxetine, 1101 treated with compa-rable products and 544 in the placebo control group. For this population as well, suicidal ideation was also relatively insignificant at the moment of inclusion (1.3). After 6 weeks of treatment with active products, suicidal ideation decreased significantly as compared with the placebo control group. Increases in suicidal ideation during the trial were more common in the placebo control group.

Another meta-analysis that included 1205 depressed patients treated with the benzodiazepine alprazolam (Jonas and Hearron, 1996), 1318 treated with comparable products and 694 in the placebo control group, was car-ried out (Table 17.7). Alprazolam and the comparable products had a more favorable effect on the total depression score than did the placebo.

As far as the 'suicide' item is concerned, the frequency of emergence of suicidal ideation is the same for all three groups. The two groups treated with active products showed more improvement on the 'suicide' item that did the placebo control group. However, the comparable prod-ucts (mainly antidepressants) have more of an effect (that is statistically significant) than does alprazolam, in terms of the percentages of the pop-ulation improved as well as aggravated. This study shows, therefore, that a powerful meta-analysis is able to detect the different effects of two types of treatment as measured by changes in the suicide item, improv-ing the global score. Traditional antidepressants improve responses to the suicide item more than do benzodiazepines, in spite of the effects

Table 17.7   Meta-analysis of alprazolam (Jones et al, 1991).

	n	Improvement (%)	Worsening (%)	Emergence (%)
Placebo	694	57.7	21.5	3.5
Alprazolam	1205	71.9[a]	18.8	4.1
Comparators	1318	76.0[b]	13.2[c]	2.5

Significant difference; relative risk (95% CI).
[a]Alprazolam versus placebo : 1.22 (1.11–1.34).
[b]Alprazolam versus comparators : 0.94 (0.88–0.99).
[c]Alprazolam versus comparators : 1.36 (1.13–1.64).

that benzodiazepines have on the symptoms measured by a large number of the items in the depression scale.

Based on these meta-analyses, it can be concluded that antidepressants (selective serotonin reuptake inhibitors (SSRIs) as well as tricyclics) improve responses to the 'suicidal ideation' item in a way that is proportional to overall improvement. There do not seem to be large differences between antidepressants. The differences described seem to be anecdotal in nature and could not be reproduced. It must be noted, however, that the majority of these studies were conducted with subjects experiencing relatively low levels of suicidal ideation. The results might be different if populations with a high level of suicidal ideation were studied.

In addition, suicidal ideation emerges 1–3% of the time, regardless of the treatment used, and aggravation of suicidal ideation is observed 15–20% of the time regardless of the group of subjects in question, a figure which is approximately equal to the failure to respond to treatment.

Pharmacoepidemiology

Pharmacoepidemiologic studies have assessed the incidence of suicide and the factors that influence it among patients treated with antidepressants. These studies have also attempted to evaluate treatment differences. The largest study of this type was published by Jick et al (1995). It included 172 598 patients treated with antidepressants in the UK for various lengths of time. For this population, 143 suicides were reported, which is equal to 0.085% (CI 0.072, 0.1).

In this large population, it was possible to assess several risk factors

Table 17.8   Adjusted relative risk (95% CI)* (Jick et al, 1995).

Age	<40**	1
	40–59	1.2 (0.7, 1.9)
	>60	0.8 (0.5, 1.3)
Sex	Female**	1
	Male	2.8 (1.9, 4.0)
Dose	Low**	1
	High	2.3 (1.4, 3.7)
History of suicidal behavior	No**	1
	Yes	19.2 (9.5, 38.7)
Previous prescription of antidepressants	No**	1
	Yes	2.8 (1.8, 4.3)

*Adjusted for age, sex and calendar year.
**Reference group.

(Table 17.8). The risk of suicide was found to increase for men (2.8), for subjects who have made prior suicide attempts (19.2) and for those who have already been treated with antidepressants (2.8). Surprisingly, this study does not find that age is a risk factor, although many other studies have shown that the rate of suicide increases with age. Furthermore, the risk is higher for subjects treated with higher doses of antidepressants (2.3). It is likely that subjects receiving higher doses are more severely depressed, and this result shows that, even when they are treated with high doses, severely depressed patients maintain a risk of suicide that is higher than that of mildly depressed patients treated with low doses of antidepressants. The relative risk for patients who have already attempted suicide is much higher in this study (19) than was reported by Goldstein (about 2) (Goldstein et al, 1991). However, the incidence of suicide among severely depressed patients seems about the same in these two powerful studies, since the incidence for patients, severely depressed or not, is very different: 1 per 1000 in Jick's study and 1 per 100 over a 1-year interval in Goldstein's (Table 17.4)

From this large cohort, a case-control study was carried out on 143 cases and 1000 controls. This allowed risks to be compared for the different anti-depressants (Table 17.9). When the observed risk for the most commonly prescribed antidepressant in the UK (dothiepin) is set to 1, it becomes pos-sible to calculate a relative risk for the others, adjusting for age, sex, and calendar year. Few significant differences were observed. However, the risks reported for the tricyclics (amitryptiline, clomipramine, imipramine, lofepramine) are all less than 1. If all tricyclics are grouped together so as to decrease the confidence interval, the suicide risk might decrease for patients treated with tricyclics by 30% as compared to dothiepin.

For patients treated with fluoxetine, the relative risk is 3.8, which is

Table 17.9   Adjusted relative risk estimates of suicide for prescribed antidepressants in cases and controls (Jick et al, 1995).

Antidepressant prescribed	(%) of cases ($n = 143$)	(%) of controls ($n = 1000$)	Adjusted relative risk (95% CI)[a]
Dothiepin[b]	36	36	1.0
Amitriptyline	20	28	0.7 (0.4–1.2)
Clomipramine	6	7	0.8 (0.4–1.8)
Imipramine	5	6	0.7 (0.3–1.7)
Flupenthixol	9	6	1.5 (0.7–3.0)
Lofepramine	3	6	0.5 (0.2–1.6)
Mianserin	8	5	1.6 (0.7–3.3)
Fluoxetine	8	3	3.8 (1.7–8.6)
Doxepin	2	2	1.0 (0.3–3.7)
Trazodone	3	2	1.2 (0.4–4.0)

[a]Adjusted for age, sex, and calendar year; [b]Reference group.

Table 17.10   Antidepressants and suicide (Avery and Winokur, 1978).

	ECT $n = 257$	Adequate antidepressants $n = 71$	Total antidepressants $n = 192$	Neither nor group $n = 71$
Suicide attempts at 6 months of follow-up				
n	2	5	10	2
%	0.8	7	5.2	2.8

ECT, electroconvulsive therapy.

statistically significant. Various authors have suggested that a prescription bias might be occurring, since fluoxetine is prescribed for severely depressed patients for whom the suicide risk is high. Thus, they analyzed a low-risk subgroup (first-time prescription for an antidepressant, no prior suicidal behavior). For this group, the relative risk is equal to 2.1, which is no longer significant.

The authors conclude that there is no difference of risk between antidepressants, but there is still some doubt about this, especially for severely depressed patients. It might also be interesting to compare all tricyclics with fluoxetine for all patients or just for a subgroup.

An older study (Avery and Winokur 1978) that lasted 6 months followed a cohort of patients hospitalized and treated (without randomization) by electroshock therapy, antidepressants or a combination of the two. The incidence of suicide attempts in this probably severely depressed population is high. Of particular interest are the figures for suicide attempts by patients treated by electroshocks. In this group of extremely depressed patients, only two suicide attempts were reported for the 257 patients, or 0.8% (Table 17.10).

Other epidemiologic studies have focused on the percentage of suicides that were committed by patients treated with antidepressants. Isacsson et al (1992a) studied 74 suicides by subjects diagnosed a posteriori to suffer from depression. Fifty-five per cent of these patients were seen by a medical doctor within the 90 days preceding their suicide. A diagnosis of depression was made for 36%, antidepressants were prescribed for 22% and subjects were positive for antidepressants in toxicology.

Other studies with larger numbers of subjects, 3400 (Isacsson et al, 1994b) and 1600 (Marzuk et al 1995) have found toxic doses of antidepressants in 16%. All these figures demonstrate the extent to which patients do not seek medical aid, the lack of a proper diagnosis of depression, inadequately prescribed antidepressants even when depression is diagnosed, and difficulties in monitoring the patient once an antidepressant is prescribed.

There have been many studies that have tried to evaluate the relative toxicity of antidepressants. It is not possible, in the scope of this chapter, to review them all. Just to mention one briefly, Kapur et al (1992) assessed the relative risk of a prior suicide attempt and that of dying from an overdose. There were no differences found between various antidepressants and the risk associated with prior suicide attempts, but there was, however, a significant difference between antidepressants. This risk of overdose increased 16 times for desipramine with respect to a less toxic antidepressant like trazodone.

Suicide methods vary from one country to another, but in most countries suicide by overdose is relatively rare. There is still some risk, however, and thus differences in toxicity must be taken into account.

Conclusion

While the effectiveness of antidepressants in the short- and long-term treatment of depression has been demonstrated, proof of their efficacy in preventing suicide and attempted suicide is lacking.

For technical and ethical reasons, it seems difficult to imagine a study using a placebo control group with a large number of depressed subjects that would make it possible to answer this question. It is likely that a meta-analysis grouping together all available studies would make it possible to shed some light on this issue, even if the placebo control group is made up of low-risk subjects.

It might be easier in the long run to try to understand the different effects of various antidepressants. In this case, high-risk patients could be included without raising an ethical dilemma.

In the absence of actual proof, the current figures are rather reassuring. Even non-significant meta-analyses provide results that concur. Antidepressants for which information is available have been shown to decrease suicidal ideation, which is one of the factors that can predict suicide.

Eventually, other factors, such as impulsiveness, can be taken into account. In fact, given the available information, it would seem that some psychotropic medicines (antidepressants and benzodiazepines) could modify impulsiveness and influence suicide attempts independent of their effect on mood.

In reality, the adequate assessment of the different effects of various antidepressants on severely depressed patients who have the highest suicide risk may be more important in terms of providing useful information than large studies of low-risk patients.

Furthermore, even if the problems caused by a lack of knowledge are not discussed here (they will be developed in a different chapter), a study conducted on Gotland Island (Rutz et al, 1989) should come to mind, as it demonstrated that a well-managed program of education for the majority of medical doctors can make it possible to reduce the incidence of suicide significantly in subsequent years.

References

Avery D, Winokur G (1978) Suicide, attempted suicide, and relapse rates in depression, *Arch Gen Psychiatry* **35:**749–53.

Beasley CM, Dornseif BE, Bosomworth JC et al (1991) Fluoxetine and suicide: a meta-analysis of controlled trials of treatment for depression, *Br Med J* **303:**685–92.

Fawcett J, Scheftner A, Fogg L et al (1990) Time-related predictors of suicide in major affective disorder, *Am J Psychiatry* **147:**1189–94.

Goldstein RB, Black DW, Nasrallah A, Winokur G (1991) The prediction of suicide. Sensitivity, specificity, and predictive value of a multivariate model applied to suicide among 1906 patients with affective disorders, *Arch Gen Psychiatry* **48:**418–22.

Isacsson G, Bergman U, Rich CL (1994a) Antidepressants, depression and suicide: an analysis of the San Diego study, *J Affect Disord* **32:** 277–86.

Isacsson G, Holmgren P, Wasserman D, Bergman V (1994b) Use of antidepressants among people committing suicide in Sweden, *Br Med J* **308:**506–9.

Jick SS, Dean AD, Jick H (1995) Antidepressants and suicide, *Br Med J* **310:**215–18.

Jonas JM, Hearron AE (1996) Alprazolam and suicidal ideation: a meta-analysis of controlled trials in the treatment of depression, *J Clin Psychopharmacol* **16:**208–11.

Kapur S, Mieczkowski T, Mann JJ (1992) Antidepressant medications and the relative risk of suicide attempt and suicide, *JAMA* **268:**3441–45.

Marzuk PM, Tardiff K, Leon AC et al (1995) Use of prescription psychotropic drugs among suicide victims in New York city, *Am J Psychiatry* **152:**1520–2.

Montgomery SA, Dunner DL, Dunbar GC (1995) Reduction of suicidal thoughts with paroxetine in comparison with reference antidepressants and placebo, *Eur Neuropsychopharmacol* **5:**5–13.

Rouillon F, Phillips R, Serrurier D, Ansart E, Gérard MJ (1989) Rechutes de dépression unipolaire et efficacité de la maprotiline, *Encephale* **XV:** 527–34.

Rutz W, Von Knorring L, Walinder J (1989) Frequency of suicide on Gotland after systematic postgraduate education of general practitioners, *Acta Psychiatr Scand* **80:**151–4.

Tollefson GD, Fawcett J, Winokur G et al (1993) Evaluation of suicidality during pharmacologic treatment of mood and nonmood disorders, *Ann Clin Psychiatry* **5:**209–24.

18

Resistant depression: the need for better antidepressants

Lars von Knorring and Kerstin Bingefors

Introduction

Despite the fact that the tricyclic antidepressants (TCAs) have been available for more than 40 years and the selective serotonin reuptake inhibitors (SSRIs) for more than a decade, the long-term outcome of depressive disorders has not changed (Editorial, 1992). In an early review by Guze and Robins (1970), the authors reported that in 17 studies concerning death and suicide, the affective disorders were associated with very high suicide rates. In no study did suicide account for less than 12% of all deaths. In nine studies the suicides accounted for between 12% and 19% of the deaths, while in the other eight studies the suicides accounted for between 35% and 60% of all deaths. In three reports in the late 1980s (Kiloh et al, 1988; Lee and Murray, 1988; Lehmann et al, 1988) little had changed.

However, in early studies (Perris, 1966) it was also noted that depressed patients tended to have an increased mortality even if the deaths by suicide were disregarded. In a later study by Bingefors et al (1996a) the situation was still about the same.

Although mortality is the most commonly used measure of health status in populations (Westerling, 1993), morbidity is also important. In a 16-year follow-up, Lee and Murray (1988) reported that only one-third of the patients were free of recurrent moderate or severe psychiatric morbidity during the follow-up period. In the same way, Bingefors and Isacson (1996) reported that more than half of the patients identified in the general population, followed for 8 years after the first treatment episode with antidepressants, had one or several periods of antidepressant treatment after the index year. The relapse rate was between 23% and 33% for each year after the index year, and 11% experienced continuous use of antidepressants every year after the index year.

In one study comprising patients with major depressive disorders, the course of depressive symptoms was followed during an 18-month naturalistic follow-up period. The patients were treated in the National Institute of Mental Health Treatment of Depression Collaborative Research Program. The treatment phase consisted of 16 weeks of randomly assigned treatment with cognitive therapy, interpersonal therapy, imipramine or placebo. At the 18-month follow-up, 19–30% of the patients remained well. Among patients who had recovered, rates of major depressive disorder relapses were 33–50% (Shea et al, 1992).

Efficacy of the antidepressants

Efficacy in randomized controlled studies

In randomized controlled trials, both the TCAs and the SSRIs have a significantly higher efficacy than placebo. However, the effect size is limited. In the eight placebo-controlled trials available when fluoxetine was licensed in Sweden (Medical Products Agency, 1995), the mean difference in change between placebo and fluoxetine was 3.9 points on the Hamilton Depression Rating Scale. Overall, 43% of the patients responded to fluoxetine and 22% to placebo. The response rate for fluoxetine varied from 31.2% to 70.4%, while the placebo responder rate varied from 8.8% to 42.9% (Figures 18.1 and 18.2).

There are several studies comparing fluoxetine with TCAs and placebo. In general, fluoxetine has been found to be superior to placebo on all major efficacy parameters and comparable to imipramine with respect to the primary indicators of depression. However, a significantly smaller percentage of fluoxetine than imipramine patients terminated therapy because of adverse experiences (Stark and Hardison, 1985). All the SSRIs have also demonstrated antidepressant efficacy greater than that of placebo and similar to that of the standard TCAs amitriptyline and imipramine. In a meta-analysis, it has also been demonstrated that the SSRIs do have a significantly lower discontinuation rate than the old

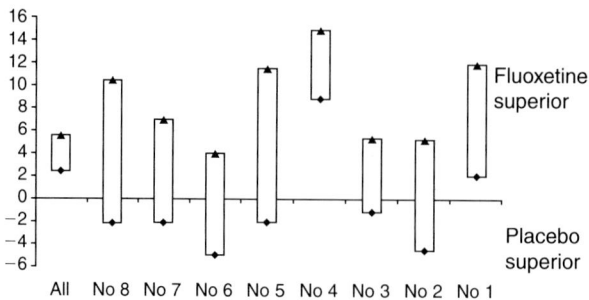

Figure 18.1

Ninety-five per cent confidence intervals for differences in change in Hamilton Depression Scale total mean scores between fluoxetine and placebo in eight controlled, randomized trials (Medical Products Agency, 1995).

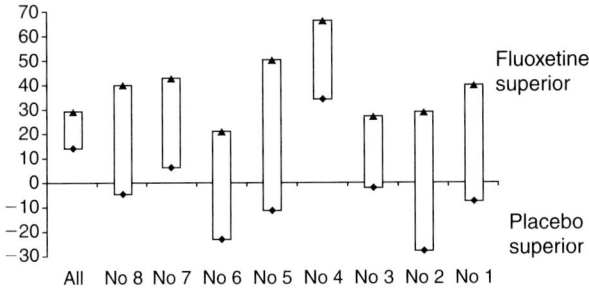

Figure 18.2

Ninety-five per cent confidence interval for differences in responder rates between fluoxetine and placebo in eight controlled, randomized trials (Medical Products Agency, 1995).

TCAs (amitriptyline and imipramine) but a similar discontinuation rate as that of newer TCAs (including clomipramine) and heterocyclic antidepressants (including mianserin, maprotiline and nomifensin) (Hotopf et al, 1997). In another meta-analysis of controlled trials, it was found that the efficacy of the SSRIs is about equivalent to that of amitriptyline and imipramine. However, because of small patient numbers included in most studies that compare SSRIs with other antidepressants, no definitive statements about relative efficacy can be made (Kasper et al, 1992).

Other new antidepressants are usually found to be superior to placebo and equivalent, as concerns efficacy, with the TCAs. For example, nefazodone has been found to be an effective antidepressant drug with overall efficacy similar to that of imipramine in three out of four phase 3 active and placebo-controlled studies. The remaining study did not differentiate either active drug from placebo controls (Rickels et al, 1995). Venlafaxine has also been found to be superior to placebo and comparable to imipramine (Morton et al, 1995). The selective monoamine oxidase group A (MAO-A) inhibitor moclobemide has been compared to placebo and imipramine, clomipramine and amitriptyline in four three-way comparison trials. Two studies indicated that the efficacy of moclobemide was significantly greater than that of placebo and similar to that of other antidepressants (imipramine and amitriptyline) (Silverstone, 1993).

There are, however, some problems involved when equal efficacy is discussed. Leon et al (1993) demonstrated that alprazolam, imipramine and placebo in a clinical trial for patients meeting criteria for both panic disorder and depression resulted in a significant difference between active medication and placebo on the Hamilton Rating Scale for Depression (Ham-D), but no difference between the antidepressant effects of the active medications despite their diverse psychopharmacological properties. Examination of effect sizes for each Ham-D item revealed distinct symptom-specific effects of each active medication. Thus, equal number of responders or equal reduction of the total score of the Ham-D does not necessarily mean equal antidepressant efficacy, at least not equal efficacy on all symptoms or all subgroups of patients.

In three well-controlled studies by the Danish University Antidepressant Group (DUAG) (Danish University Antidepressant Group, 1986, 1990, 1993), it was demonstrated that in well-designed and rigorously executed multisite drug trials three representatives (citalopram, paroxetine and moclobemide) from two classes of recent antidepressant drugs were less effective than the standard reference drug (clomipramine). The most important reasons for the superiority of clomipramine were probably that clomipramine was given in a high and fixed dose (150 mg/day) throughout the entire treatment period and that patient compliance was ensured through drug monitoring (Vestergaard et al, 1993).

Another possibility might be that the three studies comprised only inpatients. In other studies performed at the same time where outpatients were included, paroxetine, citalopram and moclobemide were found to have efficacies similar to that of imipramine and clomipramine (Ohrberg et al, 1992; Rosenberg et al, 1994; Kragh-Sörensen et al, 1995). Thus, it has been suggested that there are clinical differences between inpatients and outpatients which are of importance for the clinical response. In a separate analysis where the inpatients and outpatients included in the clinical trials were compared, inpatients were found to have more pronounced depressed mood, more suicidal ideas and more inhibition and retardation. Significantly more hospitalized patients (76% of the hospitalized patients as compared to 40% of the outpatients) fulfilled the criteria for 'endogenous depression' according to the Newcastle index (Gram and Stage, 1997). Thus, one possibility might be that clomipramine is more efficacious in inpatients with major depression with melancholia, especially if high and fixed doses are used and if compliance is controlled.

In response to a recent inquiry sent to Swedish psychiatrists by the board of the Swedish Serotonin Society (Mårtensson and Åberg-Wistedt, 1996), only 20% of the Swedish psychiatrists considered the SSRIs to be as effective as the TCAs in severely depressed patients. A higher dosage was considered necessary by 34.1% when treating severe depressions. A majority, 61.8%, reported that they had experience with patients who had previously responded well to TCAs but did not respond adequately when treated for a new episode of depression with SSRIs. On the question of whether there are indications more suited for treatment with TCAs than with SSRIs, 56.3% answered yes. Major depression with melancholia was mentioned as an example by many.

Doses used in clinical practice

In real life, the doses used are not the same as those used in randomized, controlled clinical trials. In the Swedish Diagnosis and Therapy

Table 18.1   Doses of antidepressants used in clinical practice in Sweden 1995 according to the Swedish Diagnosis and Therapy Survey (Läkemedelsstatistik AB, 1996).

	Defined daily doses (DDD)	Prescribed daily doses (PDD)
Clomipramine	100	65
Amitriptyline	75	46
Citalopram	20	28
Paroxetine	20	26
Sertraline	50	55
Moclobemide	300	345
Mianserin	60	45

Survey 1995 (Läkemedelsstatistik AB, 1996), it can be seen that while the defined daily doses (DDDs) for the TCAs were, for example, clomipramine 100 mg and amitriptyline 75 mg, the prescribed daily doses (PDDs) were lower, 65 mg and 46 mg, respectively. As concerns the SSRIs, the differences are in the opposite direction. The DDDs for citalopram and paroxetine were 20 mg, while the PDDs were 28 mg and 26 mg, respectively (Table 18.1). In the same way, the selective, reversible MAO-A inhibitor moclobemide was used in higher doses than the DDDs, while mianserin was used in lower doses. However, if therapeutic drug monitoring (TDM) is applied, even higher doses than the DDDs are needed. In patients monitored by means of plasma concentrations, the median daily doses for amitriptyline and imipramine were 150 mg and 200 mg, respectively (Rosholm, 1997).

There are no randomized controlled studies comparing the efficacy of, for example, clomipramine 65 mg a day versus, for example, citalopram 28 mg a day, i.e. the doses commonly used in everyday clinical practice, but it is reasonable to believe that comparisons of this kind would reveal results different to the ones usually found in clinical trials.

Efficiency of the antidepressants

Treatment-resistant depression

There are no agreed criteria for treatment-resistant depression, but failure to respond adequately to two successive courses of monotherapy with pharmacologically different antidepressants, given in adequate doses for sufficient time, is one pragmatic definition. Inherent within this definition are notions of what constitutes an adequate dose of the drug, the length of treatment and pharmacological specificity of the treatments. When these factors are accounted for, treatment resistance may be encountered in 15–20% of patients (Burrows et al, 1994). There have also been attempts to provide more specific and detailed definitions. Thus Kuhs (1995) has suggested that first-degree treatment resistance implies non-response to standard antidepressive therapy (two successive adequate treatments with antidepressants, combined with induced-wakefulness therapy). Second-degree treatment resistance is defined by non-response to alternative treatment strategies (MAO inhibitors, lithium augmentation, electroconvulsive therapy, infusion therapy). Criteria for third-degree treatment resistance should not be based on non-response to specific further therapeutic trials but on the duration of the treatment (at least 2 years). However, in clinical practice the definition of treatment resistance is not easy. In a study by Nelson and Dunner (1995), it was revealed that there were frequent misdiagnoses of depression subtype, relatively infrequent treatment with electroconvulsive therapy, and pharmacotherapy trials which often were too brief or characterized by inadequate dosing to be effective.

It is also obvious that the time period studied is of great importance. In an Australian study, 107 patients referred to a mood disorders unit with an episode of treatment-resistant major depression were followed for a mean period of 37.5 months. At the end of the follow-up period, 41% of the patients were fully recovered and a further 43% were partially improved (Wilhelm et al, 1994). The concept of treatment-resistant depression has thus been criticized (Dyck, 1994). The methodological problems include: (1) the failure to adequately conceptualize and/or specifically define treatments; (2) the extreme variety of treatments evaluated in the absence of methodological controls; (3) inadequate sampling procedures; (4) the heterogeneity of the patient samples; (5) the bias in favour of reporting positive results; (6) the misrepresentation of outcome in published reports; and (7) the neglect of considering spontaneous remission as a viable alternative explanation.

Thus, although it has been claimed that treatment-resistant depression is a clinical complication that not infrequently affects a certain number of patients (Berlanga and Ortega-Soto, 1995), a problem of as much concern is the low efficiency of the antidepressants when used in clinical practice in the community (Bingefors, 1996).

Antidepressants in clinical practice

Patients with depressive disorders are known to have high health services utilization (Johnson et al, 1992). Likewise, affective disorders are common in chronically ill patients. In epidemiological studies, depressive disorders have been demonstrated in 5–9% of outpatients with somatic disease and in up to 50% of inpatients (Rodin et al, 1991). In a recent cross-sectional study of prescription drug use during 1 year, patients treated with antidepressants had a significantly greater use of ambulatory care, hospital care and prescription drugs than those who did not take

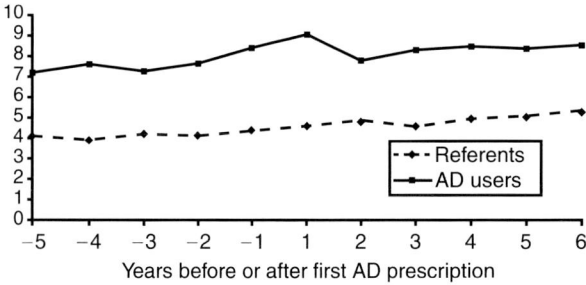

Figure 18.3

Average use of non-psychotropic drugs during 5 years before and 6 years after the index episode (first episode with antidepressant (AD) treatment) (Bingefors et al, 1996a).

antidepressants. They also had an increased frequency of use of prescription drugs from virtually all pharmacological classes (Bingefors et al, 1995). It can be questioned whether the depressive syndromes are a consequence of the medical diseases or whether they precede the medical diagnosis (Rodin et al, 1991). It has also been suggested that both the medical diseases and the depressive syndromes are due to a generalized vulnerability (Perris, 1966).

When the patients identified as first-time antidepressant users in the general population were followed 5 years before and 6 years after the index (first) treatment, it could be demonstrated that the antidepressant-treated patients used considerably more non-psychotropic drugs during the whole study period than the referent group (Bingefors et al, 1996b) (Figure 18.3). They also made a significantly greater use of somatic primary care during the whole study period, with a significant increase in the year before antidepressants were first prescribed. They also had a significantly higher risk of receiving a diagnosis in most ICD categories (Bingefors, 1996).

The long-term morbidity was also considerable, despite the use of antidepressant medication (Bingefors and Isacson, 1996). When the patients were followed for 8 years, more than half of them had one or several periods of antidepressant treatment after the index year. The relapse rate was between 23% and 33% for each year after the index year, and 11% made continuous use of antidepressants every year after the index year. Patients with one or more relapses had a significantly higher number of other prescription drugs compared to those treated only once.

As a result of the rather low efficiency of the antidepressants in general practice, mortality is still high in antidepressant-treated patients. In an early study (Perris, 1966), it was demonstrated that mortality was also increased if the suicides were disregarded. Later studies have indicated increased short-term (Bruce and Leaf, 1989) and long-term (Murphy et al, 1987) mortality. In a separate study by Bingefors et al (1996b), all first-incidence antidepressant users in the defined population during a 5-year

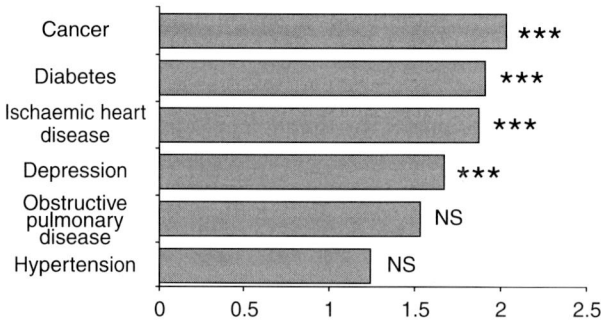

Figure 18.4

Adjusted mortality rate in a Cox regression analysis relating age, sex and baseline morbidity to 9-year mortality in depressed outpatients treated with antidepressants (Bingefors et al, 1996b).

period were identified. Their total mortality during a 9-year follow-up was analysed. Antidepressant treatment at the index date was a statistically significant predictor for increased long-term mortality, even when controlling for pre-existing chronic medical diseases. Baseline ischaemic heart disease and concurrent antidepressant treatment significantly predicted mortality from cardiovascular disease (Bingefors et al, 1996a) (Figure 18.4).

During the last decade, and especially after the introduction of the SSRIs, the sales of antidepressants have increased rapidly in most countries. In Sweden, there was a gradual increase in the sales from 7.4 DDD/1000 inhabitants per day in 1983 to 10.7 DDD/1000 inhabitants per day in 1992. During that period, the frequency of suicides in Sweden also decreased from 25.1 suicides/100 000 inhabitants per year to 21.2 suicides/100 000 inhabitants per year. However, after 1992 there was a rapid increase in the sales of antidepressants, and the market has

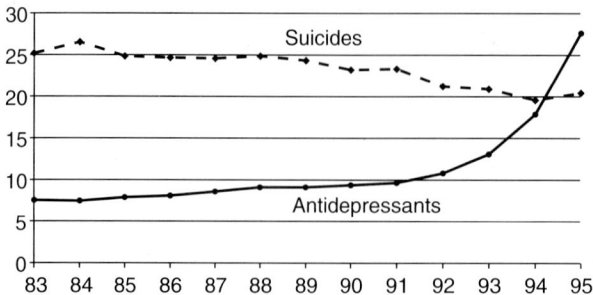

Figure 18.5

Sales of antidepressants in Sweden (DDD/1000 inhabitants per day) and the frequency of suicides (per 100 000 inhabitants/year) during the years 1983–1996.

changed from predominantly TCAs to predominantly SSRIs. In 1992 clomipramine and amitriptyline together had about 50% of the Swedish antidepressant market (shares of DDD prescribed) and the SSRIs had about 8%. Three years later, the SSRIs had 75% of the market. The dominating single compound was citalopram. During this time period, no further decrease can be seen in the frequency of suicides (Figure 18.5). Thus, although we cannot exclude the possibility that the gradual increase in the sales of antidepressants 1983–1991 may have had some beneficial effects on the frequency of suicides, it is obvious that the rapid increase in the sales of the SSRIs during the last years is not reflected in a similar reduction in the frequency of suicides.

Documented efficiency of antidepressants

Although the long-term course of depressive disorders in the general population has not changed considerably since the introduction of the antidepressants, and although the antidepressants thus seem to have a low efficiency despite the fact that they are superior to placebo in randomized controlled trials, there are also some examples of documented efficiency of the antidepressants. In an early study by Avery and Winokur (1976), it was demonstrated that while patients treated with electroconvulsive therapy (ECT) or antidepressants in an adequate way, i.e. correct doses and correct length of treatment, had a 3-year mortality of 2.2–2.8%, patients treated with antidepressants in an inadequate way—too low doses or too short a time—had a 3-year mortality of 9.1%. Thus, the treatment situation and the way the antidepressants are handled is of considerable importance. In the same way, maintenance treatment with adequate compliance and adequate doses can be of considerable importance (Frank et al, 1990). Whereas patients treated with imipramine 200 mg a day had a mean time before relapse of 131 weeks, the corresponding figure for the placebo group was 45 weeks. Coppen et al (1991) also reported a low standardized mortality ratio in patients treated at a mood disorders clinic in which compliance was good and drop-out rate was low.

However, to have an effect in the general population, the correct patients have to be identified. In a report from the DEPRES Steering Committee 1996 (Tylee, 1996), it was demonstrated that out of 100 depressed patients in the general population, 69 will consult the healthcare system. Forty-one will receive prescription drugs but only 18 will receive antidepressants. Depending on compliance, the doses prescribed and the efficacy of the antidepressants, 9–12 out of the 100 depressed patients in the community will benefit from antidepressant drugs. Thus, increased efficiency at a population level will include better diagnostic routines as well as better antidepressants.

In an evaluation of an educational programme on depressive disorders

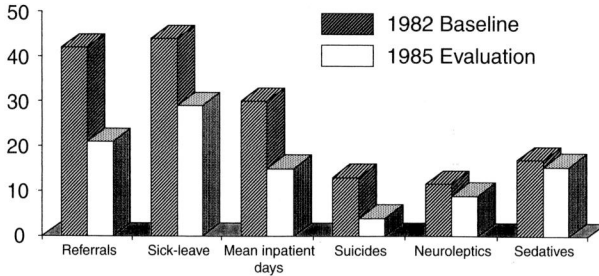

Figure 18.6

Evaluation of an educational programme on depressive disorders given to general practitioners on Gotland by the Swedish PTD Committee during the years 1983–1984 (Eberhard et al, 1986; Rutz et al, 1989, 1995).

given to general practitioners at Gotland in 1983 and 1984 (Eberhard et al, 1986; Rutz et al, 1989, 1990, 1992a,b, 1995, 1997), it could be demonstrated that increased knowledge of diagnosis and treatment of depressive disorders resulted in a decreased number of referrals from the general practitioners to psychiatry, decreased sick-leave due to depression, decreased number of suicides and decreased prescription of sedatives and major tranquillizers (Figure 18.6). During the studied time period, the amounts of antidepressants prescribed increased somewhat, but also, at the end of the study period, the prescription rate on Gotland was only 77% of that in Sweden as a whole. Thus, increased prescription of antidepressants may be beneficial when combined with increased knowledge on diagnosis and treatment.

In a later intensive study of all suicides before and after the educational programme was given to the general practitioners on Gotland (Rihmer et al, 1995), it was demonstrated that, after the PTD programme, the proportion of depressive suicides was significantly lower than before. This finding strongly suggests that the significant decrease in the suicide rate after the PTD programme is a direct result of the robust decrease in depressive suicides in the area served by trained general practitioners.

In a Hungarian study (Rihmer et al, 1993), a strong positive correlation was found between the number of working physicians and the rate of diagnosed depression, and both parameters showed a strong negative correlation with the suicide rate. Thus, the more physicians, the better is the recognition of depression and the lower is the suicide rate in the given region.

Conclusions

Treatment-resistant depression has been estimated to occur in 15–20% of the patients when pragmatic criteria are used (Burrows et al, 1994).

However, there are several problems concerning the delineation of and definition of treatment-resistant depression (Dyck, 1994), and the concept can be questioned. It can also be demonstrated that the diagnosis of treatment-resistant depression is often given to patients who have been misdiagnosed, or inadequately treated (Nelson and Dunner, 1995), and that about 50% of the patients defined as treatment resistant are fully or partially recovered 3 years later (Willhelm et al, 1994).

Of greater concern is the fact that depressed patients in the general community, treated with antidepressants and followed up for 6 years still have a high prescription rate of psychotropic and non-psychotropic drugs, and still have more visits to general practitioners due to somatic main diagnosis; if followed over a 9-year period, they still have an increased mortality of about the same size as that seen in cancer and ischaemic heart disease (Bingefors, 1996; Bingefors and Isacson, 1996; Bingefors et al, 1995, 1996a,b). The increased mortality, not only from suicide but from other medical disorders, was observed 30 years ago (Perris, 1966) and is still as pronounced (Bingefors et al, 1996a), despite new diagnostic criteria, new antidepressants and more knowledge concerning the importance of long-term treatment (Editorial, 1992).

One problem is that although both old and new antidepressants have a documented efficacy as compared to placebo in randomized, controlled studies, the effect size is limited. In placebo-controlled studies, 43% of patients responded to fluoxetine versus 21.6% to placebo (Medical Products Agency, 1995). In most meta-analyses and reviews, the old and the new antidepressants tend to have about the same efficacy (Kasper et al, 1992). However, when, for example, clomipramine is given in a high, fixed dose and when compliance is guaranteed, clomipramine can be demonstrated to be more efficacious than citalopram, paroxetine and moclobemide (Danish University Antidepressant Group, 1986, 1990, 1993). The majority of Swedish psychiatrists responding to an inquiry were also convinced that the TCAs are more effective than the SSRIs in the treatment of severe depression. However, the new antidepressants are usually better tolerated and the frequency of drop-outs is lower (Stark and Hardison, 1985; Silverstone, 1993; Rickels et al, 1995). Thus, to have an effect in clinical practice we would need new antidepressants as effective as the TCAs, and with as few side effects and as well tolerated as the SSRIs.

There are also some examples where the antidepressants have influenced morbidity and mortality in the community. One example is the Gotland project (Eberhard et al, 1986; Rutz et al, 1989, 1990, 1992a,b, 1995) and another is the Hungarian experience (Rihmer et al, 1993). However, it should be kept in mind that to have an effect with antidepressants on a community level, it is important for the patients to consult the health-care system and for the doctors to be trained in the diagnosis and treatment of depression. According to the DEPRES data (Tylee, 1996), 82% of the patients are missed before an antidepressant drug is even prescribed. Thus, even an antidepressant drug tolerated by all subjects and with 100% efficacy will result in no more than 18 cured patients out of 100 in the community if the treatment strategy does not include educational programmes for patients, relatives and people working in the health-care system.

References

Avery D, Winokur G (1976) Mortality in depressed patients treated with electroconvulsive therapy and antidepressants, *Arch Gen Psychiatry* **33:** 1029–37.

Berlanga C, Ortega-Soto HA (1995) A 3-year follow up of a group of treatment-resistant depressed patients with a MAOI/tricyclic combination, *J Affect Disord* **34:**187–92.

Bingefors K (1996) *Antidepressant-treated Patients. Population-based Longitudinal Studies* (Uppsala University: Uppsala).

Bingefors K, Isacson D (1996) Continued use of antidepressants among patients in ambulatory care, *Nord J Psychiatry* **50:**217–24.

Bingefors K, Isacson D, von Knorring L, Smedby B (1995) Prescription drug and health care use among Swedish patients treated with antidepressants, *Ann Pharmacother* **29:**566–72.

Bingefors K, Isacson D, von Knorring L, Smedby B, Wicknertz K (1996a) Antidepressant-treated patients in ambulatory care. Mortality during a nine-year period after first treatment, *Br J Psychiatry* **169:**647–54.

Bingefors K, Isacson D, von Knorring L, Smedby B, Ekselius L, Kupper L (1996b) Antidepressant-treated patients in ambulatory care. Long-term use of non-psychotropic and psychotropic drugs, *Br J Psychiatry* **168:**292–8.

Bruce M, Leaf P (1989) Psychiatric disorders and 15 month mortality in a community sample of older adults, *Am J Public Health* **79:**727–30.

Burrows GD, Norman TR, Judd FK (1994) Definition and differential diagnosis of treatment-resistant depression, *Int Clin Psychopharmacol* **9:** 5–10.

Coppen A, Standish-Berry H, Bailey J, Houston G, Silcocks P, Hermon C (1991) Does lithium reduce the mortality of recurrent mood disorders? *J Affect Disord* **23:**1–7.

Danish University Antidepressant Group (1986) Citalopram. Clinical effect profile in comparison with clomipramine: a controlled multicenter trial, *Psychopharmacology* **90:**131–8.

Danish University Antidepressant Group (1990) Paroxetine: a selective serotonin reuptake inhibitor showing better tolerance, but weaker antidepressant effect than clomipramine in a controlled multicenter trial, *J Affect Disord* **18:**289–99.

Danish University Antidepressant Group (1993) Moclobemide: a reversible MAO-A-inhibitor showing weaker antidepressant effect than clomipramine in a controlled multicenter study, *J Affect Disord* **28:**105–16.

Dyck MJ (1994) Treatment-resistant depression: a critique of current approaches, *Aust NZ J Psychiatry* **28:** 34–41.

Eberhard G, Holmberg G, von Knorring A-L et al (1986) Evaluation of postgraduate medical education given by the Swedish PTD-Committee, *Nord J Psychiatry* **40:**185–92.

Editorial (1992) Depression and suicide: are they preventable? *Lancet* **340:**700–1.

Frank E, Kupfer D, Perel J et al (1990) Three-year outcomes for maintenance therapies in recurrent depression, *Arch Gen Psychiatry* **17:**1093–9.

Gram LF, Stage K (1997) Dose, drop-out and symptomatology. Important methodological problems in testing new antidepressants, *Nord J Psychiatry* **51**(suppl 38):27–31.

Guze S, Robins E (1970) Suicide and primary affective disorders, *Br J Psychiatry* **117:**437–8.

Hotopf M, Hardy R, Lewis G (1997) Discontinuation rates of SSRI's and tricyclic antidepressants: a meta-analysis and investigation of heterogeneity, *Br J Psychiatry* **170:**120–7.

Johnson J, Weissman M, Klerman GL (1992) Service utilization and social morbidity associated with depressive symptoms in the community, *J Am Med Assoc* **267:**1478–83.

Kasper S, Fuger J, Möller H-J (1992) Comparative efficacy of antidepressants, *Drugs* **43:**11–23.

Kiloh L, Andrews G, Neilson M (1988) The long-term outcome of depressive illness, *Br J Psychiatry* **153:**752–7.

Kragh-Sörensen P, Muller B, Andersen JV, Buch D, Stage KB (1995) Moclobemide versus clomipramine in depressive patients in general practice. A randomized, double-blind parallel, multicentre study, *J Clin Psychopharmacol* **15/4:**245–305.

Kuhs H (1995) Stages of treatment resistance in depressive disorders, defined after somatotherapeutic methods, *Nervenarzt* **66:**561–7.

Läkemedelsstatistik AB (1996) *Medical Index Sweden* (Läkemedelsstatistik AB: Stockholm).

Lee A, Murray R (1988) The long-term outcome of Maudsley depressives, *Br J Psychiatry* **153:**741–51.

Lehmann H, Fenton F, Deutsch M, Feldman S, Engelsmann F (1988) An 11-year follow-up study of 110 depressed patients, *Acta Psychiatr Scand* **78:**57–65.

Leon AC, Shear MK, Portera L, Klerman GL (1993) Effect size as a measure of symptom specific drug change in clinical trials, *Psychopharmacol Bull* **29:**163–7.

Mårtensson B, Åberg-Wistedt A (1996) The use of selective serotonin reuptake inhibitors among Swedish psychiatrists, *Nord J Psychiatry* **50:**443–50.

Medical Products Agency (1995) Läkemedelsmonografier. Fontex (fluoxetin), *Info från Läkemedelverket* **6:**397–401.

Morton WA, Sonne SC, Verga MA (1995) Venlafaxine: a structurally unique and novel antidepressant, *Ann Pharmacother* **29:**387–95.

Murphy J, Monson R, Olivier D et al (1987) Affective disorders and mortality, *Arch Gen Psychiatry* **44:**473–80.

Nelson MR, Dunner DL (1995) Clinical and differential diagnostic aspects of treatment-resistant depression, *J Psychiatr Res* **29:**43–50.

Ohrberg S, Christiansen PE, Severin B (1992) Paroxetine and imipramine in the treatment of depressive patients in psychiatric practice, *Acta Psychiatr Scand* **86:**437–44.

Perris C (1966) A study of bipolar (manic-depressive) and unipolar recurrent depressive psychoses X. Mortality, suicide and life-cycles, *Acta Psychiatr Scand* **42:**172–83.

Rickels K, Robinson DS, Schweizer E, Marcus RN, Roberts DL (1995) Nefazodone: aspects of efficacy, *J Clin Psychiatry* **56:**43–6.

Rihmer Z, Rutz W, Barsi J (1993) Suicide rate, prevalence of diagnosed depression and prevalence of working physicians in Hungary, *Acta Psychiatr Scand* **88:**391–94.

Rihmer Z, Rutz W, Pihlgren H (1995) Depression and suicide on Gotland. An intensive study of all suicides before and after a depression-training programme for general practitioners, *J Affect Disord* **35:**147–52.

Rodin G, Craven J, Littlefield C (1991)

Depression in the Medically Ill (Brunner/Mazel: New York, NY).

Rosenberg C, Damsbo N, Fuglum E, Jacobsen LV, Horsgård S (1994) Citalopram and imipramine in the treatment of depressive patients in general practice. A Nordic multicenter clinical trial, *Int Clin Psychopharmacol* **9**(suppl 1):41–8.

Rosholm J-U (1997) Antidepressants in general practice—too much or too little? *Nord J Psychiatry* **51** (suppl 38):53–6.

Rutz W, Wålinder J, Eberhard G et al (1989) An educational program on depressive disorders for general practitioners on Gotland: background and evaluation, *Acta Psychiatr Scand* **79**:19–26.

Rutz W, von Knorring L, Wålinder J, Wistedt B (1990) Effect of an educational program for general practitioners on Gotland on the pattern of prescription of psychotropic drugs, *Acta Psychiatr Scand* **82**:399–403.

Rutz W, Carlsson P, von Knorring L, Wålinder J (1992a) Cost-benefit analysis of an educational program for general practitioners by the Swedish Committee for the Prevention and Treatment of Depression, *Acta Psychiatr Scand* **85**:457–64.

Rutz W, von Knorring L, Wålinder J (1992b) Long-term effects of an educational program for general practitioners given by the Swedish Committee for Prevention and Treatment of Depression, *Acta Psychiatr Scand* **85**:83–8.

Rutz W, von Knorring L, Pihlgren H, Rihmer Z, Wålinder J (1995) An educational project on depression and its consequences: is frequency of major depression among Swedish men underrated, resulting in high suicidality? *Primary Care Psychiatry* **1**:59–63.

Rutz W, Wålinder J, von Knorring L, Rihmer Z, Pihlgren H (1997) Prevention of depression and suicide: Gotland Study update, *Int J Psychiatr Clin Prac* **1**:39–46.

Shea MT, Elkin I, Imber SD et al (1992) Course of depressive symptoms over follow-up. Findings from the National Institute of Mental Health Treatment of Depression Collaborative Research Program, *Arch Gen Psychiatry* **49**:782–7.

Silverstone T (1993) Moclobemide—placebo-controlled trials, *Int Clin Psychopharmacol* **7**:133–6.

Stark P, Hardison CD (1985) A review of multicenter controlled studies of fluoxetine versus imipramine and placebo in outpatients with major depressive disorder, *J Clin Psychiatry* **46**:53–8.

Tylee A (1996) *The Patients' Perspective of Depression* (Association of European Psychiatrists: London).

Vestergaard P, Gram LF, Kragh-Sörensen P, Bech P, Reisby N, Bolwig TG (1993) Therapeutic potentials of recently introduced antidepressants. Danish University Antidepressant Group, *Psychopharmacol Ser* **10:** 190–8.

Westerling R (1993) *The 'Avoidable' Mortality Method. Empirical Studies Using Data from Sweden* (Uppsala University: Uppsala).

Wilhelm K, Mitchell P, Sengoz A, Hickie I, Brodaty H, Boyce P (1994) Treatment resistant depression in an Australian context II: Outcome of a series of patients, *Aust NZ J Psychiatry* **28**:23–33.

19

Which antidepressant for which depression?

Stuart A Montgomery

Over the last twenty years, a considerable number of new antidepressants have been introduced which have brought important progress in the treatment of depression. The pharmacological rationale underlying the development of these antidepressant compounds is broadly related to the presumed basis of the mechanism of antidepressant action of the early tricyclic antidepressants (TCAs) i.e. the activity of these compounds in blocking the reuptake of the neurotransmitters noradrenaline and serotonin. There has been no radical shift in concept, therefore, with recent antidepressants but major advances have nevertheless been made.

Well-tolerated antidepressants

Attention has been focused on the shortcomings of the traditional TCAs, in particular their poor tolerability profile and potential toxicity. In response, drug development programmes have emphasized the need to reduce unwanted pharmacological effects. The TCAs have a broad range of pharmacological actions, including affinity for muscarinic and histaminergic receptors, in addition to their noradrenaline and serotonin reuptake-blocking actions related to therapeutic effect. These unwanted effects account for the toxicity of some of the older TCAs when taken in overdose which has been a cause for considerable concern. They also produce the side effects which comprise the usefulness of the older TCAs for many patients who find them difficult to tolerate.

The disadvantages of treatments that are associated with a high level of side effects are three-fold. Initiating treatment at an adequate dose may be difficult if patients are unable to tolerate the side effects and, indeed, some patients may never reach a therapeutic dose; there is a decreased likelihood that patients will take their medication as prescribed; patients are likely to be discouraged by the side effects and be unwilling to continue treatment. This lack of compliance with medication is a particular problem in long-term illnesses like depression, where long-term treatment is needed to prevent relapse after response and to reduce the risk of further episodes in recurrent depression.

The introduction of antidepressants that are better tolerated than the traditional TCAs is an important step in improving the outcome of depressed patients. These newer antidepressants, which have fewer side effects, are associated with better compliance and fewer premature withdrawals from treatment. The direct result is that there are fewer treatment failures, which has implications beyond the immediate benefit to the treated patients. Premature discontinuation of treatment increases the overall costs of health care, which include such factors as increased hospital admissions, outpatient visits, etc. It has been shown, for example, that there is a pharmacoeconomic advantage to be gained from the use of the newer, better tolerated antidepressants, as the cost of a failed treatment outweighs any apparently higher unit cost of a newly introduced antidepressant.

Currently, the selective serotonin reuptake inhibitors (SSRIs) are the most widely known of these better tolerated antidepressants. Developed, as their class name suggests, to be selective pharmacologically, they have largely avoided the anticholinergic effects that limit the TCAs. Ideally, studies that make direct head-to-head comparisons are needed to establish whether there are differences in tolerability between drugs, but usually the size of study carried out in the development programmes is insufficient to permit this type of analysis. However, assessments have been made of the relative tolerabilities of the SSRIs and the TCAs based on meta-analyses of published papers and, sometimes, on both published and unpublished data. These meta-analyses have shown overwhelmingly that there are fewer withdrawals from treatment attributed to side effects during treatment with SSRIs compared with TCAs (Jenner, 1992; Pande and Sayler, 1993; Montgomery et al, 1994a; Anderson and Tomenson, 1995; Montgomery and Kasper, 1995).

Antidepressants with superior efficacy

Improving the efficacy of antidepressants remains a legitimate goal of drug development, since current treatments are slow to work and up to a third of patients have little or only modest response. The SSRIs are better tolerated but, in terms of overall efficacy, do not appear to be better than the existing TCAs. Similar levels of efficacy were reported for SSRIs compared with TCAs in the meta-analysis of efficacy in the generality of patients included in trials with major depression (Anderson and Tomenson, 1995). Nor is there a consistent body of evidence for any advantage in the onset of response: the SSRIs appear to require the usual 4–6 weeks of treatment before a response is reliably observed.

There is, however, evidence to support the view that there may be differences between antidepressants in their efficacy in particular sub-groups of patients. While there are relatively few direct comparisons between drugs, several groups have suggested that clomipramine may be more effective than some of the newer drugs in treating hospitalized patients or those with severe depression (Andersen et al, 1986; Danish University Antidepressant Group, 1990). The very high level of side effects associated with clomipramine makes it difficult to maintain blind conditions in studies, so some caution is needed in interpreting the results.

However, many clinicians hold the view that clomipramine is a particularly potent antidepressant, and the advantage reported in these studies in relation to newer antidepressants has tended to strengthen the perception of clomipramine as a better antidepressant than other TCAs, endowed with some special attribute which allows increased efficacy in many patients and even efficacy in some depressions where other treatments have failed. However, the dose levels where best efficacy is thought to be obtained are very high, with a consequent increase in associated side effects. A convulsion rate of 1.5% was found in a large study carried out in the USA (De Veaugh Geiss et al, 1991) and this has led to restrictions on the maximum permitted dose.

Nevertheless, the potential superiority of clomipramine over other antidepressants has greatly strengthened the notion that antidepressants can be developed which have superior efficacy, either in general effect, or in producing a more rapid response, or in showing efficacy in subgroups where the efficacy of existing conventional antidepressants appears to be compromised.

Subgroups of depression with selective efficacy

One avenue of enquiry in the quest to maximize the effect of antidepressants is the identification of subgroups of depressed patients who may respond selectively to particular antidepressants. The main divisions, which have been based on the possibility of differential response, are dysthymia and subsyndromal depression, bipolar depression, severe depression, major depression with concomitant conditions, and recurrent brief depression.

Severe depression

Severe depression is generally perceived as part of a continuum from mild, to moderate, to severe major depression. Severe depression is not a separate disorder but there is some evidence to suggest that treatment may require different strategies. For example, higher dosages of some antidepressants may be required. Because of the lack of proper fixed-dose studies of the efficacy of TCAs, it is difficult to be sure of the correct dose, let alone which dose is more appropriate in severe depression. However, the clinical trial databases with newer antidepressants tend to lead to the conclusion that higher doses may be needed to achieve response. The meta-analysis of the citalopram placebo-controlled efficacy data suggests that higher doses are needed for severe than for moderate depression, and similar data, though less striking, are revealed in a meta-analysis of paroxetine (Montgomery et al, 1994b; Tignol et al, 1992). The fixed-dose studies of venlafaxine also suggest that better efficacy is obtained with the higher doses. In moderate depression, efficacy was shown with the low dose of 75 mg/day, but in severe depression, in hospitalized depression and possibly in resistant depression a dose of above 200 mg/day would seem to be more effective (Guelfi et al, 1995; Rudolph et al, 1997).

In the severely depressed population, particularly in a hospital setting, a number of studies have demonstrated superior efficacy for particular antidepressants. Venlafaxine has been shown to be more effective than fluoxetine in two studies (Clerc et al, 1996); mirtazapine has been shown to have an advantage compared with fluoxetine (Montgomery, 1996) and trazodone (van Moffaert et al, 1995); superior efficacy was shown for milnacipram compared with fluoxetine and fluvoxamine (Lopez-Ibor et al, 1996). The studies of the Danish University Antidepressant Group (DUAG) have reported that clomipramine in a dose of 150 mg/day was more effective than citalopram, paroxetine, and moclobemide, although these comparators were all used in relatively low doses (Andersen et al, 1986; Danish University Antidepressant Group, 1990, 1993). Although the evidence is patchy and definitive studies have not yet been carried out, there are enough data to suggest that some antidepressants, including venlafaxine, mirtazapine, milnacipram and clomipramine, when used in the right doses might well have advantages in treating severe depression.

Dysthymia and subsyndromal depression

There is little evidence to suggest that major depression and dysthymia are different disorders. Their defining symptoms overlap and the only substantive difference is that dysthymia is chronic mild depression. However, for the most part it appears that the chronic depression that is the characteristic feature of dysthymia fluctuates in severity. In most cases of labelled dysthymia, the definition of comorbid major depression and dysthymia, the so-called double depression, is the more appropriate description. The number of cases who can be clearly defined as suffering from pure dysthymia appears, from the epidemiological studies, to be very small (Angst, 1992).

Antidepressants, both old and new, that are effective in major depression appear to be effective also, as would be expected, in double depression. As far as one can tell, they are also effective in pure dysthymia, though relatively few studies have tested efficacy in this narrow population.

The consistency of response indicates that the diagnostic category of dysthymia is not of great importance from the treatment point of view. It is, however, clear that both major depression and dysthymia are associated with substantial dysfunction and impairment, and a measure of the dysfunction would usefully be included in the definition of major depression, which may currently be too narrowly set. Whether a patient fulfils diagnostic criteria requiring a certain number of symptoms is affected by cultural factors, and it has also become apparent that men report fewer symptoms for the same degree of dysfunction as women, which may account for the higher prevalence of major depression in women. A more realistic view would be to take chronicity and dysfunction as measures of severity. In this case, persistent depressions which cause dysfunction but are otherwise regarded as subsyndromal could be appropriately included in the definition of major depression.

Given the evidence that major depression, dysthymia, double depression and subsyndromal depression are likely to respond well to a variety of antidepressants, the choice of which treatment to use will be made on the basis of safety and tolerability. The selective serotonin reuptake inhibitors (SSRIs) and most of the newer antidepressants, which include nefazadone, milnacipran, venlafaxine in low doses of 75 mg/day, mirtazapine and moclobemide, would have the advantage of improved tolerability compared with older TCAs.

Bipolar depression—Bipolar I and II mixed states

It is generally recognized that many antidepressants are associated with the precipitation of hypomanic or manic episodes. This occurs at a low level in patients with unipolar depression, but in patients with bipolar disorder this risk is an important complicating factor in the treatment of depressive episodes. There is evidence from the antidepressant treatment studies (Prien et al, 1973) that TCAs provoke manic switches in an unacceptable number of bipolar depression patients, estimated at between 11% and 38% of those treated. The switch rate appears to be dose related, as the rate rises when high doses are used.

There is a certain rate of spontaneous switches and this has to be borne in mind when establishing the risk of treatment. The meta-analyses of large placebo-controlled clinical trial databases with the newer antidepressants have given more precise information on the extent to which these drugs may precipitate mania. The switch rate appears to be lower with some SSRIs than with the TCAs. For example, in the meta-analysis of the data on paroxetine, used at relatively high doses, the rate was reported to be 2–3% (Montgomery, 1992a). This compared with the rate of 11% on the TCAs used in the studies. More modest doses of 20 mg of paroxetine may be preferred to try to reduce further the risk of switches to mania. Low switch rates have been reported for other newer antidepressants, e.g. moclobemide (not available in the USA) and buproprion (not available in Europe).

Some clinicians recommend lithium for treating bipolar depression or for reducing the risk of switches to mania by using lithium to cover the use of an antidepressant. While the place of lithium in the prophylaxis of manic episodes is established, there is considerable doubt about its ability to treat the acute episode of depression. Positive effects were reported from a few placebo-controlled studies but these were small and included mixed samples of bipolar and unipolar patients (Goodwin and Jamison, 1990). There is increasing evidence from the long-term studies that lithium is effective in reducing the risk of episodes of mania but that it has much less effect on the depressive episodes (Secunda et al, 1985; Prien et al, 1973, 1984). This is a cause of concern, since lithium, with its well-known toxicity problems, is in any case a far from ideal drug. Moreover, it appears that withdrawal from lithium may have the effect of provoking an increase in the rate of manic episodes.

The efficacy of sodium valproate in mania has been established in a series of studies carried out in the USA. It appears to be superior to placebo and as effective as lithium as monotherapy, without the difficulties of monitoring levels (Pope et al, 1991; Bowden et al, 1994). It also appears to be a more acceptable and better tolerated drug, with fewer discontinuations due to side effects reported in the comparison studies (lithium 11%, valproate 6%) (Bowden et al, 1994).

There is some evidence to suggest that valproate may be more effective than lithium in treating the depressive symptoms in bipolar patients (Montgomery and Cassano, 1996). Where major depression and mania co-exist, the so-called mixed states, valproate has been shown to be effective (Freeman et al, 1992; Calabrese et al, 1993), and those patients with both mania and a high score registered on depression rating scales seem to respond better to valproate than to lithium (Freeman et al, 1992). A superior effect of valproate on depressive symptoms compared with lithium is also indicated in prophylactic treatment. Open studies pointed to the ability of valproate to prevent both mania and depressive episodes, and in controlled studies, while both mood stabilizers appeared to be effective in preventing episodes of mania (Lambert and Venaud, 1992; Bowden et al, 1994), there was an advantage for valproate compared with lithium in reducing mania if patients exhibited even minimal depressive symptoms. The presence of depressive symptoms was a predictor of poor response to lithium (Swann et al, 1997).

Carbamazepine is widely used in the prophylaxis of bipolar disorder, although it is conceded that it is less effective than lithium and is largely used for lithium non-responders. The therapeutic effect of carbamazepine seems to be in the prophylaxis of mania rather than depression.

Of the other potential stabilizers, verapamil, a calcium channel blocker, has been reported to be effective in acute mania, but a study carried out in 1989 reported little effect in depression (Hoschl and Kozeny, 1989). Lamotrigine has been used in small open treatment studies, where it is reported to be useful in chronic depression and bipolar depression. There are as yet no controlled studies to support these open observations which, although subject to the usual biases, remain promising.

Major depression with mild mood swings

Although lithium is sometimes recommended for those patients who suffer from major depression but who are characterized also by minor mood swings, this has not been systematically studied, and soundly based evidence to support its therapeutic advantage is lacking. TCAs are probably also better avoided because of the associated increased risk of switches to hypomania, and particularly because in these patients hypomanic episodes may have been poorly diagnosed. Antidepressants that have been shown to have a lower switch rate, such as the SSRIs, are the more appropriate treatment. Because of the high toxicity and low evidence of efficacy, the risk–benefit assessment would not seem to favour the use of mood stabilizers in this population.

Depression with obsessive-compulsive disorder

Obsessive-compulsive disorder (OCD) is a distinct disorder which shows a selective response to antidepressants that have a potent effect in inhibiting the reuptake of 5-hydroxytryptamine (5-HT). This differential efficacy was first observed and established in treatment studies of clomipramine and has been clearly demonstrated with the SSRIs (review: Montgomery, 1994a). Antidepressants lacking important serotonergic activity do not appear to exert an anti-obsessional effect. The clinical findings of a differential pharmacological response in OCD led to the perception of a disturbance in the serotonin system being involved in the pathogenesis; the many neurobiological studies carried out have tended to support this hypothesis.

OCD is frequently accompanied by depressive symptoms, and half of OCD patients may fulfil diagnostic criteria for major depression at some point (Myers et al, 1984). However, these depressive symptoms differ in response to treatment from conventional major depression. The depressive symptoms associated with OCD are seen to respond slowly, following the same slow time course of response as the other OCD symptoms. Nor do they appear to respond to antidepressants which are not also effective anti-obsessional agents. The habit enshrined in DSM-III and DSM-IV of registering the depressive symptoms in OCD as part of major depression is misleading to clinicians. There are powerful arguments supporting the view that the depression manifested by many patients with OCD is part of the OCD and should be treated with anti-obsessional agents (Goodman et al, 1990; Montgomery, 1992b). The choice of pharmacological treatment lies between clomipramine and the SSRIs, which are the only drugs to have been found consistently to be effective in this group.

Depression with panic disorder

Only a few antidepressants have received adequate investigation in panic disorder, and to date the best evidence of efficacy is found with the SSRIs. Paroxetine is the only SSRI with clear-cut efficacy and a licence for treating the condition (Oehrberg et al, 1995), although the evidence for fluvoxamine is also substantial (den Boer et al, 1987). A distinction should be drawn between treatments, pharmacological or psychological, which suppress the anxiety associated with panic disorder, and those which suppress or extinguish both the anxiety and panic attacks in panic disorder. There is reasonable evidence to support the view that the benefit of benzodiazepines is focused mainly on the anxiety, with a lesser effect in reducing panic attacks (Basoglu et al, 1994), whereas cognitive-behavioural therapy is of more doubtful efficacy with the panic attacks and paroxetine is effective across the spectrum.

The separation of panic attacks, which are a natural part of depression, and panic disorder with comorbid depression is difficult, and for this reason anti-panic agents such as SSRIs with established efficacy in depression are mostly recommended. The use of alprazolam, which is effective on panic symptoms, is contraindicated in depression, because of the reports of raised suicidality risk and aggression and the general failure to show efficacy in depression (Gardner and Cowdry, 1985).

Depression and social phobia

Social phobia, which is a distressing and debilitating condition, carries a high risk of other comorbid psychiatric disorders. The lifetime risk of comorbid major depression has been reported to be 14.6% (Davidson et al, 1993). The presence of depression, in addition to increasing morbidity and the impairment of the individual with social phobia, complicates treatment.

The most thoroughly studied treatments for social phobia are the RIMAs moclobemide and brofaromine, and both are clearly effective (van Vliet et al, 1992; Versiani et al, 1992). For moclobemide, there is evidence of efficacy at 600 mg daily in three placebo-controlled studies, and to date it is the only antidepressant to have a licence for the treatment of social phobia. An alternative treatment is provided by the monoamine oxidase inhibitor (MAOI) phenelzine, which has been shown to be effective although it has been less thoroughly studied, and which is a more difficult drug because of the risk of associated toxicity (Liebowitz et al, 1992). The early results of treatment of social phobia with SSRIs are also promising. The beta-blockers are widely used for performance tremors but they do not appear to be effective in treating the social phobia. It is important to select an antidepressant that has been shown to be effective in social phobia, particularly where depression is present, and to avoid beta-blockers not only because they lack antidepressant effects but also because they have been reported to worsen the depression.

Recurrent brief depression

One category of depression for which effective treatments have not yet been found is recurrent brief depression. This serious condition, characterized by brief episodes of depression which have a mean duration of around 3 days but which are often very severe, is very common, with a prevalence equalling or exceeding that of major depression (Angst et al, 1990; Montgomery, 1994b).

Some reports have held out the promise that low-dose neuroleptics might offer an effective treatment, though these drugs have not been investigated specifically in recurrent brief depression (Montgomery and Montgomery, 1982). Antidepressants which would have been the obvious treatment modality for a depressive disorder do not appear to be effective. Antidepressants from different pharmacological classes have been tried in this condition, but placebo-controlled long-term studies have failed to show efficacy for SSRIs, reversible selective MAO-A inhibitors (RIMAs) or TCAs (Montgomery et al, 1994b). Anecdotal reports suggest that lithium, valproate and nimodopine may have some effect, but these reports have not yet been followed up with blinded studies.

The general failure to show that antidepressants which are effective in major depression are also effective in recurrent brief depression is disappointing and leads inevitably to the thought that recurrent brief depression has a different pharmacology to that of major depression.

A roughly equal proportion of those with major depression or recurrent brief depression later develop the comorbid disorder known as combined depression. This appears to complicate the picture, and it is generally thought that the major depression in these cases is difficult to treat.

Improving antidepressants

Faster onset of antidepressant response

The lag time to response of depressive symptoms is a limitation of conventional antidepressants. Although most antidepressants exert some therapeutic effect early, the full response is often only seen after several weeks. Antidepressants with a rapid onset of action would have a number of important clinical advantages: patients would experience more rapid relief of symptoms, and the risk of suicide might be reduced, as might morbidity and mortality from comorbid physical illness. Rapid onset of antidepressant effect has therefore become a focus of development effort.

The usual clinical efficacy study to investigate a putative antidepressant makes a comparison with placebo in a 6-week treatment study to allow time for a possible drug–placebo difference to evolve. This approach is recommended by the European Community guidelines on the investigation of antidepressant drugs (European Community, 1994). A different methodological approach is needed to demonstrate that an antidepressant has a slower or faster response (Montgomery, 1995). The specific interest of these studies is detecting the point at which improvement emerges in the early stage of treatment during the first 2 weeks, when a more frequent assessment schedule will be needed than the weekly ratings that are the norm in conventional efficacy studies. It is for this reason that it is difficult to test for early response in conventionally designed studies which lack frequent early assessments.

Pindolol augmentation strategies

One of the approaches that has been taken to the improvement of antidepressant efficacy has been the augmentation of treatment with SSRIs with pindolol, a beta-blocker with $5\text{-}HT_{1A}$ antagonist properties, on the basis that this could lead to an increase in 5-HT neuronal firing and counteract the attentuation following chronic administration of SSRIs thought to be due to the negative feedback via the $5\text{-}HT_{1A}$ autoreceptors.

Early open studies of augmentation strategies using pindolol added to SSRIs reported positive findings with a faster onset of antidepressant response and, in some cases, a response in resistant depression (Artigas et al, 1994; Blier and Bergeron, 1995). Because these were small open studies with all the well-known potential for bias, double-blind placebo-controlled studies were needed to confirm the enthusiastically positive results. These, as could be expected, have been slower to complete, but an increasing body of evidence has supported the positive effect of the addition of pindolol to SSRIs (Perez et al, 1997; Tome de la Granja et al, 1997).

The addition of pindolol to paroxetine has been shown to reduce the time to response compared with treatment with paroxetine alone, and, interestingly, it was possible to show in this study that the accelerated response was apparent in patients who were followed up in a community setting and who had fewer prior depressive episodes but not in those with the more chronic, resistant depression in a hospital-based practice

(Tome de la Granja et al, 1997). There was also some indication that the effect might be attenuated in patients who had received prior antidepressant treatment. A relatively small study of fluoxetine compared with fluoxetine plus pindolol did not find a significant acceleration, and this may have been due to the fairly chronic population studied (Berman et al, 1997). A larger study of the addition of pindolol to fluoxetine compared with fluoxetine alone in a community sample that included relatively few recurrent depressives reported a clear accelerated response in the augmented group (Blier and Bergeron, 1995). These positive studies were both moderately sized, with between 80 and 110 patients, but are smaller than one would normally expect to be necessary to detect a difference between active treatments. These studies support the view that response to treatment with SSRIs is not rapid and can be accelerated by pharmacological manipulation.

One of the important findings from these exploratory studies has been that the observed early response is reflected in superior response rates seen at the end of treatment. This accords with the findings of Stassen and colleagues, who analysed large clinical trial databases to determine the time to response with different treatments (Stassen et al, 1993). They also reported that early improvement is closely related to final response.

Dual-action antidepressants

The positive results with pindolol augmentation point the way to successful targeted treatment using antidepressants designed for faster response. A somewhat different approach has been taken in postulating that antidepressants that are selective reuptake inhibitors of both noradrenaline and serotonin might be more successful, or faster-acting, antidepressants.

An accelerated onset of response was reported for venlafaxine, the selective noradrenaline and serotonin reuptake inhibitor (SNRI), in a study in hospitalized inpatients suffering from severe melancholia (Guelfi et al, 1995). In this study a significantly better response compared with placebo was seen as early as the fourth day of treatment. This study used rapid dose increments to reach a high dose early in treatment, and it appears that a high dose may be necessary to achieve the rapid response. In the fixed-dose study of venlafaxine, the high dose was effective compared with placebo at 1 week, whereas the low dose was effective only after 6 weeks, suggesting that high doses were needed for accelerated response (Rudolph et al, 1997). A significant acceleration of response has also been observed on some measures in a study comparing venlafaxine with imipramine, again in severely depressed inpatients (Benkert et al, 1996).

Venlafaxine appears from these data to be a fast-acting antidepressant and it is possible that a contributing factor is its selective double action on noradrenaline and serotonin. Further support comes from the studies of augmentation of fluoxetine treatment with desipramine (Nelson et al, 1991). This augmentation strategy was reported in an open study to produce both a faster and superior effect compared to fluoxetine alone, and suggests that action on both the noradrenaline and serotonin reuptake might be the mechanism by which the extra efficacy is achieved. If so, SNRIs as a class might be more effective than single-action drugs such as the SSRIs, at least in certain subgroups of depressions.

Superior efficacy

The studies of augmentation of SSRI treatment with pindolol have shown the way to a strategy for improving the efficacy of these antidepressants. In those populations where an accelerated response was evident, a superior response at the end of treatment was also seen. This supports the idea of a probable link between the two measures of efficacy, though the nature of the relationship is not clear. The prediction of outcome from response early in treatment is a valuable tool in the management of depressed patients.

When two active antidepressants are compared, in general, significant differences in efficacy have not been observed. However, there is evidence to suggest that some antidepressants may be superior to others, as the studies comparing the efficacy of the SNRIs with that of SSRIs have shown. For example, an advantage was shown for venlafaxine compared to fluoxetine in hospitalized patients suffering from severe depression (Dierick et al, 1996; Clerc et al, 1996). Milnacipran, a more recently introduced SNRI, also appears to be more effective than the SSRIs, as was seen in comparisons with fluoxetine and with fluvoxamine (Lopez-Ibor et al, 1996). Again, this superiority was tested in severe, mainly hospitalized depression. It is not known whether there was also an accelerated response associated with the advantage of the SNRIs, since none of these studies undertook the extra ratings early in the treatment period which would have allowed a proper test of early onset of response. Nor were they strictly powered to test for superior efficacy. Venlafaxine has also been reported to show superior efficacy in a short-term study, and in a long-term extension study, compared with the TCA imipramine. Taking these data together, a picture begins to emerge suggesting that SNRIs are more effective than more conventional antidepressants, particularly in hospitalized patients with severe depression.

Consistent with the concept of the superiority of dual-action antidepressants is the evidence of superior efficacy of mirtazapine compared with trazadone (van Moffaert et al, 1995) and fluoxetine in short-term studies, and amitriptyline in a long-term study. Mirtazapine also exerts an effect on both noradrenaline and serotonin, albeit by quite different mechanisms.

Conclusion

The research effort to develop new and better antidepressants is at last yielding results. Antidepressants have already been developed which have superior efficacy compared with existing treatments. The superior efficacy is seen either as improved response at the end of treatment, or as faster onset of action, depending on the design of the trial and the nature of the drug. At the same time, advances in our understanding of depression have identified subgroups of depression, where particular antidepressants are more appropriate than others. Using psychopharmacology as a diagnostic tool is likely to produce refinements in these subdivisions of depression which will allow better targeting of treatment and the development of specific antidepressants for particular purposes.

References

Andersen J, Bech P, Benjaminsen S et al (1986) Citalopram: clinical effect profiles in comparison with clomipramine. A controlled muticentre study, *Psychopharmacology* **90:**131–8.

Anderson IM, Tomenson BM (1995) Treatment discontinuation with selective serotonin reuptake inhibitors compared with tricyclic antidepressants: a meta-analysis, *Br Med J* **310:**1433–8.

Angst J (1992) How recurrent and predictable is depressive illness? In: Montgomery SA, Rouillon F, eds, *Long-term Treatment of Depression* (Wiley: Chichester) 1–14.

Angst J, Merinkangas K, Scheidegger P (1990) Recurrent brief depression: a new subtype of affective disorder, *J Affect Disord* **19:**87–98.

Artigas F, Perez V, Alvarez E (1994) Pindolol induces a rapid improvement of depressed patients treated with serotonin reuptake inhibitors, *Arch Gen Psychiatry* **51:**248–51.

Basoglu M, Marks IM, Kilic C et al (1994) Relationship of panic, anticipatory anxiety, agoraphobia and global improvement in panic disorder with agoraphobia treated with alprazolam and exposure, *Br J Psychiatry* **164:** 647–52.

Benkert O, Grunder G, Wetzel H,

Hackett D (1996) A randomized, double-blind comparison of a rapidly escalating dose of venlafaxine and imipramine in inpatients with major depression and melancholia, *J Psychiatr Res* **30:**441–52.

Berman RM, Darnell AM, Anand A, Charney DS (1997) Effect of pindolol in hastening response to fluoxetine in the treatment of major depression: a double-blind placebo-controlled trial, *Am J Psychiatry* **154:**37–43.

Blier P, Bergeron R (1995) Effectiveness of pindolol with selected antidepressant drugs in the treatment of major depression, *J Clin Psychopharmacol* **15:**217–22.

Bowden CL, Brugger AM, Swann AC et al (1994) Efficacy of divalproex vs lithium and placebo in the treatment of mania, *JAMA* **271:**918–24.

Calabrese JR, Woyshville MJ, Kimmel SE, Rapport DJ (1993) Mixed states and bipolar rapid cycling and their treatment with VPA, *Psychiatr Ann* **23:**70–8.

Clerc GE, Ruimy P, Verdeau Pailles J (1996) A double-blind comparison of venlafaxine and fluoxetine in patients hospitalized for major depression and melancholia, *Int Clin Psychopharmacol* **9:**139–43.

Danish University Antidepressant Group (1990) Paroxetine: a selective serotonin reuptake inhibitor showing better tolerance, but weaker antidepressant effect than clomipramine in a controlled multicenter study, *J Affect Disord* **18:**289–99.

Danish University Antidepressant Group (1993) Moclobemide: a reversible MAO-A-inhibitor showing weaker antidepressant effect than clomipramine in a controlled multicenter study, *J Affect Disord* **28:** 105–16.

Davidson JRT, Hughes DL, George LK, Blazer DG (1993) The epidemiology of social phobia: findings from the Duke Epidemiologic Catchment Area Study, *Psychol Med* **23:**709–18.

De Veaugh Geiss J, Katz RJ, Landau P et al (1991) Clomipramine in the treatment of patients with obsessive-compulsive disorder, *Arch Gen Psychiatry* **48:**730–8.

den Boer JA, Westenberg HGM, Kamerbeek WD, Verhoeven WM, Kahn RS (1987) The effect of serotonin uptake inhibitors in anxiety disorders: a double-blind comparison of clomipramine and fluvoxamine, *Int Clin Psychopharmacol* **2:**21–32.

Dierick M, Ravizza L, Realini R, Martin A (1996) A double-blind comparison of venlafaxine and fluoxetine for treatment of major depression in outpatients, *Prog Neuropsychopharmacology Biol Psychiatry* **20:**57–71.

European Community (1994) Guidelines on psychotropic drugs for the European Community, *Eur Neuropsychopharmacol* **4:**61–77.

Freeman TW, Clothier JL, Passaglia, P, Lesem MD, Swann AC (1992) A double blind comparison of VPA and LI in the treatment of acute mania, *Am J Psychiatry* **149:**108–11.

Gardner D, Cowdry R (1985) Alprazolam-induced dyscontrol in borderline personality disorder, *Am J Psychiatry* **141:**98–100.

Goodman, WK, Price LH, Delgado PL et al (1990) Specificity of serotonin reuptake inhibitors in the treatment of obsessive compulsive disorder: comparison of fluvoxamine and desipramine, *Arch Gen Psychiatry* **47:**577–85.

Goodwin FK, Jamison KR (1990) *Manic-depressive Illness* (Oxford University Press: New York).

Guelfi JD, White AC, Hackett D, Guichoux JV (1995) Effectiveness of venlafaxine in hospitalized patients with major depression and melancholia, *J Clin Psychiatry* **56:**450–8.

Hoschl C, Kozeny J (1989) Verapamil in affective disorders: a controlled, double-blind study, *Biol Psychiatry* **25:**128–40.

Jenner PN (1992) Paroxetine: an overview of dosage, tolerability, and safety, *Int Clin Psychopharmacol* **6**(suppl 4):69–80.

Lambert PA, Venaud G (1992) Comparative study of valpromide versus LI in treatment of affective disorders, *Nervure* **5**(2):57.

Liebowitz MR, Schneier FR, Campeas R et al (1992) Phenelzine vs atenolol in social phobia: a placebo-controlled comparison, *Arch Gen Psychiatry* **49:**290–300.

Lopez-Ibor JJ, Guelfi JD, Pletan Y, Tournoux A, Prost JF (1996) Milnacipran and selective serotonin reuptake inhibitors in major depression, *Int Clin Psychopharmacol* **11**(suppl 4): 41–6.

Montgomery SA (1992a) The advantages of paroxetine in different subgroups of depression, *Int Clin Psychopharmacol* **6**(suppl 4):91–100.

Montgomery SA (1992b) The place of obsessive compulsive disorder in the diagnostic hierarchy, *Int Clin Psychopharmacol* **7**(suppl 1):19–23.

Montgomery SA (1994a) Pharmacological treatment of obsessive compulsive disorder. In: Hollander E, Zohar J, Marazziti D, Olivier B, eds, *Current*

Insights in Obsessive Compulsive Disorder (Wiley: Chichester) 215–25.

Montgomery SA (1994b) Recurrent brief depression. In: Montgomery SA, Corn TH, eds, *Psychopharmacology of Depression* (Oxford Medical Publications: Oxford) 129–40.

Montgomery SA (1995) Are 2 week trials sufficient to indicate efficacy? *Psychopharmacol Bull* **31:**41–4.

Montgomery SA, Cassano GB (1996) *Management of Bipolar Disorder* (Martin Dunitz: London).

Montgomery SA, Kasper S (1995) Comparison of compliance between serotonin reuptake inhibitors and tricyclic antidepressants: a meta-analysis, *Int Clin Psychopharmacol* **9**(suppl 4):33–40.

Montgomery SA, Montgomery DB (1982) Pharmacological prevention of suicidal behaviour, *J Affect Disord* **4:**291–8.

Montgomery SA, Rasmussen JGC, Lyby K, Connor P, Tanghoj P (1992) Dose response relationship of citalopram 20 mg, citalopram 40 mg, and placebo in the treatment of moderate and severe depression, *Int Clin Psychopharmacol* **6**(suppl 5):65–70.

Montgomery DB, Roberts A, Green M, Bullock T, Baldwin D, Montgomery SA (1994) Lack of efficacy of fluoxetine in recurrent brief depression and suicidal attempts, *Eur Arch Psychiatry Clin Neurosci* **244:**211–15.

Montgomery SA, Henry J, McDonald G et al (1994a) Selective serotonin reuptake inhibitors: meta-analysis of discontinuation rates, *Int Clin Psychopharmacol* **9:**47–53.

Montgomery SA, Pedersen V, Tanghoj P et al (1994b) The optimal dosing regimen for citalopram—a meta-analysis of nine placebo-controlled studies, *Int Clin Psychopharmacol* **9**(suppl 1):35–40.

Montgomery SA, Brown RE, Clark M (1996) Economic analysis of treating depression with nefazodone v. imipramine, *Br J Psychiatry* **168:** 768–71.

Myers JK, Weissman MM, Tischler GL et al (1984) Six-month prevalence of psychiatric disorders in three communities 1980–1982, *Arch Gen Psychiatry* **41:**959–67.

Nelson JC, Mazure C, Bowers MB, Jatlow P (1991) A preliminary, open study of the combination of fluoxetine and desipramine for rapid treatment of major depression, *Arch Gen Psychiatry* **48:**303–6.

Oehrberg S, Christiansen PE, Behnke K et al (1995) Paroxetine in the treatment of panic disorder: a randomised, double-blind, placebo-controlled study, *Br J Psychiatry* **167:**374–9.

Pande AC, Sayler ME (1993) Adverse events and treatment discontinuations in fluoxetine clinical trials, *Int Clin Psychopharmacol* **8:**267–70.

Perez V, Gilaberte I, Faries D, Alvarez E, Artigas F (1997) Pindolol augments the antidepressant efficacy of fluoxetine. Results of a double-blind, randomized trial, *Lancet* (in press).

Pope HGJ, McElroy SL, Keck PEJ, Hudson JI (1991) Valproate in the treatment of acute mania: a placebo controlled study, *Arch Gen Psychiatry* **48:**62–8.

Prien RF, Klett CJ, Caffey EM (1973) Lithium carbonate and imipramine in the prevention of affective episodes, *Arch Gen Psychiatry* **29:**420–5.

Prien RF, Kupfer DJ, Manskey PA et al (1984) Drug therapy in the prevention of recurrences in unipolar and bipolar affective disorders: Report of the NIMH Collaborative Study Group comparing lithium carbonate, imipramine and a lithium carbonate–imipramine carbonate combination, *Arch Gen Psychiatry* **41:**1096–104.

Rudolph RL, Fabre L, Feighner J, Rickels K (1997) A randomized, placebo-controlled, dose–response trial of venlafaxine hydrochloride in the treatment of major depression, *J Clin Psychiatry*.

Secunda SK, Katz MM, Swann A et al (1985) Mania: diagnosis, state measurement and prediction of treatment response, *J Affect Disord* **8:**113–21.

Stassen HH, Delini-Stula A, Angst J (1993) Time course of improvement under antidepressant treatment: a survival-analytical approach, *Eur Neuropsychopharmacol* **3:**127–35.

Swann AC, Bowden CL, Morris D et al (1997) Depression during mania. Treatment response to lithium or divalproex, *Arch Gen Psychiatry* **54:**37–42.

Tignol J, Stoker MJ, Dunbar GC (1992) Paroxetine in the treatment of melancholia and severe depression, *Int Clin Psychopharmacol* **7:**91–4.

Tome de la Granja MB, Harte R, Holland C, Isaac MT (1997) Paroxetine and pindolol: a randomised trial of serotonergic autoreceptor blockade in the reduction of antidepressant latency, *Int Clin Psychopharmacol* (in press).

van Moffaert M, De Wilde J, Vereecken A et al (1995) Mirtazapine is more effective than trazodone: a double-blind controlled study in hospitalized patients with major depression, *Int Clin Psychopharmacol* **10:**3–10.

van Vliet IM, den Boer JA, Westenberg HGM (1992) Psychopharmacological treatment of social phobia: clinical and biochemical effects of brofaromine, a selective MAO-A inhibitor, *Eur Neuropsychopharmacol* **2:**21–9.

Versiani M, Nardi AE, Mundim FD, Alves AB, Liebowitz MR, Amrein R (1992) Pharmacotherapy of social phobia, *Br J Psychiatry* **161:**353–60.

Index